HIV

For a catalogue of publications available from ACP–ASIM, contact:

Customer Service Center
American College of Physicians–American Society of Internal Medicine
190 N. Independence Mall West
Philadelphia, PA 19106-1572
215-351-2600
800-523-1546, ext. 2600

Visit our Web site at www.acponline.org

HIV

Howard Libman, MD
Associate Professor of Medicine
Harvard Medical School
Associate in Medicine
Division of General Medicine and Primary Care
Beth Israel Deaconess Medical Center
Boston, Massachusetts

Harvey J. Makadon, MD
Associate Professor of Medicine
Harvard Medical School
Vice President, Medical Affairs
Division of General Medicine and Primary Care
Beth Israel Deaconess Medical Center
Boston, Massachusetts

A|C|P

American College of Physicians
Philadelphia, Pennsylvania

Clinical Consultant: David R. Goldmann, MD
Manager, Book Publishing: David Myers
Administrator, Book Publishing: Diane McCabe
Production Supervisor: Allan S. Kleinberg
Production Editor: Scott Thomas Hurd
Developmental Editor: Vicki Hoenigke
Acquisitions Editor: Mary K. Ruff
Editorial Assistant: Alicia Dillihay
Interior Design: Kate Nichols
Cover Design: Elizabeth Swartz
Indexer: Nelle Garrecht

Printed in the United States of America
Composition by Fulcrum Data Services, Inc.
Printing/binding by Versa Press

American College of Physicians (ACP) became an imprint of the American College of Physicians–American Society of Internal Medicine in July 1998.

Library of Congress Cataloging-in-Publication Data

HIV / [edited by] Howard Libman, Harvey Makadon.
   p. cm.
   Includes bibliographical references and index
   ISBN 0-943126-84-3
   1. AIDS (Disease)—Handbooks, manuals, etc. I. Libman, Howard. II. Makadon, Harvey, 1947-.
   [DNLM: 1. HIV Infections—prevention & control. 2. HIV Infections—complications. 3. Neoplasms—complications. 4. Opportunistic Infections—complications. 5. Opportunistic Infections—prevention & control. WC 503.6 H6755 2000]
   RC607.A26 H57575 2000
   616.97'92—dc21

                                                                                    99-057890

The authors and publisher have exerted every effort to ensure that drug selection and dosage set forth in this book are in accord with current recommendations and practice at the time of publication. In view of ongoing research, occasional changes in government regulations, and the constant flow of information relating to drug therapy and drug reactions, the reader is urged to check the package insert for each drug for any change in indications and dosage and for added warnings and precautions. This care is particularly important when the recommended agent is a new or infrequently used drug.

00 01 02 03 04 / 9 8 7 6 5 4 3 2 1

Contributors

Tamar Barlam, MD
Assistant Professor of Medicine
Harvard Medical School
Division of Infectious Diseases
Beth Israel Deaconess Medical Center
Boston, Massachusetts

M. Anita Barry, MD, MPH
Assistant Professor of Medicine and
  Public Health
Boston University School of Medicine
Director, Communicable Disease Control
Boston Public Health Commission
Boston, Massachusetts

Colm Bergin, MD
Fellow in Infectious Diseases
Boston Medical Center
Boston, Massachusetts

Stephen L. Boswell, MD
Instructor in Medicine
Harvard Medical School
Executive Director
Fenway Community Health Center
Boston, Massachusetts

Timothy Cooley, MD
Associate Professor of Medicine
Boston University School of Medicine
Sections of Hematology and Oncology
Boston Medical Center
Boston, Massachusetts

Sara E. Cosgrove, MD
Fellow in Infectious Diseases
Beth Israel Deaconess Medical Center
Boston, Massachusetts

Judith S. Currier, MD, MSc
Associate Professor of Medicine
Center for Clinical AIDS Research and
  Education
University of California, Los Angeles
Los Angeles, California

Bruce J. Dezube, MD
Assistant Professor of Medicine
Harvard Medical School
Division of Hematology and Oncology
Beth Israel Deaconess Medical Center
Boston, Massachusetts

John P. Doweiko, MD
Assistant Professor of Medicine
Harvard Medical School
Division of Hematology and Oncology
Beth Israel Deaconess Medical Center
Boston, Massachusetts

Jon D. Fuller, MD
Associate Clinical Professor of
  Medicine
Boston University School of Medicine
Assistant Director, Adult Clinical AIDS
  Program
Boston Medical Center
Boston, Massachusetts

Robert Garofalo, MD, MPH
Instructor in Pediatrics
Harvard Medical School
Children's Hospital
Director of Adolescent Medicine
JRI Sidney Borum Health Center
Boston, Massachusetts

Jerome E. Groopman, MD
Recanati Professor of Medicine
Harvard Medical School
Division of Hematology and Oncology
Beth Israel Deaconess Medical Center
Boston, Massachusetts

Lisa R. Hirschhorn, MD, MPH
Assistant Professor of Clinical Medicine
Harvard Medical School
Director of HIV Medical Care and
  Research
Dimock Community Health Center
Roxbury, Massachusetts

Helen M. Jacoby, MD
Clinical Instructor in Medicine
Harvard Medical School
Department of Medicine
Cambridge Health Alliance
Cambridge, Massachusetts

Daniel B. Levy, MD, PhD
Fellow in Infectious Diseases
Beth Israel Deaconess Medical Center
Boston, Massachusetts

Howard Libman, MD
Associate Professor of Medicine
Harvard Medical School
Associate in Medicine
Division of General Medicine and
  Primary Care
Beth Israel Deaconess Medical Center
Boston, Massachusetts

Harvey J. Makadon, MD
Associate Professor of Medicine
Harvard Medical School
Vice President, Medical Affairs
Division of General Medicine and
  Primary Care
Beth Israel Deaconess Medical Center
Boston, Massachusetts

Jennifer Adelson Mitty, MD
Instructor in Medicine
Harvard Medical School
Attending Physician
Beth Israel Deaconess Medical Center
Boston, Massachusetts

Lori A. Panther, MD
Instructor in Medicine
Harvard Medical School
Division of Infectious Diseases
Beth Israel Deaconess Medical Center
Boston, Massachusetts

Peter J. Piliero, MD
Assistant Professor of Medicine
Director of HIV Research
Albany Medical College AIDS Program
Albany, New York

Raymond Powrie, MD
Assistant Professor of Medicine
Brown University School of Medicine
Department of Medicine
Women and Infants Hospital of
  Rhode Island
Providence, Rhode Island

Kenneth Sands, MD
Assistant Professor of Medicine
Harvard Medical School
Division of Infectious Diseases
Beth Israel Deaconess Medical Center
Boston, Massachusetts

Michael Stein, MD
Associate Professor of Medicine
Brown University School of Medicine
Division of General Medicine
Rhode Island Hospital
Providence, Rhode Island

Contents

Preface ▪ ix
Howard Libman and Harvey J. Makadon

1. Epidemiology and Transmission ▪ 1
   M. Anita Barry

2. Pathogenesis and Natural History ▪ 21
   Stephen L. Boswell and Jon D. Fuller

3. HIV Prevention in Clinical Practice ▪ 45
   Robert Garofalo and Harvey J. Makadon

4. Primary Care of HIV Disease ▪ 63
   Howard Libman, Raymond Powrie, and Michael Stein

5. Antiretroviral Therapy ▪ 95
   Timothy Cooley and Colm Bergin

6. Prevention of Opportunistic Infections ▪ 117
   Helen M. Jacoby and Judith S. Currier

7. Diagnostic Approach to Common Clinical Syndromes ▪ 135
   Lisa R. Hirschhorn and Peter J. Piliero

8. Diagnosis and Management of Opportunistic Infections ▪ 165
   Tamar Barlam and Lori A. Panther

9. Diagnosis and Management of Opportunistic Cancers ▪ 213
   Bruce J. Dezube, Jerome E. Groopman, and John P. Doweiko

10. Infection Control and Risk Reduction for Health Care Workers ▪ 243
    Kenneth Sands

Clinical Vignettes

CASE 1 HIV Infection in Pregnancy ▪ 258
Raymond Powrie

CASE 2 Initiation of Antiretroviral Therapy ▪ 261
Jennifer Adelson Mitty

CASE 3 Lipodystrophy Syndrome ▪ 263
Howard Libman

CASE 4 Co-infection with Hepatitis C Virus ▪ 266
Daniel B. Levy

CASE 5   Postexposure Prophylaxis ▪ 268
Sara E. Cosgrove

CASE 6   Antiretroviral Therapy Failure ▪ 271
Jennifer Adelson Mitty

Appendix   Drugs Used in the Treatment of HIV Infection ▪ 275

Index   ▪ 297

Preface

■　■　■

The care of HIV-infected patients has evolved dramatically over the past few years. What was previously a progressive disease manifested by frequent debilitating opportunistic infections and neoplasms is now a treatable chronic medical condition in many patients. However, the significant changes in management, including combination antiretroviral therapy and viral load testing, that prompted this transformation have resulted in important challenges for clinicians. Chief among these is the assimilation of a rapidly changing but incomplete knowledge base and its clinical application.

Although many different models of care have been effective, the medical literature has shown clearly that competence in HIV care requires, first and foremost, adequate clinical experience in the field rather than specific subspecialty training. Nursing support and access to social services, subspecialty consultations, mental health and other professionals, and clinical trials are also essential for the optimal management of patients.

This volume in the ACP Key Diseases series is intended to support physicians, nurses, and other health professionals in their efforts to provide high-quality primary medical care to HIV-infected adults. It is written mainly by staff at Boston's Beth Israel Deaconess Medical Center, which has a long tradition of clinical, teaching, and research expertise in this area. All of the authors have extensive experience in HIV care and recognize the needs of practicing primary care physicians. The text—divided into 10 chapters that address major clinical issues such as antiretroviral therapy and prophylaxis of opportunistic infections—offers up-to-date practical advice on HIV disease management. Tables, charts, and photographs make this information easily accessible to the busy clinician. Illustrative clinical vignettes and an appendix containing information about drugs used in HIV treatment supplement the text.

Our understanding of HIV disease is constantly advancing, and practice standards continue to evolve. There are many unresolved issues about the care of patients with HIV infection. We have tried to indicate where uncertainty exists and to present a reasonable approach to management based on the current medical literature and accepted standards of clinical practice.

We thank the authors for their informative contributions. We are indebted also to the American College of Physicians–American Society of Internal Medicine, especially Mary Ruff and her colleagues in the book division, for their unwavering support. Finally, we wish to acknowledge the staff and faculty of Beth Israel Deaconess Medical Center and Harvard Medical School. Their professionalism and commitment to patient care continue to inspire us.

Howard Libman, MD

Harvey J. Makadon, MD

1

■ ■ ■

Epidemiology and Transmission

M. Anita Barry, MD, MPH

ince the first description in 1981 of opportunistic infections (OIs) and unusual neoplasms associated with severe immunodeficiency, the acquired immunodeficiency syndrome (AIDS) has become a pandemic, with over 30 million people infected worldwide (1–6). Human immunodeficiency virus (HIV), the etiologic agent of AIDS, was identified in 1983. Subsequently, the virus' association with a range of clinical conditions (from asymptomatic infection to profound immunosuppression) was confirmed (7–10). By 1985, an assay to detect HIV antibody had been developed (11). The ensuing widespread use of this assay provided insights into the epidemiology of the virus. Subsequent studies demonstrated the clinical and prognostic use of other serologic markers, such as the CD4+ T-lymphocyte count, resulting in its incorporation into both clinical practice and classification systems (12–17). More recently, plasma viral load assays have been developed, which also are useful prognostically and for guidance in antiretroviral therapy management (18–22). Viral load testing has been incorporated into clinical practice guidelines but has not yet been included in disease classification schemes (23).

HIV includes two closely related retroviruses, HIV-1 and HIV-2. At least eight subtypes of HIV-1 (A through H) have been identified on the basis of genetic sequence coding within the major group (group M) of HIV-1. HIV-1 predominates worldwide, whereas HIV-2 is primarily found in West Africa. In the United States, HIV-1 subtype B is most common. In contrast, non–type B isolates are more often found in most developing countries. Whether different HIV-1 subtypes vary in their transmissibility or pathogenicity remains an unanswered question.

Classification of HIV Infection

Although a variety of classification systems have been promulgated (24–27), the one used most widely in the United States was developed by the Centers for Disease Control and Prevention (CDC) to perform national AIDS surveillance studies (28). To reflect evolving scientific knowledge and to improve the sensitivity and specificity of the case definition, the CDC classification system, originally published in 1986, has undergone several revisions (28–30). The version in 1993 added a CD4 lymphocyte count of fewer than 200 cells/mm^3 as an AIDS-defining state as well as including the clinical conditions of pulmonary tuberculosis, recurrent bacterial pneumonia (at least two episodes within 12 months), and invasive cervical cancer. Because changes in case definition may bias detection of HIV infection among certain groups, AIDS surveillance data must be adjusted to reflect accurately its longitudinal epidemiology (31).

The current CDC classification scheme for HIV/AIDS includes categories A through C, ranging from asymptomatic to minimally symptomatic infection to AIDS (Table 1.1). HIV-infected adults meet diagnostic criteria for AIDS if they have 1) a CD4 cell count of fewer than 200 cells/mm^3, 2) a CD4/total lymphocyte percentage of less than 14, or 3) any one of the clinical conditions listed in Table 1.2 (32).

Table 1.1   Classification System and Case Definition for HIV Infection and AIDS in Adults*†

CD4+ T-cell Categories	*Clinical Categories*		
	(A) *Asymptomatic* *Acute (Primary)* *HIV or PGL*	*(B)* *Symptomatic* *Not (A) or (C)* *Conditions*	*(C)* *AIDS-Indicator* *Conditions‡*
(1) ≥500 cells/mm^3	A1	B1	C1
(2) 200–499 cells/mm^3	A2	B2	C2
(3) <200 cells/mm^3	A3	B3	C3

PGL = persistent generalized lymphadenopathy.
* Criteria for HIV infection in adults, adolescents, and children aged ≥18 months: 1) positive result on a screening test for HIV antibody (e.g., repeatedly reactive enzyme immunoassay), followed by positive result on a confirmatory test for HIV antibody (e.g., Western blot or immunofluorescence antibody test); or 2) positive result or report of a detectable quantity on any of the following virologic tests: HIV nucleic acid detection, HIV p24 antigen test, or HIV isolation (viral culture). In the absence of laboratory diagnostic criteria for HIV infection, patient must have clinical condition included in AIDS case definition.
† Persons with an AIDS-indicator condition (category C) as well as those with CD4+ T-lymphocyte counts <200/mm^3 (categories A3 or B3) are reportable as AIDS cases in the United States and its territories as of January 1, 1993.
‡ AIDS-indicator conditions are listed in Table 1.2.
Adapted from Centers for Disease Control (28,30).

Table 1.2   Indicator Conditions Included in the 1993 AIDS Surveillance Case Definition

- Candidiasis of bronchi, trachea, or lungs

- Candidiasis, esophageal

- Cervical cancer, invasive*

- Coccidioidomycosis, disseminated or extrapulmonary

- Cryptococcosis, extrapulmonary

- Cryptosporidiosis, chronic intestinal (>1-month duration)

- Cytomegalovirus disease (other than liver, spleen, or lymph nodes)

- Encephalopathy, HIV-related

- Herpes simplex: chronic ulcer(s) (>1-month duration) or bronchitis, pneumonitis, or esophagitis

- Histoplasmosis, disseminated or extrapulmonary

- Isosporiasis, chronic intestinal (>1-month duration)

- Kaposi's sarcoma

- Lymphoma, Burkitt's

- Lymphoma, immunoblastic

- Lymphoma, primary (in brain)

- *Mycobacterium avium* complex or *M. kansasii*, disseminated or extrapulmonary

- *M. tuberculosis*, any site (pulmonary* or extrapulmonary)

- *Pneumocystis carinii* pneumonia

- Pneumonia, recurrent*

- Progressive multifocal leukoencephalopathy

- *Salmonella* septicemia, recurrent

- Toxoplasmosis of brain

- Wasting syndrome, HIV-related

*Added in the 1993 expansion of the AIDS surveillance case definition.
Adapted from Centers for Disease Control. 1993 revised classification system for HIV infection and expanded surveillance case definition for AIDS among adolescents and adults. *MMRW Morb Mortal Wkly Rep.* 1992;41(RR-17):15.

Laws or regulations in all 50 states require AIDS cases to be reported. However, identified cases represent only a fraction of those infected with HIV, consisting mainly of those who acquired the condition many years earlier. Although AIDS case reporting is believed to be over 90% complete, many factors are likely to influence these data, including patient access to health care, availability of HIV testing, and temporal and geographic trends in local surveillance practices (33). In addition, combination antiretroviral therapy and improved preventive regimens for OIs have reduced the proportion of people infected with HIV who meet the AIDS case surveillance definition, despite a relatively constant prevalence (34,35). Estimates of the proportion of people in various stages of HIV infection are derived from spectrum of disease studies, but little information is available on the effects of recent treatment advances.

Reporting of HIV-infected people who do not meet national surveillance criteria for AIDS, which had been advocated by some authorities, was recommended recently by the CDC (30a,36,37). Through December 1998, states requiring confidential reporting of HIV infection reported 104,411 individuals to be infected with HIV (but not AIDS) (38). The argument for this type of surveillance is that HIV-infected people who have not yet progressed to AIDS are still at risk for transmitting the infection to others. In addition, reporting HIV infection is advocated as a method to initiate earlier effective antiretroviral therapy in individual cases.

Epidemiology in the United States

Despite its limitations, the national AIDS surveillance system currently provides the most comprehensive data on HIV epidemiology in the United States. Through December 1998, a total of 664,921 AIDS cases had been reported to the CDC by state and territorial health departments, including 8060 cases among children under 13 years of age. The annual AIDS incidence rate in 1998 was 17.6 per 100,000 population, a decrease from 22.1 per 100,000 population reported in 1997. A declining trend in the number of reported AIDS cases has been noted over the past several years (Fig. 1.1). However, the total number of people with HIV/AIDS in the United States has continued to increase, with a CDC estimate of 372,586 at the end of 1998 (36,39).

Mortality and incidence of OIs among those diagnosed with AIDS also has declined (Fig. 1.2). A 23% reduction in deaths among reported AIDS cases was noted in 1996 compared with 1995, with decreases in both sexes, all racial/ethnic groups, and all risk-exposure categories. A decrease in the number of deaths also was noted in 1997. As a result, AIDS prevalence increased 12% from 1996 to 1997. Better antiretroviral therapeutic options and advances in prophylaxis of OIs probably explain the improvement in survival. AIDS resulted in 39,200 deaths overall in the United States in 1996, and it was the second leading cause of death among people aged 25 to 44 years (40). As of December 1998, the overall AIDS-case fatality rate was 59.7% (410,800 deaths per 688,200 cases).

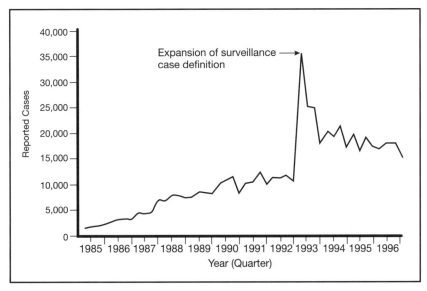

Figure 1.1   AIDS cases reported in the United States from 1985 through 1996. The expansion of the AIDS surveillance case definition in 1993 resulted in a substantial increase in reported cases during 1993, followed by declines in cases reported each year from 1994 through 1996. However, the number of reported AIDS cases in 1996 was substantially higher than the number reported in 1992, the year before the definition was changed. (Republished with permission from Centers for Disease Control and Prevention. Summary of notifiable diseases, 1996. *MMWR Morb Mortal Wkly Rep.* 1997;45:17.)

Of AIDS cases reported to date, 83% have been in adult/adolescent men, 16% in adult/adolescent women, and fewer than 1% in children under 13 years of age. Although women account for a minority of cases, the proportion in this group has increased steadily. In 1994, women accounted for 18% of adult/adolescent cases compared to 7% in 1985 (41). In 1998, women accounted for 23% of reported cases. Women from racial and ethnic minority groups have been affected disproportionately by HIV/AIDS most likely because of socioeconomic factors. From 1991 through 1995, AIDS incidence rates were highest in black women, women residing in the northeastern United States, heterosexual contacts of people with or at risk for HIV infection, and women living in metropolitan statistical areas with more than 1 million residents. The greatest increases in incidence were observed among women in the southern United States and those reporting heterosexual contact as a risk exposure (42). Among all reported AIDS cases in women to date, most can be linked to injection-drug use (IDU); 43% of cases are attributable to IDU, and another 17% to heterosexual contact with an injection-drug user. However, the importance of heterosexual

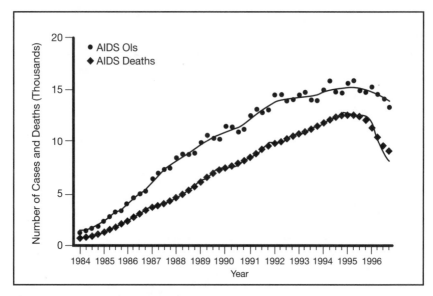

Figure 1.2   Estimated incidence of AIDS opportunistic illnesses (AIDS OIs) and estimated number of deaths among persons older than 13 years of age with AIDS (AIDS deaths) by quarter in the United States from 1984 through 1996. The figures have been adjusted for delays in reporting. (Republished with permission from Centers for Disease Control and Prevention. Update—Trends in AIDS incidence: United States, 1996. *MMWR Morb Mortal Wkly Rep.* 1997;46:862.)

transmission of HIV infection is becoming increasingly apparent over time. By 1995, the highest AIDS incidence rate in women 15 to 44 years of age occurred in those who acquired it heterosexually, surpassing IDU as a reported risk.

Men continue to comprise a majority of AIDS cases, and male-to-male sexual contact (MSM) as a single-risk behavior represents the most frequently reported HIV exposure risk (47% of total cases). Another 6% of cases report transmission by both MSM and IDU. However, the incidence of AIDS transmitted by MSM has been slowing over time; in 1998, MSM accounted for only 34% of cases. Data from 1989 through 1994 also showed a decline in the estimated incidence of OIs among cases transmitted by MSM, but changes in incidence rates vary considerably by geographic region and race/ethnicity (43). Modification of high-risk sexual practices among some groups is believed to be partially responsible for the declining numbers of AIDS cases. However, recent increases in sexually transmitted diseases (STDs) among cases transmitted by MSM have raised concerns that harm-reduction behaviors, such as safer sex practices, are not being sustained (44).

The age distribution of reported AIDS cases has remained relatively constant over time. Most cases occur in people between the ages of 25 to 44 years. However, a total of 27,860 cases have been reported in adolescents (ages 13 to 25 years), and evidence suggests that the average age at which HIV infection is acquired has declined (45). The proportion of reported AIDS cases among the elderly has been stable. People aged 50 years or over accounted for 10% of cases through 1998. However, the elderly are more often reported as having an OI or HIV encephalopathy rather than laboratory evidence of immunosuppression and are more likely than other adults to die within 1 month of diagnosis (46).

Racial/ethnic minorities have accounted for a disproportionate share of cumulative AIDS cases to date; 55% have occurred in non-Hispanic blacks and in Hispanics. In 1998, these groups represented 44% and 19% of adult/adolescent cases, respectively. These findings are even more striking among women; non-Hispanic blacks and Hispanics accounted for 80% of cases in adult/adolescent women during the same time period. Comparing 1995 with 1996 surveillance data, the greatest proportionate increases in estimated OI incidence occurred among those reporting heterosexual behavior as a risk, including non-Hispanic black men (19% increase), Hispanic men (13% increase), and non-Hispanic black women (12% increase) (47).

Reported risk behaviors also vary among different racial/ethnic groups. Among white men who report a single-risk behavior, 75% cite MSM compared to 38% in black men and 43% in Hispanic men. IDU as a single-risk behavior was reported by 9%, 35%, and 36% of white, black, and Hispanic men, respectively. Among women, IDU is reported in 42% of whites, 44% of blacks, and 41% of Hispanics, and heterosexual contact is reported in 40%, 37%, and 47% of the same groups, respectively. Among Hispanic women, reported risk also varies with birthplace. Compared with other Hispanic women, those born in the United States or Puerto Rico are more likely to have acquired HIV infection through IDU (48).

Geographic variation of AIDS cases has been observed since surveillance began, with initial cases clustered on the Northeast and West coasts of the United States; however, as the epidemic has progressed, an increasing number of cases have been reported from the South and the Midwest (49). More than half (57%) of people reported with AIDS in 1998 were from California, Florida, New Jersey, New York, and Texas. The AIDS incidence rate in 1998 ranged widely by geographic region, with the highest incidence (189.1 per 100,000 population) reported from the District of Columbia and the lowest (0.9 per 100,000 population) from North Dakota.

Although most AIDS cases have been reported from large urban areas, increased numbers from rural and small metropolitan areas, particularly in the southern and midwestern United States, have been reported over the past several years. However, recent analysis shows that the incidence of AIDS continues to be higher in large metropolitan areas compared with nonmetropolitan areas (23.0 vs. 6.3 per 100,000 population).

Estimating the Prevalence of HIV Infection

Although AIDS surveillance data provide extensive epidemiologic information, they include only those meeting specified clinical or laboratory parameters indicative of advanced immunosuppression. To estimate the prevalence of HIV infection, various methods have been used, including back-calculation from reported AIDS cases, HIV seroprevalence surveys, and HIV prevalence information from the Third National Health and Nutrition Examination Survey (NHANES III). Back-calculation is a statistical method that uses information on the progression of HIV disease to estimate the number of infections required to account for reported AIDS cases. HIV seroprevalence surveys are anonymous (unlinked) serosurveys carried out in selected populations, including people attending STD clinics, participants in drug treatment programs, childbearing women, military applicants, Jobs Corps applicants, blood donors, prisoners, and others (50–54). NHANES III, a health and nutrition survey based on a multistage area probability sample of the U.S. household population, used serum samples from selected participants for determining HIV prevalence (55). From these sources, Karon and coworkers (56) recently estimated that 650,000 to 900,000 U.S. residents (0.3%) were infected with HIV in 1992, which constitutes approximately 0.1% of adult/adolescent women and 0.6% of adult/adolescent men. The rate among non-Hispanic black men at that time was thought to be approximately 2%.

A similar estimate of 700,000 HIV-infected people living in the United States, including 565,000 in 96 large metropolitan areas, was derived by Holmberg (57) using a variety of data sources. Of an estimated 41,000 annual new infections, half were acquired through IDU. Although these estimates are lower than the 1986 CDC estimates of 1 million to 1.5 million HIV-infected U.S. residents, they indicate that HIV disease will remain a major public health and clinical issue for years to come (58).

Transmission

HIV infection can be transmitted sexually; through parenteral exposure; and perinatally during pregnancy, childbirth, or postpartum.

Sexual Transmission

Sexual behavior accounts for the majority of AIDS cases reported to date. Worldwide, 75% to 85% of cases are attributed to heterosexual contact, and, in the United States, 64% of adult/adolescent cases are acquired through either homosexual or heterosexual contact. Many variables influence the likelihood of sexual transmission (59). Key factors are HIV prevalence and stage of the epidemic within a population, number of sexual contacts, and specific sexual practices. Individual infectiousness also varies, with late-stage HIV disease associated with increased transmission risk (60–64). Data are conflicting on whether increased risk is related to high HIV levels in the semen of men with advanced HIV disease (65–68). Primary HIV infection is associated with an increased transmission risk, possibly related to higher viral concentrations in blood (69,70). An increased transmission risk also has been described in sexual contacts of those who have acquired HIV through blood transfusion (71).

The interaction between STDs (including ulcerative and nonulcerative genital tract infections) and HIV disease is well documented (72). Chancroid, syphilis, herpes, chlamydia, gonorrhea, and trichomoniasis have been associated with a higher risk of HIV acquisition (73–77). Treatment of STDs has been shown to reduce the risk of HIV transmission (78). HIV is more readily detected in the semen of men with urethritis, gonorrhea, or cytomegalovirus infections (79–81). In women, bacterial vaginosis also has been associated with acquisition of HIV infection. Although data on HIV in cervical secretions of women with STDs are conflicting, sexual partners of women with concurrent genital ulcer disease are more likely to seroconvert (82). Other factors in women that may increase the risk of sexual transmission include cervical ectopy and sexual activity during menstruation or pregnancy (83,84). Circumcision is associated with decreased risk of transmission (74,85). Consistent use of condoms is protective for both sexes (86–88). However, there are conflicting data on the effect of other contraceptive methods (e.g., nonoxynol-9–containing spermicides, intrauterine devices, hormonal contraceptives) on HIV transmission (89,90). The effectiveness of prophylactic antiretroviral therapy given after sexual exposure to reduce infection risk is unknown (91).

Parenteral Transmission

Parenteral transmission includes exposure through IDU, transfusion of HIV-infected blood or blood products, and nosocomial exposure through nonsterile medical supplies, such as needles and syringes. Among injection-drug users, HIV transmission is related to use of contaminated needles and injection supplies. Because injection-drug users are also often at risk for HIV infection through other behaviors, quantifying risk related to needle use alone has been difficult. Heterosexual activity has been demonstrated to be an independent risk behavior in this group (92). Other factors that have been associated with HIV acquisition among injection-drug users include the number of injections, frequency of needle sharing, number of needle-sharing partners, number of injections in "shooting galleries," average number of injections per month, and prevalence of HIV infection in the geographic area (93–95).

In the United States, HIV transmission from transfusion of infected blood or blood products declined rapidly following the introduction in 1985 of screening blood donations for HIV antibodies. Transfusion-related transmission of HIV infection in the United States is now rare (96). Recruitment of low-risk donors, exclusion of donors whose specimens are positive for other pathogens (e.g., hepatitis B, hepatitis C, or syphilis), and heat treatment of clotting factors also have contributed to the reduced risk. Although concern has been expressed about HIV transmission from blood donations given during the "window period" before development of HIV antibodies, a recent analysis suggests that only 18 to 27 of the 12 million donations annually in the United States would be infectious for HIV (97).

Parenteral HIV transmission related to use of nonsterile medical equipment has been reported, but its relative contribution to HIV transmission overall is likely small. At least one outbreak in Romania has been reported (98). Risk of transmission to health care workers from percutaneous exposure to blood is approximately 0.3%; following mucous membrane exposure, the risk is 0.09% (99,100). A retrospective case-control study of health care workers who sustained percutaneous exposure to HIV found that risk increased with deep injury, injury with a device visibly contaminated with blood, a procedure that involved a needle placed directly in a vein or artery, or exposure to blood from a person who died of AIDS within 2 months of the incident (101).

Perinatal Transmission

Mother-to-child transmission accounts for the majority of HIV infection in children. Exposure *in utero*, intrapartum, or through breast feeding results in infection in 15% to 40% of infants, with the lowest rates reported in North America and Europe and with the highest rates in Africa (102). Most transmission is believed to occur in late pregnancy or during labor and delivery. Factors that increase the risk of transmission include advanced maternal stage of disease, low maternal CD4 cell count, high maternal viral load, the presence of chorioamnionitis, and prolonged rupture of membranes (103–108). Recent data indicate decreased rates of transmission in women undergoing elective cesarean section. In the United States, a regimen of zidovudine given to the mother during pregnancy, labor, and delivery and to the infant postpartum has been shown to reduce the risk of vertical transmission from 25.5% to 8.3% in mothers with CD4 cell counts greater than 200 cells/mm³ (109). Breast feeding has been associated with an increased risk of transmission (110). In developing countries, it may increase the risk of transmission by 10% to 20%, with rates as high as 50% among mothers who become infected during late pregnancy or after delivery (111). A recent study demonstrated that a very short course of nevirapine also may be effective (111a). This approach may prove useful in developing countries.

Worldwide Epidemiology

The World Health Organization (WHO) estimates that 33.6 million people worldwide had been infected with HIV through 1999. At the end of 1997, an estimated 29.4 million adults and 1.1 million children under 15 years of age were living with HIV/AIDS (6). In 1997, approximately 16,000 new infections occurred each day and a total of 5.8 million infections annually. To date, approximately 9 million adults and 2.7 million children under 15 years of age have died from an HIV-related illness; 1.8 million adults and 460,000 children died in 1997 alone.

The dynamics of the HIV epidemic, including total burden of disease, have varied markedly by geographic region. In the industrialized countries of North America, Europe, and Australia, the number of AIDS cases has started to level off or decline. However, HIV infection continues to spread at an alarming rate in other parts of the world. Over two thirds of all people now living with HIV infection reside in sub-Saharan Africa; it is estimated that 3% of the population in this region are already infected. Most infections have occurred in East and Central Africa. However, rapid spread has now been identified in countries such as Nigeria, where the virus was introduced more recently (112). Seroprevalence rates as high as 43% have been reported among pregnant women in some parts of Africa, with urban areas particularly affected.

Although lower HIV infection rates have been reported in Asia, total cases are expected to exceed those in sub-Saharan Africa in the coming years because of higher population density. India alone is estimated to have 5 million HIV-infected people (113). A recent study of Indian STD clinic attendees reported an HIV incidence rate of 26.1 per 100 person-years among prostitutes (114).

Within countries, populations at risk and predominant modes of transmission have varied. In Thailand, HIV infection was noted initially among injection-drug users and female prostitutes, with subsequent spread to their heterosexual contacts and the general population. An aggressive government campaign to halt transmission of the virus by advertising, providing free condoms, and enforcing condom use in commercial sex establishments resulted in a 79% decline in STDs from 1989 to 1993 (115).

A total of 12.2 million women worldwide are living with HIV/AIDS, and the number is growing. An estimated 8.2 million children have been orphaned as a result of premature deaths of HIV-infected parents since the epidemic began (6). With no vaccine currently available and limited therapeutic options in developing countries, education, STD treatment, and general health measures offer the best hope for preventing millions of new HIV cases worldwide.

■   ■   ■

Key Points

- Since HIV was first identified in 1983, AIDS has become a global pandemic, with over 30 million people infected worldwide; most cases have been transmitted heterosexually.

- Mortality from AIDS has declined steadily in the United States since 1995, which is likely attributable to the widespread use of combination antiretroviral therapy.

- Men comprise 83% of AIDS cases in the United States. MSM remains the most frequently reported risk behavior but has accounted for a decreasing share of cases in recent years.

- Women account for a minority of AIDS cases in the United States, but the proportion of cases has been rising steadily from 7% in 1985 to 23% in 1998.

- Communities of color in the United States are affected disproportionately by AIDS, with 55% of adult cases occurring in blacks and Hispanics.

- Infection with other sexually transmitted pathogens has been associated with an increased risk of HIV acquisition.

■   ■   ■

REFERENCES

1. **Gottlieb MS, Schroff R, Schanker HM, et al.** *Pneumocystis carinii* pneumonia and mucosal candidiasis in previously healthy homosexual men: evidence of a new acquired cellular immunodeficiency. *N Engl J Med.* 1981;305:425–31.

2. **Centers for Disease Control.** Kaposi's sarcoma and *Pneumocystis* pneumonia among homosexual men: New York City and California. *MMWR Morb Mortal Wkly Rep.* 1981;30:305–8.

3. **Centers for Disease Control.** *Pneumocystis pneumonia*: Los Angeles. *MMWR Morb Mortal Wkly Rep.* 1981;30:25–32.

4. **Centers for Disease Control.** Follow-up on Kaposi's sarcoma and Pneumocystis pneumonia. *MMRW Morb Mortal Wkly Rep.* 1981;300:409–10.

5. **Quinn TC.** Global burden of the HIV pandemic. *Lancet.* 1996;348:99–106.

6. **Joint United Nations Programme on HIV/AIDS/World Health Organization.** *Report on the Global HIV/AIDS Epidemic.* Jun 1998.

7. **Barre-Sinoussi F, Chermann JC, Rey F, et al.** Isolation of a T-lymphotrophic retrovirus from a patient at risk for acquired immune deficiency syndrome (AIDS). *Science.* 1983;220:868–71.

8. **Gallo RC, Salahuddin SZ, Popovic M, et al.** Frequent detection and isolation of cytopathic retroviruses (HTLV-III) from patients with AIDS and at risk for AIDS. *Science.* 1984;224:500–3.

9. **Broder S, Gallo RC.** A pathogenic retrovirus (HTLV-III) linked to AIDS. *N Engl J Med.* 1984;311:1292–7.

10. **Farizo KM, Buehler JW, Chamberland ME, et al.** Spectrum of disease in persons with human immunodeficiency virus infection in the United States. *JAMA.* 1992;267:1798–1805.

11. **Centers for Disease Control.** Provisional Public Health Service interagency recommendations for screening donated blood and plasma for antibody to the virus causing acquired immunodeficiency syndrome. *MMWR Morb Mortal Wkly Rep.* 1985;34:1–5.

12. **Goedert JJ, Bigger RJ, Melbye M, et al.** Effect of T4 count and cofactors on the incidence of AIDS in homosexual men infected with human immunodeficiency virus. *JAMA.* 1987;257:331–4.

13. **Lang W, Perkins H, Anderson RE, et al.** Patterns of T lymphocyte changes with human immunodeficiency virus infection: from seroconversion to the development of AIDS. *J Acquir Immune Defic Syndr Hum Retrovirol.* 1989;2:63–9.

14. **Lange MA, deWolf F, Goudsmit J.** Markers for progression of HIV infection. *AIDS.* 1989;3(Suppl 1):S153–60.

15. **Masur H, Ognibene FP, Yarchoan R, et al.** CD4 counts as predictors of opportunistic pneumonias in human immunodeficiency virus (HIV) infection. *Ann Intern Med.* 1989;111:223–31.

16. **Fahey JL, Taylor JM, Detels R, et al.** The prognostic value of cellular and serologic markers in infection with human immunodeficiency virus type 1. *N Engl J Med.* 1990;322:166–72.

17. **Fernandez-Cruz E, Desco M, Garcia Montes M, et al.** Immunological and serological markers predictive of progression to AIDS in a cohort of HIV-infected drug users. *AIDS.* 1990;4:987–94.

18. **Mellors JW, Rinaldo CR Jr, Gupta P, et al.** Prognosis in HIV-1 infection predicted by the quantity of virus in plasma. *Science.* 1996;272:1167–70.

19. **Mellors JW, Munoz A, Giorgi JV, et al.** Plasma viral load and CD4+ lymphocytes as prognostic markers of HIV-1 infection. *Ann Intern Med.* 1997;126:946–54.

20. **O'Brien WA, Hartigan PM, Daar ES, et al.** Changes in plasma HIV RNA levels and CD4+ lymphocyte counts predict both response to antiretroviral therapy and therapeutic failure. *Ann Intern Med.* 1997;126:939–45.

21. **Katzenstein DA, Hammer SM, Hughes MD, et al.** The relation of virologic and immunologic markers to clinical outcomes after nucleoside therapy in HIV-

infected adults with 200 to 500 CD4 cells per cubic millimeter. *N Engl J Med.* 1996;335:1091–8.

22. **Hughes MD, Johnson VA, Hirsch MS, et al.** Monitoring plasma HIV-1 RNA levels in addition to CD4+ lymphocyte count improves assessment of antiretroviral therapeutic response. *Ann Intern Med.* 1997;126:929–38.

23. **Carpenter CCJ, Fischl MA, Hammer SM, et al.** Antiretroviral therapy in adults: updated recommendations of the International AIDS Society, USA panel. *JAMA.* 2000;283:381–90.

24. **Redfield RR, Wright DC, Tramount ED.** The Walter Reed staging classification for HTLV-III/LAV infection. *N Engl J Med.* 1986;314:131–2.

25. **Haverkos HW, Gottlieb MS, Killen JY, Edelman R.** Classification of HTLV-III/LAV-related diseases. *J Infect Dis.* 1985;152:1905.

26. **World Health Organization.** Interim proposal for a WHO staging system for HIV infection and diseases. *Wkly Epidemiol Rec.* 1990;65:221–4.

27. **Justice AC, Feinstein AR, Wells CK.** A new prognostic staging system for the acquired immunodeficiency syndrome. *N Engl J Med.* 1989;35:1388–93.

28. **Centers for Disease Control.** 1993 revised classification system for HIV infection and expanded surveillance case definition for AIDS among adolescents and adults. *MMWR Morb Mortal Wkly Rep.* 1992;41:1–19.

29. **Centers for Disease Control.** Revision of the CDC surveillance case definition for acquired immunodeficiency syndrome. *MMWR Morb Mortal Wkly Rep.* 1987;35:1–15S.

30. **Centers for Disease Control and Prevention.** CDC guidelines for national human immunodeficiency virus case surveillance, including monitoring for human immunodeficiency virus infection and acquired immunodeficiency syndrome. *MMWR Morb Mortal Wkly Rep.* 1999;48(RR-13):1–31.

31. **Centers for Disease Control and Prevention.** Update—Impact of the expanded AIDS surveillance case definition for adolescents and adults on case reporting: United States, 1993. *MMWR Morb Mortal Wkly Rep.* 1994;43:160–1, 167-70.

32. **Centers for Disease Control and Prevention.** Case definitions for infectious conditions under public health surveillance. *MMWR Morb Mortal Wkly Rep.* 1997;46:5–6.

33. **Rosenblum L, Buehler JW, Morgan MW, et al.** The completeness of AIDS case reporting, 1988: a multisite collaborative surveillance project. *Am J Public Health.* 1992;82:1495–9.

34. **Palella FJ, Delaney KM, Moorman AC, et al.** Declining morbidity and mortality among patients with advanced human immunodeficiency virus infection. *N Engl J Med.* 1998;338:853–60.

35. **D'Aquila RT, Hughes MD, Johnson VA, et al.** Nevirapine, zidovudine, and didanosine compared with zidovudine and didanosine in patients with HIV-1 infection. *Ann Intern Med.* 1996;124:1019–30.

36. **Centers for Disease Control and Prevention.** Evaluation of HIV case surveillance through the use of non–name-unique identifiers: Maryland and Texas, 1994–1996. *MMWR Morb Mortal Wkly Rep.* 1998;46:1254–8,1271.

37. **Gostin LO, Ward JW, Baker AC.** National HIV case reporting: a defining moment in the history of the epidemic. *N Engl J Med.* 1997;337:1162–7.

38. **Centers for Disease Control and Prevention.** *HIV/AIDS Surveillance Report.* 1998;10:1–43.

39. **Centers for Disease Control and Prevention.** Update—Summary of notifiable diseases: United States, 1997. *MMWR Morb Mortal Wkly Rep.* 1998;46:1–87.

40. **Ventura SJ, Peters KD, Martin JA, Maurer JD.** Births and deaths: United States, 1996. *Monthly Vital Stat Rep.* 1997;46:1–40.

41. **Centers for Disease Control and Prevention.** Update—AIDS among women: United States, 1994. *MMWR Morb Mortal Wkly Rep.* 1995;44:81–4.

42. **Wortley PM, Fleming PL.** AIDS in women in the United States. Recent trends. *JAMA.* 1997;278:911–6.

43. **Centers for Disease Control and Prevention.** Update—Trends in AIDS among men who have sex with men: United States, 1989–94. *MMWR Morb Mortal Wkly Rep.* 1995;44:401–4.

44. **Centers for Disease Control and Prevention.** Resurgent bacterial sexually transmitted disease among men who have sex with men: King County, Washington, 1997–1998. *MMWR Morb Mortal Wkly Rep.* 1999;48:773–7.

45. **Rosenberg PS, Biggar RJ, Goedert JJ.** Declining age at HIV infection in the United States (Letter). *N Engl J Med.* 1994;330:789–90.

46. **Centers for Disease Control and Prevention.** AIDS among persons aged more than 50 years: United States, 1991–1996. *MMWR Morb Mortal Wkly Rep.* 1998;47:21-7.

47. **Centers for Disease Control and Prevention.** Update—Trends in AIDS incidence: United States, 1996. *MMWR Morb Mortal Wkly Rep.* 1997;46:861–7.

48. **Diaz T, Buehler JW, Castro KG, Ward JW.** AIDS trends among Hispanics in the United States. *Am J Public Health.* 1993;83:504–9.

49. **Centers for Disease Control and Prevention.** First 500,000 AIDS cases: United States, 1995. *MMWR Morb Mortal Wkly Rep.* 1995;44:849–53.

50. **Centers for Disease Control and Prevention.** *National HIV Prevalence Surveys: 1997 Summary.* Atlanta, GA: Centers for Disease Control and Prevention; 1998.

51. **Conway GA, Epstein MR, Hayman CR, et al.** Trends in HIV prevalence among disadvantaged youth. Survey results from a national job training program, 1988–1992. *JAMA.* 1993;269:2887–9.

52. **Gwinn M, Pappaioanou M, George JR, et al.** Prevalence of HIV infection in childbearing women in the United States: surveillance using newborn blood samples. *JAMA.* 1991;265:1704–8.

53. **Weinstock HS, Sidhu J, Gwinn M, et al.** Trends in HIV seroprevalence among persons attending sexually transmitted disease clinics in the United States, 1988–1992. *J Acquir Immune Defic Syndr Hum Retrovirol.* 1995;9:514–22.

54. **Prevots DR, Allen DM, Lehman JS, et al.** Trends in HIV seroprevalence among injection drug users entering drug treatment centers: United States, 1988–1993. *Am J Epidemiol.* 1996;143:733–42.

55. **McQuillan GM, Khare M, Ezzati-Rice TM, et al.** The seroepidemiology of human immunodeficiency virus in the United States household population:

NHANES III, 1988–1991. *J Acquir Immune Defic Syndr Hum Retrovirol.* 1994;7: 1195–1201.

56. **Karon JM, Rosenberg PS, McQuillan G, et al.** Prevalence of HIV infection in the United States, 1984–1992. *JAMA.* 1996;276:126–31.

57. **Holmberg SD.** The estimated prevalence and incidence of HIV in 96 large US metropolitan areas. *Am J Public Health.* 1996;86:642–54.

58. Coolfont report: a PHS plan for prevention and control of AIDS and the AIDS virus. *Public Health Rep.* 1986;101:342–8.

59. **Royce RA, Sena A, Cates W, Cohen MS.** Sexual transmission of HIV. *N Engl J Med.* 1997;336:1072–8.

60. **Lazzarin A, Saracco A, Musicco M, Nicolosi A.** Man-to-woman sexual transmission of the human immunodeficiency virus: risk factors related to sexual behavior, man's infectiousness, and woman's susceptibility. *Arch Intern Med.* 1991; 151:2411–6.

61. **DeVincenzi I.** A longitudinal study of human immunodeficiency virus transmission by heterosexual partners. *N Engl J Med.* 1994;331:341–6.

62. **European Study Group on Heterosexual Transmission of HIV.** Comparison of female to male and male to female transmission of HIV in 563 stable couples. *BMJ.* 1992;304:809–13.

63. **Seidlin M, Vogler M, Lee E, et al.** Heterosexual transmission of HIV in a cohort of couples in New York City. *AIDS.* 1993;7:1247–54.

64. **Caceres, CF, van Griensven GJ.** Male homosexual transmission of HIV-1. *AIDS.* 1994;8:1051–61.

65. **Vernazza PL, Eron JJ, Cohen MS, et al.** Detection and biologic characterization of infectious HIV-1 in semen of seropositive men. *AIDS.* 1994;8:1325–9.

66. **Anderson DJ, O'Brien TR, Politch JA, et al.** Effects of disease stage and zidovudine therapy on the detection of human immunodeficiency virus type 1 in semen. *JAMA.* 1992;267:2769–74.

67. **Krieger JN, Coombs RW, Collier AC, et al.** Recovery of human immunodeficiency virus type 1 from semen: minimal impact of stage of infection and current antiviral chemotherapy. *J Infect Dis.* 1991;163:386–8.

68. **Hamed KA, Winters MA, Holodniy M, et al.** Detection of human immunodeficiency virus type 1 in semen: effects of disease stage and nucleoside therapy. *J Infect Dis.* 1993; 167:798–802.

69. **Daar ES, Moudgil T, Meter RD, Ho DD.** Transient high levels of viremia in patients with primary human immunodeficiency virus type 1 infection. *N Engl J Med.* 1991;324:961–4.

70. **Kinloch-De Loes S, Hirschel BJ, Hoen B, et al.** A controlled trial of zidovudine in primary human immunodeficiency virus infection. *N Engl J Med.* 1995; 333:408–13.

71. **Lee TH, Sakahara N, Fiebig E, et al.** Correlation of HIV-1 RNA levels in plasma and heterosexual transmission of HIV-1 from infected transfusion recipients. *J Acquir Immune Defic Syndr Hum Retrovirol.* 1996;12:427–8.

72. **Wasserheit JN.** Epidemiological synergy: interrelationships between human immunodeficiency virus infection and other sexually transmitted diseases. *Sex Transm Dis.* 1992;19:61–77.

73. **Mastro TD, Satten GA, Nopkesorn T, et al.** Probability of female-to-male transmission of HIV-1 in Thailand. *Lancet.* 1994;343:204–7.

74. **Kreiss J, Hopkins SG.** The association between circumcision status and human immunodeficiency virus infection among homosexual men. *J Infect Dis.* 1993; 168:1404–8.

75. **Plummer FA, Simonsen JN, Cameron DW, et al.** Cofactors in male-to-female transmission of human immunodeficiency virus type 1. *J Infect Dis.* 1991;163: 233–9.

76. **Laga M, Manoka A, Kivuvu M, Malele B, et al.** Non-ulcerative sexually transmitted diseases as risk factors for HIV-1 transmission in women: results from a cohort study. *AIDS.* 1993; 7:95–102.

77. **Kapiga SH, Shao JF, Lwihula GK, Hunter DJ.** Risk factors for HIV infection among women in Dar-es-Salaam, Tanzania. *J Acquir Immune Defic Syndr Hum Retrovirol.* 1994;7:301–9.

78. **Grosskurth H, Mosha F, Todd J, et al.** Impact of improved treatment of sexually transmitted diseases on HIV infection in rural Tanzania: randomised controlled trial. *Lancet.* 1995;346:530–6.

79. **Atkins MC, Carlin EM, Emery VC, et al.** Fluctuations of HIV load in semen of HIV positive patients with newly acquired sexually transmitted diseases. *BMJ.* 1996;313:341–2.

80. **Krieger JN, Coombs RW, Collier AC, et al.** Seminal shedding of human immunodeficiency virus type 1 and human cytomegalovirus: evidence for different immunologic controls. *J Infect Dis.* 1995;171:1018–22.

81. **Moss GB, Overbaugh J, Welch M, et al.** Human immunodeficiency virus DNA in urethral secretions in men: association with gonococcal urethritis and CD4 cell depletion. *J Infect Dis.* 1995;172:1469–74.

82. **Cameron DW, Simonsen JN, D'Costa LJ, et al.** Female to male transmission of human immunodeficiency virus type 1: risk factors for seroconversion in men. *Lancet.* 1989;2:403–7.

83. **Nicolosi A, Correa Leite ML, Musicco M, et al.** The efficiency of male-to-female and female-to-male sexual transmission of the human immunodeficiency virus: a study of 730 stable couples. *Epidemiology.* 1994;5:570–5.

84. **Clemetson DB, Moss GB, Willerford DM, et al.** Detection of HIV DNA in cervical and vaginal secretions. Prevalence and correlates among women in Nairobi, Kenya. *JAMA.* 1993;269:2860–4.

85. **Bongaarts, J, Reining P, Way P, Conant F.** The relationship between male circumcision and HIV infection in African populations. *AIDS.* 1989;3:373–7.

86. **Feldblum PJ, Morrison CS, Roddy RE, Cates W Jr.** The effectiveness of barrier methods of contraception in preventing the spread of HIV. *AIDS.* 1995;9:S85–93.

87. **Saracco A, Musicco M, Nicolosi A, et al.** Man-to-woman sexual transmission of HIV: longitudinal study of 343 steady partners of infected men. *J Acquir Immune Defic Syndr Hum Retrovirol.* 1993;6:497–502.

88. **Fischl MA, Dickinson GM, Scott GB, et al.** Evaluation of heterosexual partners, children and household contacts of adults with AIDS. *JAMA.* 1987;257:640–4.

89. **Daly CC, Helling-Giese GE, Mati JK, Hunter DJ.** Contraceptive methods and the transmission of HIV: implications for family planning. *Genitourin Med.* 1994;70:110–7.

90. **Sinei SK, Fortney JA, Kigondu CS, et al.** Contraceptive use and HIV infection in Kenyan family planning clinic attenders. *Int J STD AIDS.* 1996;7:65–70.

91. **Katz MH, Gerberding JL.** Postexposure treatment of people exposed to the human immunodeficiency virus through sexual contact or injection drug use. *N Engl J Med.* 1997;336:1097–100.

92. **Schoenbaum EE, Hartel D, Selwyn PA, et al.** Risk factors for human immunodeficiency virus infection in intravenous drug users. *N Engl J Med.* 1989;321:874–9.

93. **Allen DM, Onorato IM, Green TA.** HIV infection in intravenous drug users entering drug treatment, United States, 1988–1989. *Am J Public Health.* 1992;82:541–6.

94. **Chaisson RE, Bacchetti P, Osmond D, et al.** Cocaine use and HIV infection in intravenous drug users in San Francisco. *JAMA.* 1989;261:561–5.

95. **Lange WR, Synder FR, Lozovsky D, et al.** Geographic distribution of human immunodeficiency virus markers in parenteral drug abusers. *Am J Public Health.* 1988;78:443–6.

96. **Selik RM, Ward JW, Buehler JW.** Demographic differences in cumulative incidence rates of transfusion-associated acquired immunodeficiency syndrome. *Am J Epidemiol.* 1994;140:105–12.

97. **Lackritz EM, Satten GA, Aberle-Grasse J, et al.** Estimated risk of transmission of the human immunodeficiency virus by screened blood in the United States. *N Engl J Med.* 1995;333:1721–5.

98. **Hersh BS, Popovici F, Apetrei RC, et al.** Acquired immunodeficiency syndrome in Romania. *Lancet.* 1991;1:645–9.

99. **Bell DM.** Occupational risk of human immunodeficiency virus infection in healthcare workers: an overview. *Am J Med.* 1997;102(Suppl 5B):9–15.

100. **Ippolito G, Puro V, DeCarli G, the Italian Study Group on Occupational Risk of HIV Infection.** The risk of occupational human immunodeficiency virus infection in health care workers. *Arch Intern Med.* 1993;153:1451–8.

101. **Cardo DM, Culver DH, Ciesielski CA, et al.** A case control study of HIV seroconversion in health care workers after percutaneous exposure. *N Engl J Med.* 1997;337:1485–90.

102. **Peckham C, Gibb D.** Mother-to-child transmission of the human immunodeficiency virus. *N Engl J Med* 1995;333:298–302.

103. **Dickover RE, Garratty EM, Herman SA, et al.** Identification of levels of maternal HIV-1 RNA associated with risk of perinatal transmission: effect of maternal zidovudine treatment on viral load. *JAMA.* 1996;275:599–605.

104. **European Collaborative Study.** Risk factors for mother-to-child transmission of HIV-1: European Collaborative Study. *Lancet.* 1992;339:1007–12.

105. **Ryder RW, Nsa W, Hassig SE, et al.** Perinatal transmission of the human immunodeficiency virus type 1 to infants of seropositive women in Zaire. *N Engl J Med.* 1989;320:1637–42.

106. **St. Louis ME, Kamenga M, Brown C, et al.** Risk for perinatal HIV-1 transmission according to maternal immunologic, virologic, and placental factors. *JAMA.* 1993;269:2853–9.

107. **Nair P, Alger L, Hines S, et al.** Maternal and neonatal characteristics associated with HIV infection in infants of seropositive women. *J Acquir Immune Defic Syndr Hum Retrovirol.* 1993;6:298–302.

108. **Landesman SH, Kalish LA, Burns DN, et al.** Obstetrical factors and the transmission of human immunodeficiency virus type 1 from mother to child. *N Engl J Med.* 1996;334:1617–23.

109. **Connor EM, Sperling RS, Gelber R, et al.** Reduction of maternal-infant transmission of human immunodeficiency virus type 1 with zidovudine treatment. *N Engl J Med.* 1994;331:1173–80.

110. **Van de Perre P, Simonon A, Msellati P, et al.** Postnatal transmission of human immunodeficiency virus type 1 from mother to infant: a prospective cohort study in Kigali, Rwanda. *N Engl J Med.* 1991;325:593–8.

111. **Dunn DT, Newell ML, Ades AL, Peckham CS.** Risk of human immunodeficiency virus type 1 transmission through breastfeeding. *Lancet.* 1992;340:585–8.

111a. **Guay LA, et al.** Intrapartum and neonatal single dose nevirapine compared to zidovudine in the prevention of mother-to-child transmission of HIV-1 in Kampala, Uganda: HIVNET 012 randomized trial. *Lancet.* 1999;354:795–802.

112. **Dada AJ, Oyewole F, Onofowokan R, et al.** Demographic characteristics of retroviral infections (HIV-1, HIV-2, and HTLV-I) among female professional sex workers in Lagos, Nigeria. *J Acquir Immune Defic Syndr Hum Retrovirol.* 1993; 6:1358–63.

113. **Bollinger RC, Tripathy SP, Quinn TC.** The human immunodeficiency virus epidemic in India: current magnitude and future projections. *Medicine.* 1995;74: 97–106.

114. **Mehendale SM, Rodrigues JJ, Brookmeyer RS, et al.** Incidence and predictors of human immunodeficiency virus type 1 seroconversion in patients attending sexually transmitted disease clinics in India. *J Infect Dis.* 1995;72:1486–91.

115. **Hanenberg RS, Rojanapithayakorn W, Kunasol P, Sokal DC.** Impact of Thailand's HIV-control programme as indicated by the decline of sexually transmitted diseases. *Lancet.* 1994;344:243–5.

2

■ ■ ■

Pathogenesis and Natural History

Stephen L. Boswell, MD

Jon D. Fuller, MD

ubstantial progress has been made in understanding the disease process that leads to AIDS. New assays have made it possible to quantify HIV replication accurately and have improved understanding of the mechanisms of HIV pathogenesis. These same tools also have become indispensable in the clinical management of HIV disease for assessing the risk of disease progression and gauging the effectiveness of antiretroviral therapy. The simultaneous development of highly potent inhibitors of HIV and an appreciation for how to use them to forestall resistance have led to strategies that have resulted in prolonged suppression of viral replication in many HIV-infected patients.

Pathogenesis

HIV is a cytopathic virus. It is composed of a central cylindrical core of RNA surrounded by a spherical lipid envelope. The viral antigen p24 is located in the core and serves as a serologic marker of replication. Through the binding of the HIV envelope glycoprotein gp120 to the receptor present on the surface of CD4+ T lymphocytes, the virus is able to fuse with the cell membrane (Fig. 2.1). Once within the cytoplasm of the host cell, the envelope of the virus is shed and its contents are released. It is then that reverse transcription occurs: DNA is made from the viral RNA template. Infected cells remain in a dormant state for a variable period of time. When

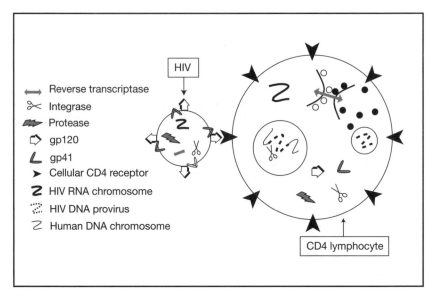

Figure 2.1   Interaction between HIV and CD4 lymphocyte.

activation occurs, the proviral DNA transcribes genomic and messenger RNA. After viral proteins are synthesized, new virions are assembled and bud from the infected cell. For budding virions to become functional, processing by a viral protease is required. Once this processing has been accomplished, the virions circulate until they identify new target cells.

Transmission

HIV is transmitted through sexual contact, from exposure to infected blood, or from an infected mother to her fetus or breast-fed infant. To establish infection, the virus targets cells with the CD4 surface molecule. When gp120 binds to CD4, it facilitates virus entry and initiates the viral replication cycle. Additional cell-surface molecules that normally function as receptors for chemokines also have been identified as important coreceptors required for the process of HIV entry. Although numerous chemokine receptors are capable of serving this function, the most important of these seem to be CCR5 and CXCR4; both are members of the seven G-transmembrane protein family of chemokine receptors. The CCR5 molecule, present on macrophages and CD4 cells, is the principal coreceptor used by macrophage-tropic (nonsyncytium-inducing [NSI]) viral strains that predominate in early stages of HIV infection (1–5). CXCR4 is found on T lymphocytes and laboratory-adapted T-cell lines and is the main coreceptor used by T-tropic (syncytium-inducing [SI]) viral strains that often predominate in the later stages of HIV disease (6).

Transmitted virus seems to have a predilection to bind CCR5. These viruses recently have been named R5 viruses in reference to their coreceptor requirement, whereas viruses that require CXCR4 are referred to as X4 viruses. Recent data suggest that within the mucosa, HIV first targets dendritic cells (e.g., Langerhans' cells). These harbor the CD4 receptor and the coreceptor CCR5 but do not seem to express CXCR4. This observation may explain the predominance of R5 viruses in acute HIV infection (7–9); furthermore, it proffers an explanation for the observation that individuals who are homozygous for a 32-base-pair deletion in CCR5 are more resistant to infection with R5 strains (10,11). Heterozygous individuals also may have a decreased risk of HIV disease progression and possibly a decreased risk of becoming infected (12,13). Mutations in stromal-derived factor 1 (SDF1), the natural ligand for the CXCR4 receptor, also have been associated with delayed disease progression (14). Among people of western European descent, it has been estimated that 18% are heterozygous and 1% homozygous for the mutant CCR5 allele. Studies of serum bank specimens have found a heterozygous prevalence of 2% to 15% among blacks in the United States but 0% among Africans, Venezuelans, and Japanese (10, 11).

Several other macrophage-tropic coreceptors also have been identified, including CCR2 and CCR3 (15). Mutations in CCR2 also may confer protection against transmission and progression but to a lesser degree than for the 32-base-pair deletion in CCR5 (14,16,17).

Host Immune Response

Neutralizing antibodies likely contribute to viral suppression, but an increasing body of evidence suggests that development of a cytotoxic T-lymphocyte response appears before reduction in viremia and may be the stronger suppressive factor (18–23). Antibody production also occasionally may lead to enhancement of viral replication (24).

Immune Destruction

Left untreated, HIV infection leads to a gradual diminution of immune function in the vast majority of infected people. The culmination of this immune deterioration is AIDS, a state of profound immune depletion characterized by a significant decrease in the number and function of CD4 lymphocytes, resulting in susceptibility to opportunistic infections and malignancies. The main characteristic of this immune disruption is the progressive destruction of the CD4 lymphocyte population.

Many causes of CD4 lymphocyte destruction have been posited, chief of which is the cytopathic effect of viral replication. Early studies had suggested that HIV was latent for an extended period in many individuals, casting doubt on the notion that CD4 cell depletion occurred as a direct consequence of HIV replication. Initial studies of patients in clinical latency using *in situ* hybridization techniques reported only rare infected circulating lymphocytes (1 in 100,000). However, more sensitive polymerase chain reaction (PCR) methods subsequently demonstrated much higher levels of circulating infected cells, ranging as high as 1 in 1000 cells in asymptomatic patients and 1 in 100 cells in patients with AIDS (25–26).

It is currently estimated that approximately 10 billion viral particles are produced each day in the untreated HIV-infected individual. This observation adds credence to the notion that the cytopathic effect of viral replication is the likely cause of CD4 lymphocyte loss and of the progressive immune deterioration that characterizes HIV disease. The means by which HIV exerts this effect have not been characterized fully but probably include both direct and indirect mechanisms.

The preponderance of replicating virus resides in lymph tissue, even in early HIV infection. HIV-specific probes of reactive lymph nodes during clinical latency have demonstrated well-delineated germinal centers whose follicular dendritic cells trap and retain the virus (27–29). It is at these sites of CD4 lymphocyte activation that cells responding to antigenic challenge become vulnerable to HIV infection and depletion. This localization of HIV to the lymph node also is associated with a progressive disruption of node architecture, which may contribute further to immunodeficiency by interfering with proper lymph node functioning. The germinal centers and the nodes themselves gradually involute, leading to a diminishment of lymphadenopathy and to the release of large quantities of virus into the plasma (27,29–32). This increase in plasma viral load also has been associated with decline in the CD4 count and with the onset of opportunistic diseases.

Clinicians and patients refer to the concentration of HIV RNA in the plasma as the viral load. Recent data indicate that the level of HIV RNA measured in plasma is also an accurate marker of viral replication in other tissue compartments and is one of the most important markers of the risk of disease progression (Fig. 2.2).

Plasma viremia reflects the net result of two opposing forces: virus production and virus clearance. During primary HIV infection, when activated CD4 lymphocytes are plentiful and the host immune response is minimal or absent, viral load can exceed 10^7 copies/mL. With the development of HIV-specific CD4 lymphocyte and cytotoxic T-lymphocyte (CTL) responses, the concentration of plasma HIV RNA declines precipitously and after a period of 6 to 12 months stabilizes at a set point (Fig. 2.3). Factors that may play a role in determining this set point include viral phenotype (e.g., SI vs. NSI virus, replication competence, other viral characteristics), effectiveness of

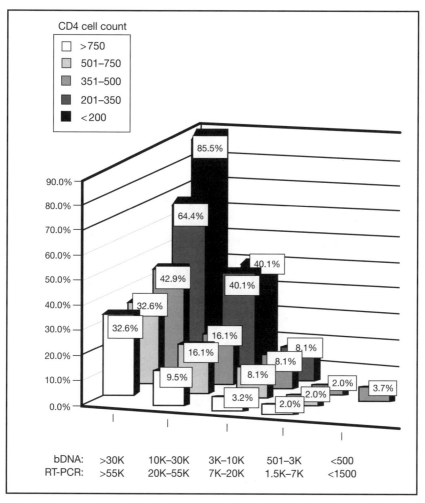

Figure 2.2 Risk of developing AIDS within 3 years based on CD4 cell count and viral load. bDNA = branchal-chain DNA; RT-PCR = reverse transcriptase–polymerase chain reaction. (Adapted from Centers for Disease Control and Prevention. Report of the NIH panel to define principles of therapy of HIV infection and guidelines for the use of antiretroviral agents in HIV-infected adults and adolescents. *MMWR Morb Mortal Wkly Rep.* 1998;47:1–82.)

host antiviral immune responses, the degree of host immune system activation, and route of transmission. HIV RNA concentration can range from fewer than 20 copies/mL to greater than 10^7 copies/mL, with set points characteristically ranging between 10^3 and 10^6 copies/mL. Population-based studies have demonstrated an inverse correlation between CD4 cell counts and plasma HIV RNA concentrations. However, although this correlation is

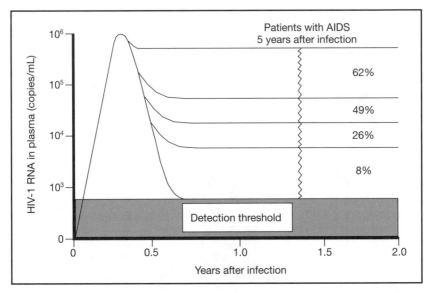

Figure 2.3   Viral set point and risk of progression to AIDS. (Reprinted with permission from Ho DD. Viral counts count in HIV infection. *Science*. 1996;272:1124–5.)

statistically significant, there is a wide variation among patients in HIV RNA concentration for any given CD4 cell count.

Viral Reservoirs

The development of powerful drugs to slow HIV replication has led to an improved understanding of viral dynamics in the infected host. Measuring the slope of the initial fall in viremia after initiating potent antiviral therapy has permitted estimation of the plasma half-life of HIV virions to be 6 hours, implying a dynamic process of viral production and clearance. Data indicate that neither HIV plasma half-life nor rate of virus clearance varies substantially between people with different CD4 cell counts or plasma HIV RNA concentrations. Thus, the principal determinants of the steady-state concentration of HIV in an infected individual are the amount of virus produced and the rate of viral clearance, which is estimated to range from 10^8 to 10^9 virions each day.

The decline of plasma HIV RNA in response to potent antiretroviral therapy seems to occur in phases (33). An initial rapid decline occurs over approximately 2 weeks, which is characterized by a 1- to 2-log drop in viral load. This is believed to represent the rapid clearance of productively infected CD4 lymphocytes. A second decay phase that responds more slowly to potent antiretroviral therapy may represent virus produced by longer-lived, chronically infected cells or by latently infected cells that have been activated to produce virus. Recent data suggest that viral replication still can occur at low levels in individuals receiving potent antiretroviral therapy, despite undetectable plasma levels. This suggests the possibility of sanctuary sites in which cells such as macrophages, dendritic cells, and persistently infected CD4 cells can maintain viral production even in the face of potent antiretroviral therapy (34). These observations have tempered initial enthusiasm for the notion of viral eradication.

Viral Phenotype

Resistance

Resistance to antiretroviral drugs is mediated by mutations in viral genes. Current agents bind to and interfere with either reverse transcriptase or protease—two viral enzymes required for replication. Mutations of viral genes that code for these proteins can diminish the activity of antiretroviral drugs, usually by interfering with binding. The number of mutations required to diminish drug activity significantly can vary considerably between classes, with only one mutation needed to develop high-level resistance to nonnucleoside reverse-transcriptase inhibitors. In contrast, multiple mutations may be necessary to achieve the same effect with protease inhibitors and with some nucleoside reverse-transcriptase inhibitors.

The high rate of viral replication that characterizes HIV infection serves as one of the conditions that enable the development of drug resistance. This rapid replication, in conjunction with a relatively high error rate associated with reverse transcription, can lead to many mutations in viral genes. As a result, viruses with single and (sometimes) double mutations that code for drug resistance may exist in an infected individual even before exposure to antiretroviral therapy. Mutant viruses (even multi–drug-resistant variants) also may be transmitted from one individual to another (35). These mutations compromise the effectiveness of antiretroviral drugs and may result in only partial suppression of viral replication. Treatment with an antiretroviral regimen that only partially suppresses virus replication allows additional mutations to accumulate. Over time, high-level resistance develops, viral replication increases substantially, and HIV disease progression occurs.

Syncytium-Inducing Virus

Most individuals are infected with a wild-type NSI strain of HIV that does not lead to the formation of multinucleated giant cells (syncytia) in cell culture. However, a single amino acid mutation in the third variable region (V3 loop) of gp120 can cause infected cells to form syncytia, leading to the development of a mutant SI strain (36). Individuals infected with SI strains are more likely to experience rapid CD4 cell loss and progression to AIDS than in those with NSI strains (37–42). NSI strains also can mutate to SI strains over time, with a more rapid depletion in CD4 lymphocytes being observed after the change in phenotype.

Immune Reconstitution

The institution of potent antiretroviral therapy can reduce dramatically the viral load and increase CD4 lymphocyte counts. Also, immune function can improve, as demonstrated by enhanced responses to antigen stimulation and by a decrease in opportunistic infections. To date, however, experience with potent antiretroviral therapy suggests that immune-function improvement may be incomplete in some individuals. A broad disruption of CD4 lymphocyte function occurs as a consequence of HIV infection, and subpopulations of these cells may be lost and irrecoverable, despite treatment with antiretroviral therapy. The large increase in CD4 lymphocytes that is observed in some patients on potent antiretroviral therapy may represent an expansion of a limited number of CD4 cell clones, resulting in only partial reconstitution of the host immune system.

A central issue in immune reconstitution is the recovery of memory versus naive subsets of CD4 lymphocytes. Naive CD4 cells can recognize new antigens and marshal a variety of other immune cells to respond to a wide range of pathogens. In contrast, memory CD4 lymphocytes—even though they circulate widely and can respond rapidly on rechallenge—can only respond to those antigens to which they have been sensitized.

The thymus plays an important role in the initial development of immunity. Thymic maturation is necessary for the production of naive CD4 lymphocytes, which can then be sensitized by antigen-presenting cells to respond to a specific pathogen. Evidence also suggests that the thymus may play an important role in the reconstitution of immunity in a number of pathologic states, including HIV infection. If the thymus is necessary for the regeneration of naive CD4 cell clones, immune reconstitution may be limited significantly in chronically infected adults because thymic function declines with age.

Natural History

Primary Infection

Symptoms associated with acute HIV infection were first described in 1984 in the case of a British nurse who sustained a needlestick injury from an HIV-seropositive patient who died shortly thereafter. Thirteen days later she experienced fever, sore throat, lymphadenopathy, headache, myalgia, facial neuralgia, malaise, and a macular rash involving the chest, trunk, neck, and face; 7 weeks later, she became HIV seropositive (43). Two series reported in 1985 helped define the clinical picture of this syndrome, which precedes HIV seroconversion (44,45), and numerous prospective and retrospective series have expanded our understanding of it (46–58). This acute HIV syndrome has been observed after HIV transmission that occurred as a result of 1) having heterosexual and/or homosexual intercourse; 2) having oral sex; 3) sharing drug-injection equipment; and 4) being given a transfusion of infected blood, factor VIII, and/or platelets (51,59–61). It has been proposed that the syndrome's protean clinical manifestations are the consequence of 1) viral replication within the reticuloendothelial system, 2) circulating immune complexes, 3) the development of a CD8-mediated immune response, and 4) the lymphocytopathic and neuropathic nature of HIV itself (51,61–63).

Clinical Manifestations

The acute HIV syndrome has been documented between 6 and 56 days after a known exposure, with an average incubation of approximately 2 weeks. The duration of symptoms has ranged from <5 to >60 days, with reported averages ranging from 2 to 4 weeks (44–46,51,57,64). Symptoms are usually acute in onset, and manifestations include fever, generalized lymphadenopathy, pharyngitis, headache, rash, myalgia, and arthralgia (Table 2.1). There is considerable variability in the clinical presentation.

Table 2.1   Clinical Manifestations of Primary HIV Syndrome

General	*Gastrointestinal*
• Fever	• Pharyngitis
• Lymphadenopathy	• Diarrhea
• Lethargy	• Nausea/vomiting
• Myalgia	• Hepatosplenomegaly
• Arthralgia	
	Other
Neurologic	• Thrombocytopenia
• Headache	• Leukopenia
• Meningoencephalitis	• Increased liver function tests
• Peripheral neuropathy	• Opportunistic infections
Dermatologic	
• Truncal maculopapular rash	
• Mucocutaneous ulcers	

DERMATOLOGIC

The rash of acute HIV syndrome is a roseola-like, diffuse, erythematous, nonpruritic maculopapular eruption that can involve the trunk and extremities and occasionally the face, palms, and soles (65,66). A vesicular, pustular exanthem also has been reported, as have urticaria and genital and anal ulcers (67–69). On histologic examination, a mononuclear cell infiltrate of the superficial dermal vessels can be seen, largely involving CD4 cells; Langerhans' cells and p24 antigen also have been identified in the perivascular infiltrate. It has been suggested that the rash represents a delayed-type hypersensitivity reaction from presentation of HIV antigen by Langerhans' cells to CD4 lymphocytes (70).

GASTROINTESTINAL

Oral manifestations may include enanthema (2–5 mm erythematous, round patches on the hard and soft palate), angular stomatitis, exudative tonsillitis, and oral ulcers (71–74). HIV-associated ulcers are similar in appearance to aphthous ulcers but with a surrounding zone of erythema. They may involve the lips, tongue, floor of the mouth, palate, tonsils, and uvula.

Esophageal ulcers also have been described. In one series of 16 homosexual men who presented with symptoms of the acute syndrome and odynophagia, between one and eight esophageal ulcers ranging in size from 0.3 to 1.5 cm were seen in each patient on endoscopy. Lesions were distributed over the entire length of the esophagus, were usually round or oval in shape, and often had well-demarcated margins. HIV was isolated from biopsy in one case (72,75). Other gastrointestinal manifestations may include abdominal pain and cramping, diarrhea, nausea and vomiting, anorexia, pancreatitis, and hepatitis (76,77).

RENAL

Nephrosis has been reported in acute HIV syndrome, both associated with and independent of rhabdomyolysis, with kidney biopsy in one case demonstrating acute tubular necrosis and mesangioproliferative glomerulonephritis (73,78).

PULMONARY

A predominantly CD8 lymphocytic alveolitis has been reported, initially presenting as a nonproductive cough associated with dyspnea. Also observed were leukocytosis, mildly increased interstitial markings on chest radiography, and decreased carbon dioxide diffusing capacity (79).

NEUROLOGIC

Numerous neurologic symptoms have been described in association with the acute syndrome, with their onset sometimes occurring several weeks after the appearance of other manifestations. In contrast to the usually short-lived nature of most symptoms, neurologic abnormalities may take months to resolve. Aseptic meningitis has been well described, sometimes in association with seizures and often with HIV demonstrable in the cerebrospinal fluid (CSF). In one such case, HIV could be cultured from CSF but not from blood (63,64,68). Other neurologic manifestations have included retro-orbital pain, confusion and irritability, depression, dementia, polyneuropathy, meningopolyradiculoneuritis, brachial neuritis, facial palsy, generalized weakness, myelopathy, and hypoesthesia (80–82). Two cases of Guillain–Barré syndrome have been reported, with onset at 1 week and 20 days, respectively, after other acute symptoms. In one case, 12 weeks of assisted ventilation were required and leg weakness persisted at 5 months (83).

OTHER

Other manifestations of the acute HIV syndrome have included myalgia, arthralgia, petechiae, splenomegaly, hepatomegaly, conjunctivitis, and myopericarditis (84). Opportunistic infections also have been reported, including cytomegalovirus colitis, esophageal candidiasis, and *Pneumocystis carinii* pneumonia (65,85–88).

Prevalence

Determining the prevalence of symptomatic disease during acute HIV syndrome is made difficult by its nonspecific nature and because studies of seroconverting patients may rely on historical recall of symptomatology over periods as long as 6 months. One study of 35 seroconverting persons found that 38% of subjects could recall at least one symptom persisting for 3 to 14 days during the seroconversion interval, but only 20% experienced a symptom that lasted at least 2 weeks (50). In contrast, a retrospective study of 39 seroconverting patients reported that 92.3% had an acute illness for which 87% sought medical attention, leading to hospital admission in 12% (52). Another retrospective study of 86 seroconverting patients estimated that 53% had acute symptoms (49).

Laboratory Findings

VIRAL STUDIES

Virus has been cultured from plasma and peripheral blood mononuclear cells (PBMCs) as early as 4 days after onset of symptoms, with titers ranging from 10 to 10,000 infectious doses per milliliter for cell-free virus and 100 to 10,000 doses per million PBMCs. Both cell-free and cell-associated infectious titers decline precipitously, often becoming nondetectable by 2 to 16 weeks after the onset of symptoms. Viral antigen, which also is detectable during early symptomatic disease, undergoes a similar rapid decline. Decreases in antigenemia and infectious virus are associated with the development of anti-HIV antibodies, HIV-specific cytotoxic T lymphocytes, and circulating immune complexes (18,46,64,89–93).

T Lymphocytes

T-lymphocyte subsets are perturbed frequently as a result of acute HIV infection. Initially, a reduction in CD4 and CD8 cell counts is followed by an increase in CD8 cells and an inversion of the CD4-to-CD8 ratio. The CD4 count then may increase gradually but without achieving normalization of the ratio; eventually the number of CD8 cells also drops (94–98). Severe and prolonged CD4 cell dysfunction, manifested as decreased responsiveness to both mitogens and antigens, also has been documented.

Seroconversion

Studies of seroconversion have demonstrated that immunoglobulin (Ig)M (usually directed against gp160) is the first antibody response to appear. Detectable an average of 5 days after onset of symptoms, IgM peaks at a mean of 24 days and disappears by an average of 81 days. IgG levels have been detected as early as 11 days after the onset of symptoms, but conventional enzyme-linked immunosorbent assays (ELISAs) may take 3 to 12 weeks to become positive (99).

Other Abnormalities

Leukopenia, atypical lymphocytosis, thrombocytopenia, hypergammaglobulinemia, and increased hepatic transaminases and alkaline phosphate have been reported. Lymph node biopsy specimens have contained a high number of CD4 cells, a reduction in B lymphocytes, and the presence of gp120 and gp160 proteins in leukocytes and dendritic cells.

Prognostic Factors for Progression

Numerous studies have documented faster progression to AIDS in symptomatic compared with asymptomatic seroconverting patients, in subjects whose symptoms are particularly severe or prolonged, and in those who develop fever or neurologic symptoms as part of the primary presentation (56,100–108). In contrast, one prospective study of 35 seroconverting patients found that subjects with symptomatic seroconversion tended to drop their CD4 counts and progress to AIDS more slowly than did asymptomatic seroconverting patients (50). The qualitative nature of the pattern of T-cell–receptor expansion in response to acute infection also has been predictive of progression (109).

Importance of Making an Early Diagnosis

When a diagnosis of HIV infection may be made during the acute stage of the disease, earlier and therefore more effective intervention is possible. Rosenberg and coworkers (110) have described three patients with the acute HIV syndrome who were treated with potent antiretroviral therapy before seroconversion. All developed and maintained an HIV-specific CD4 response, which previously had been observed only rarely in long-term nonprogressing patients. This finding suggests the possibility that antiretroviral therapy initiated during acute HIV syndrome has the potential of conserving an effective immune response.

Identification of patients with acute HIV infection also has important public health implications. Because up to 50% of HIV transmissions may occur around the time of the acute syndrome, providing individuals with appropriate educational interventions could have a significant impact on the spread of the epidemic (111–114).

The diagnosis of acute HIV syndrome can be made in the context of suggestive clinical findings by a positive viral RNA assay in the presence of a negative screening antibody test (e.g., ELISA) or a negative or indeterminate Western blot test (see Chapter 4 for more on HIV antibody testing). However, false-positive viral RNA assays in low titer have been described rarely with acute non–HIV-related illnesses. Although p24 antigen assays are also usually positive during the early period of symptomatology, the rapid reduction of antigenemia to undetectable levels makes this a less sensitive marker than plasma RNA levels.

The differential diagnoses of acute HIV syndrome are included in Table 2.2 (113). A number of clinical features can help to distinguish acute HIV infection from EBV-related mononucleosis (Table 2.3).

Progression to Symptomatic HIV Disease

When the high viral levels associated with acute HIV syndrome are suppressed by the initial immunologic response, an infected person generally moves into an asymptomatic period that may range from several months to more than 10 years (Fig. 2.4). Although symptoms are not present during this period of clinical latency, viral replication is ongoing, leading to a loss of approximately 10% of CD4 cells per year in most individuals.

Table 2.2   Differential Diagnosis of Primary HIV Syndrome

• Infectious mononucleosis*	• Disseminated gonococcal infection
• Toxoplasmosis	• Herpes simplex virus
• Rubella	• Typhus
• Syphilis	• Crohn's disease
• Viral hepatitis	• Other viral and spriochete infections

*Caused by either Epstein–Barr virus or cytomegalovirus

Table 2.3   Features Distinguishing Epstein–Barr Virus Infection from Primary HIV Infection

Features	Epstein-Barr Virus	HIV
Onset	Insidious	Acute
Oral	Tonsillar hypertrophy; enanthema on border of hard and soft palates; exudative pharyngitis common; no oral ulcers	Little or no hypertrophy; enanthema on hard palate; exudative pharyngitis uncommon; oral ulcers common
Rash	Rare unless antibiotics given	Common
Jaundice	Infrequent	Rare
Diarrhea	Does not occur	Occurs
Atypical lymphocytosis	80%–90%	<50%

Republished with permission from Tindall B, Cooper DA. Primary HIV infection: host responses and intervention strategies. *AIDS*. 1991;5:1–14.

Minor infections may develop as the CD4 count drops to fewer than 500 cells/mm^3, with increasingly severe infections associated with lower counts. Initial presentations may include bacterial cellulitis, herpes simplex and varicella zoster virus infections, and candidal infections of the mouth or the vagina. As the count drops to fewer than 200 cells/mm^3, more serious infections such as *P. carinii* pneumonia, cerebral toxoplasmosis, and cryptococcal meningitis may occur. If the CD4 count drops to fewer than 75–50 cells/mm^3, systemic infections with cytomegalovirus and *Mycobacterium avium* complex may occur.

In addition to opportunistic infections, malignancies (e.g., Kaposi's sarcoma and lymphoma) may develop with progressive immunologic dysfunction. HIV-infected individuals also may experience constitutional symptoms such as fever and night sweats. With advanced HIV disease, chronic diarrhea, wasting syndrome, and neurocognitive dysfunction symptomatic of HIV encephalopathy may occur.

Antiretroviral therapy and prophylaxis against opportunistic infections are clearly important at appropriate stages of the infection. However, some patients with advanced HIV disease may place a higher priority on quality rather than quantity of life and may want to withdraw antiretroviral therapy as well as other more specific treatments in favor of comfort measures.

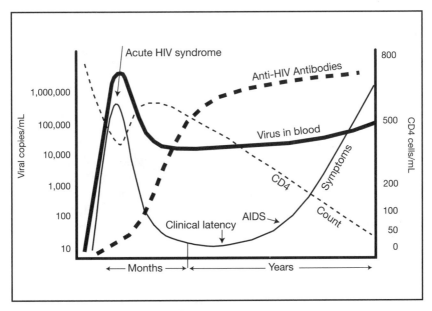

Figure 2.4   Natural history of HIV disease.

Progression to AIDS

Numerous studies have estimated the average time from HIV infection to an AIDS diagnosis in various transmission risk groups. In a study of 489 homosexual and bisexual men in the San Francisco City Clinic Cohort, 51% were estimated to have been diagnosed with AIDS at 10 years following infection (115). A similar result was reported by an international registry of homosexual men in which 39.8% were estimated to be diagnosed at 7 years, whereas only 27.3% of hemophiliacs had progressed to AIDS over the same time period (116). Studies of transfusion recipients have noted faster progression than other groups, with 49% of one group being diagnosed by 7 years (117–119).

Long-Term Nonprogression

A small percentage of HIV-infected persons will remain asymptomatic for 10 or more years. Many have CD4 lymphocyte counts in the normal range and have low or undetectable viral loads. These individuals are immunologically and epidemiologically diverse. Some seem to be infected with a strain of virus that is less virulent, whereas others seem to have unusually robust anti-HIV immune responses.

Several long-term nonprogressing patients seem to have controlled viral replication successfully in the absence of antiretroviral therapy, despite being HIV infected for 14 years or more. These individuals are asymptomatic and have maintained normal CD4 cell counts and low but detectable viral loads. A central feature of their immune responses is a specific proliferative CD4 lymphocyte response to HIV antigens. These responses are reproducible over extended periods and inversely correlate with the viral load (110). As discussed above, treating acutely infected individuals may lead to the preservation of this HIV-specific CD4 cell response. In addition, prolonged treatment of chronically infected individuals recently has been reported to be associated with the detection of a similar immune response (120,121), raising the theoretical possibility of discontinuing or interrupting treatment following immune reconstitution.

■ ■ ■

Key Points

- HIV infection is established by virus entry into cells and initiation of its replication cycle.

- The deterioration of immune function that is characteristic of HIV infection occurs through CD4 lymphocyte depletion, which is caused primarily by viral replication.

- HIV replicates rapidly in untreated individuals, with estimates of up to 10 billion viral particles produced each day. Random-point mutations, some of which confer resistance to antiretroviral agents, are common.

- High-level viral resistance may develop over time in patients receiving antiretroviral therapy. The rapid turnover of HIV leads to mutations in viral genes that code for drug resistance. Such mutations may exist in some viral strains even before patients are exposed to antiretroviral drugs.

- Symptomatic primary HIV syndrome (characterized by fever, pharyngitis, rash, and diarrhea) is associated with faster progression to AIDS than is asymptomatic infection.

- Early diagnosis of HIV infection is important because potent antiretroviral therapy initiated during primary HIV syndrome may help conserve an effective immunologic response to the virus.

- Primary HIV syndrome is followed by an asymptomatic period ranging from several months to 10 years, during which, if the infection is not treated, viral replication continues, resulting in decline in CD4 cell count over time, symptomatic disease, and ultimately AIDS.

■ ■ ■

REFERENCES

1. **Samson M, Labbe O, Mollereau C, et al.** Molecular cloning and functional expression of a new human CC-chemokine receptor gene. *Biochemistry.* 1996;35: 3362–7.

2. **Wu L, Gerard NP, Wyatt R, et al.** CD4-induced interaction of primary HIV-1 gp120 glycoproteins with the chemokine receptor CCR-5. *Nature.* 1996;384: 179–83.

3. **Alkhatib G, Combadiere, Broder CC, et al.** CC CKR5: a RANTES, MIP-1alpha, MIP-1beta-receptor as a fusion cofactor for macrophage-tropic HIV-1. *Science.* 1996;272:1955–58.

4. **Dragic T, Litwin V, Allaway GP, et al.** HIV-1 entry into CD4+ cells is mediated by the chemokine receptor CC-CKR-5. *Nature.* 1996;381:667–73.

5. **Deng H, Liu R, Ellmeier W, et al.** Identification of the major co-receptor for primary isolates of HIV-1. *Nature.* 1996;381:661–66.

6. **Feng Y, Broder CC, Kennedy PE, Berger EA.** HIV-1 entry co-factor: Functional cDNA clone of a seven-transmembrane, G protein-coupled receptor. *Science.* 1996;272:872–77.

7. **Kahn JO, Walker BD.** Acute human immunodeficiency virus type 1 infection. *N Engl J Med.* 1998;339:33–9.

8. **Veenstra J, Schuurman R, Cornelissen M, et al.** Transmission of zidovudine-resistant human immunodeficiency virus type 1 variants following deliberate injection of blood from a patient with AIDS: characteristics and natural history of the virus. *Clin Infect Dis.* 1995;21:556–60.

9. **Zaitseva M, Blauvelt A, Lee S, et al.** Expression and function of CCR5 and CXCR4 on human Langerhans cells and macrophages: implications for HIV primary infection. *Nat Med.* 1997;3:1369–75.

10. **Liu R, Paxton WA, Choe S, et al.** Homozygous defect in HIV-1 coreceptor accounts for resistance of some multiply exposed individuals to HIV-1 infection. *Cell.* 1996;86:367–77.

11. **Samson M, Libert F, Doranz BJ, et al.** Resistance to HIV-1 infection in caucasian individuals bearing mutant alleles of the CCR-5 chemokine-receptor gene. *Nature.* 1996; 382:722–25.

12. **Dean M, Carrington M, Winkler, et al.** Genetic restriction of HIV-1 infection and progression to AIDS by a mutant allele of the CKR5 structural gene. *Science.* 1996;273:1856–62.

13. **Smith MW, Dean M, Carrington M, et al.** Contrasting genetic influence of CCR2 and CCR5 variants on HIV-1 infection and disease progression. *Science.* 1997: 277:959–65.

14. **Winkler C, Modi W, Smith MW, et al.** Genetic restriction of AIDS pathogenesis by an SDF-1 chemokine gene variant. *Science.* 1998;279:389–93.

15. **Choe H, Farzan M, Sun Y, et al.** The beta-chemokine receptors CCR3 and CCR5 facilitate infection by primary HIV-1 isolates. *Cell.* 1996;85:1135–48.

16. **Rizzardi G, Morawetz RA, Vicenzi E, et al.** CCR2 polymorphism and HIV disease. *Nat Med.* 1998;4:252–3.

17. **Michael NL, Louie LG, Rohrbaugh AL, et al.** The role of CCR5 and CCR2 polymorphisms in HIV-1 transmission and disease progression. *Nat Med.* 1997;3: 1160–2.

18. **Ariyoshi K, Harwood E, Chiengsong-Popov R, Weber J.** Is clearance of HIV-1 viraemia at seroconversion mediated by neutralizing antibodies? *Lancet.* 1992;340: 1257–8.

19. **Koup RA, Safrit JT, Cao Y, Andrews CA, McLeod G, Borkowsky W, Farthing C, et al.** Temporal association of cellular immune responses with the initial control of viremia in primary human immunodeficiency virus type 1 syndrome. *J Virol.* 1994;68:4650–5.

20. **Lathey JL, Pratt RD, Spector SA.** Appearance of autologous neutralizing antibody correlates with reduction in virus load and phenotype switch during primary infection with human immunodeficiency virus type 1. *J Infect Dis.* 1997;175: 231–2.

21. **Ogg GS, Jin X, Bonhoeffer S, et al.** Quantitation of HIV-1-specific cytotoxic T lymphocytes and plasma load of viral DNA. *Science.* 1998;279:2103–8.

22. **Haynes BF, Pantaleo G, Fauci AS.** Toward an understanding of the correlates of protective immunity to HIV infection. *Science.* 1996;271:324–32.

23. **Pantaleo G, Demarest JF, Soudeyns H, et al.** Major expansion of CD8+ T cells with a predominant V-B usage during the primary immune response to HIV. *Nature.* 1994;370:463–7.

24. **Morens DM.** Antibody-dependent enhancement of infection and the pathogenesis of viral disease. *Clin Infect Dis.* 1994;19:500–12.

25. **Harper ME, Marselle LM, Gallo RC, Wong-Staal F.** Detection of lymphocytes expressing human T-lymphotropic virus type III in lymph nodes and peripheral blood from infected individuals by in situ hybridization. *Proc Natl Acad Sci U S A.* 1986;83:772–6.

26. **Schnittman SM, Greenhouse JJ, Psallidopoulos MC, et al.** Increasing viral burden in CD4+ T cells from patients with human immunodeficiency virus (HIV) infection reflects rapidly progressive immunosuppression and clinical disease. *Ann Intern Med.* 1997;113:438–443.

27. **Fox CH, Tenner-Racz K, Racz P, et al.** Lymphoid germinal centers are reservoirs of human immunodeficiency virus type 1 RNA. *J Infect Dis.* 1991;164:1051–7.

28. **Haase AT, Henry K, Zupancic M, et al.** Quantitative image analysis of HIV-1 infection in lymphoid tissue. *Science.* 1996;274:985–9.

29. **Pantaleo G, Cohen OJ, Schacker T, et al.** Evolutionary pattern of human immunodeficiency virus (HIV) replication and distribution in lymph nodes following primary infection: implications for antiviral therapy. *Nat Med.* 1998;4:341–5.

30. **Embretson J, Zupancic M, Ribas JL, et al.** Massive covert infection of helper T lymphocytes and macrophages by HIV during the incubation period of AIDS. *Nature.* 1993;362:359–62.

31. **Pantaleo G, Graziosi C, Demarest JF, et al.** HIV infection is active and progressive in lymphoid tissue during the clinically latent stage of disease. *Nature.* 1993; 362:355–8.

32. **Pantaleo G, Graziosi C, Butini L, et al.** Lymphoid organs function as major reservoirs for human immunodeficiency virus. *Proc Natl Acad Sci U S A.* 1988;88: 9838–42.

33. **Ho DD, Neumann AU, Perelson AS, et al.** Rapid turnover of plasma virions and CD4 lymphocytes in HIV-1 infection. *Nature.* 1995;373:123–6.

34. **Ho D.** *Turnover of HIV.* Plenary session (167) presented at the XII International AIDS Conference, June 29 to July 2, 1998, Geneva.

35. **Hecht FM, Grant FM, Petropoulos CJ, et al.** Sexual transmission of an HIV-1 variant resistant to multiple reverse transcriptase and protease inhibitors. *N Engl J Med.* 1998;339:307–10.

36. **Willey RL, Theodore TS, Martin MA.** Amino acid substitutions in the human immunodeficiency virus type 1 gp120 V3 loop that change viral tropism also alter physical and functional properties of the virion envelope. *J Virol.* 1994;68: 4409–19.

37. **Keet IPM, Kirjnen P, Koot M, et al.** *Fever with Skin Rash and Absence of Anti-HIV Core in HIV Seroconverters are Predictors of Rapid Progression to AIDS.* VIIIth International AIDS Conference, July 19 to 24, Amsterdam (MoC 0085).

38. **Roos MTL, Lange JMA, de Goede REY, et al.** Viral phenotype and immune response in primary human immunodeficiency virus 1 infection. *J Infect Dis.* 1992; 165:427–32.

39. **Koot M, Keet IPM, Vos AHV, et al.** Prognostic value of HIV-1 syncytium-inducing phenotype for rate of CD4+ depletion and progression to AIDS. *Ann Intern Med.* 1993;118:681–8.

40. **Bozzette SA, McCutchan JA, Spector SA, et al.** A cross-sectional comparison of persons with syncytium- and non–syncytium-inducing human immunodeficiency virus. *J Infect Dis.* 1993;168:1374–9.

41. **Nielsen C, Pedersen C, Lundgren JD, Gerstoft J.** Biological properties of HIV isolates in primary HIV infection: Consequences for the subsequent course of infection. *AIDS.* 1993;7:1035–40.

42. **Keet IPM, Krol A, Koot M, et al.** Predictors of disease progression in HIV-infected homosexual men with CD4+ cells <200 x 10^6/l but free of AIDS-defining clinical disease. *AIDS.* 1994;8:1577–83.

43. **Anonymous.** Needlestick transmission of HTLV-III from a patient infected in Africa. *Lancet.* 1984;2:1376–7.

44. **Ho DD, Sarngadharan G, Resnick L, et al.** Primary human T-lymphotropic virus type III infection. *Ann Intern Med.* 1985;103:880–3.

45. **Cooper DA, Gold J, Maclean P, et al.** Acute AIDS retrovirus infection: definition of a clinical illness associated with seroconversion. *Lancet.* 1985;1:537–40.

46. **Gaines H.** Primary HIV infection: clinical and diagnostic aspects. *Scand J Infect Dis.* 1989;S61:1–46.

47. **Wantzin GRL, Lindhardt BO, Weismann K, Ulrich K.** Acute HTLV-III infection associated with exanthema, diagnosed by seroconversion. *Br J Derm.* 1986;115: 601–6.

48. **Lindskov R, Lindhardt BO, Weismann K, et al.** Acute HTLV-III infection with roseola-like rash. *Lancet.* 1986;1:447.

49. **Pedersen C, Lindhardt BO, Jensen BL, et al.** Clinical course of primary HIV infection: consequences for subsequent course of HIV infection. *BMJ.* 1989;299: 154–7.

50. **Phair JP, Margolick JB, Jacobson LP, et al.** Detection of infection with human immunodeficiency virus type I before seroconversion: correlation with clinical symptoms and outcome. *J Infect Dis.* 1997;175:959–62.

51. **Sinicco A, Palestro G, Caramello P, et al.** Acute HIV-1 infection: clinical and biological study of 12 patients. *J Acquir Immune Defic Syndr Hum Retrovirol.* 1990; 3:260–5.

52. **Tindall B, Barker S, Donovan B, et al.** Characterization of the acute clinical illness associated with human immunodeficiency virus infection. *Arch Intern Med.* 1988;148:945–9.

53. **Schacker T, Collier AC, Hughes J, et al.** Clinical and epidemiologic features of primary HIV infection. *Ann Intern Med.* 1996;125:257–64.

54. **Valle SL.** Febrile pharyngitis as the primary sign of HIV infection in a cluster of cases linked by sexual contact. *Scand J Infect Dis.* 1987;19:13–7.

55. **Kinloch-de Loes S, de Saussure P, Saurat JH, et al.** Symptomatic primary infection due to human immunodeficiency virus type 1: review of 31 cases. *Clin Infect Dis.* 1993;17:59–65.

56. **Veugelers PJ, Kaldor JM, Strathdee SA, et al.** Incidence and prognostic significance of symptomatic primary human immunodeficiency virus type 1 infection in homosexual men. *J Infect Dis.* 1997;176:112–7.

57. **Vanhems P, Allard R, Cooper DA, et al.** Acute human immunodeficiency virus type 1 disease as a mononucleosis-like illness: Is the diagnosis too restrictive? *Clin Infect Dis.* 1997;24:965–70.

58. **Bollinger RC, Brookmeyer RS, Mehendale SM, et al.** Risk factors and clinical presentation of acute primary HIV infection in India. *JAMA.* 1997;278:2085–9.

59. **Ruutu P, Suni J, Oksanen K, Ruutu T.** Primary infection with HIV in a severely immunosuppressed patient with acute leukemia. *Scand J Infect Dis.* 1987;19: 369–72.

60. **White GC, Matthews TJ, Weinhold, et al.** HTLV-III seroconversion associated with heat-treated factor VIII concentrate. *Lancet.* 1986;1:611–2.

61. **Daar ES, Bai J, Hausner MA, et al.** Acute HIV syndrome after discontinuation of antiretroviral therapy in a patient treated before seroconversion. *Ann Intern Med.* 1998;128:827–9.

62. **Tindall B, Cooper DA.** Primary HIV infection: host responses and intervention strategies. *AIDS.* 1991;5:1–14.

63. **Carne CA, Tedder RS, Smith A, et al.** Acute encephalopathy coincident with seroconversion for anti-HTLV-III. *Lancet.* 1985;2:1206–8.

64. **Scully RE, Mark EJ, McNeely WF, McNeely BU.** Case records of the Massachusetts General Hospital: case 33–1989. *N Engl J Med.* 1989;321:454-63.

65. **Gupta KK.** Acute immunosuppression with HIV seroconversion. *N Engl J Med.* 1993;328:288–9.

66. **Rustin MHA, Ridley CM, Smith MD, et al.** The acute exanthem associated with seroconversion to human T-cell lymphotropic virus III in a homosexual man. *J Infect.* 1986;12:161–3.

67. **Calabrese LH, Proffitt MR, Levin KH, et al.** Acute infection with the human immunodeficiency virus (HIV) associated with acute brachial neuritis and exanthematous rash. *Ann Intern Med.* 1987;107:849–51.

68. **Ho DD, Rota TR, Schooley RT, et al.** Isolation of HTLV-III from cerebrospinal fluid and neural tissues of patients with neurologic syndromes related to the acquired immunodeficiency syndrome. *N Engl J Med.* 1985;313:1493–7.

69. **Calza AM, Kinloch S, Mainetti C, et al.** Primary human immunodeficiency virus infection mimicking syphilis. *J Infect Dis.* 1991;164:615–6.

70. **McMillan A, Bishop PE, Aw D, Peutherer JF.** Immunohistology of the skin rash associated with acute HIV infection. *AIDS.* 1989;3:309–12.

71. **Wall RA, Denning DW, Amos A.** HIV antigenaemia in acute HIV infection. *Lancet.* 1987;1:566.

72. **Rabeneck L, Popovic M, Gartner S, et al.** Acute HIV infection presenting with painful swallowing and esophageal ulcers. *JAMA.* 1990;263:2318–22.

73. **Lawrenson J, Chapman P, Geffen L, et al.** Proteinuria and the acute mononucleosis-like illness associated with seroconversion in HIV infection. *S Afr Med J.* 1991;79:625–6.

74. **Biggs B, Newton-John HF.** Acute HTLV-III infection: a case followed from onset to seroconversion. *Med J Austr.* 1986;144:545–7.

75. **Fusade T, Liony C, Joly P, et al.** Ulcerative esophagitis during primary HIV infection. *Am J Gastroenterol.* 1992;87:1523–4.

76. **Molina JM, Welker Y, Ferchal F, et al.** Hepatitis associated with primary HIV infection. *Gastroenterology.* 1992;102:739–746.

77. **Rizzardi GP, Tambussi G, Lazzarin A.** Acute pancreatitis during primary HIV-1 infection. *N Engl J Med.* 1997;336:1836–1837.

78. **del Rio C, Soffer O, Widell JL, et al.** Acute human immunodeficiency virus infection temporally associated with rhabdomyolysis, acute renal failure, and nephrosis. *Rev Infect Dis.* 1990;12:282–5.

79. **Longworth DL, Spech TJ, Ahmad M, et al.** Lymphocytic alveolitis in primary HIV infection. *Cleve Clin J Med.* 1997:57:379–82.

80. **Piette AM, Tusseau F, Vignon D, et al.** Acute neuropathy coincident with seroconversion for anti-LAV/HTLV-III. *Lancet.* 1986;1:852.

81. **Denning DW, Anderson J, Rudge P, Smith H.** Acute myelopathy associated with primary infection with human immunodeficiency virus. *BMJ.* 1987;294:143–4.

82. **Holland DJ, Dwyer DE, Saksena NK, et al.** Dementia and pancytopenia in a patient who died of AIDS within one year of primary human immunodeficiency virus infection. *Clin Infect Dis.* 1996;22:1121–2.

83. **Hagberg L, Malmvall BE, Svennerholm L, et al.** Guillain-Barre syndrome as an early manifestation of HIV central nervous system infection. *Scand J Infect Dis.* 1986;18:591–2.

84. **Guillaume MP, Van Beers D, Delforge ML, et al.** Primary HIV infection presenting as myopericarditis and rhabdomyolysis. *Clin Infect Dis.* 1995;21:451–2.

85. **Clotet B.** Oesophageal candidiasis in people with primary HIV infection. *AIDS.* 1991;5:1034.

86. **Decker CF, Tiernan R, Paparello SF.** Esophageal candidiasis associated with acute infection due to human immunodeficiency virus. *Clin Infect Dis.* 1992;14: 791.

87. **Pena JM, Martinez-Lopez MA, Arnalich F, et al.** Esophageal candidiasis associated with acute infection due to human immunodeficiency virus: case report and review. *Rev Infect Dis.* 1991;13:872–5.

88. **Vento S, Di Perri G, Garofano T, et al.** *Pneumocystis carinii* pneumonia during primary HIV-1 infection. *Lancet.* 1993;342:24–5.

89. **Daar ES, Moudgil T, Meyer RD, Ho DD.** Transient high levels of viremia in patients with primary human immunodeficiency virus type III infection. *N Engl J Med.* 1991;324:961–4.

90. **Clark SJ, Saag MS, Don Decker W, et al.** High titers of cytopathic virus in plasma of patients with symptomatic primary HIV-1 infection. *N Engl J Med.* 1991; 324:954–60.

91. **Gaines H, Albert J, Von Sydow M, et al.** HIV antigenaemia and virus isolation from plasma during primary HIV infection. *Lancet.* 1987;1:1317–8.

92. **Roos MTL, de Leeuw NASM, Claessen FAP, et al.** Viro-immunological studies in acute HIV-1 infection. *AIDS.* 1994;8:1533–8.

93. **Musey L, Hughes J, Schacker T, et al.** Cytotoxic-T-cell responses, viral load, and disease progression in early human immunodeficiency virus type I infection. *N Engl J Med.* 1997;337:1267–74.

94. **Cooper DA, Tindall B, Wilson EJ, et al.** Characterization of T lymphocyte responses during primary infection with human immunodeficiency virus. *J Infect Dis* 1988; 157:889–96.

95. **Pedersen C, Dickmeiss E, Gaub J, et al.** T-cell subset alterations and lymphocyte responsiveness to mitogens and antigen during severe primary infection with HIV: a case series of seven consecutive HIV seroconverters. *AIDS.* 1990;4:523–6.

96. **Gaines H, von Sydow MAE, von Stedingk LV, et al.** Immunological changes in primary HIV-1 infection. *AIDS.* 1990;4:995–9.

97. **Cossarizza A, Ortolani C, Mussini C, et al.** Massive activation of immune cells with an intact T-cell repertoire in acute human immunodeficiency virus syndrome. *J Infect Dis.* 1995;172:105–12.

98. **Tucker J, Ludlam CA, Craig A, et al.** HTLV-III infection associated with glandular-fever-like illness in a haemophiliac. *Lancet.* 1985;1:585.

99. **Cooper DA, Imrie AA, Penny R.** Antibody response to human immunodeficiency virus after primary infection. *J Infect Dis.* 1987;155:1113–8.

100. **Keet IPM, Krijnen P, Koot M, et al.** Predictors of rapid progression to AIDS in HIV-1 seroconverters. *AIDS.* 1993;7:51–7.

101. **Pedersen C, Gerstoft J, Lundgren J, et al.** *Development of AIDS and Low CD4 Cell Counts in a Cohort of 180 HIV Seroconverters.* IXth International AIDS Conference, June 6 to 11, 1993, Berlin (PO-B01–0862).

102. **Pedersen C, Katzenstein T, Nielsen C, et al.** Prognostic value of serum HIV-RNA levels at virologic steady state after seroconversion: relation to CD4 cell

count and clinical course of primary infection. *J Acquir Immune Defic Syndr Hum Retrovirol.* 1997;16:93–9.

103. **Lindback S, Brostrom C, Karlsson A, Gaines H.** Does symptomatic primary HIV-1 infection accelerate progression to CDC stage IV disease, CD4 count below 200 x 10^6/l, AIDS, and death from AIDS? *BMJ.* 1994;309:1535–7.

104. **Bachmeyer C, Boufassa F, Sereni D, et al.** *Prognostic Value of Acute Symptomatic HIV-1 Infection.* IXth International AIDS Conference, June 6 to 11, 1993, Berlin (PO-B01–0870).

105. **Vanhems P, Lambert J, Cooper DA, et al.** Severity and prognosis of acute human immunodeficiency virus type I illness: A dose-response relationship. *Clin Infect Dis.* 1998;26:323–9.

106. **Dorrucci M, Rezza G, Vlahov D, et al.** Clinical characteristics and prognostic value of acute retroviral syndrome among injecting drug users. *AIDS.* 1995:9: 597–604.

107. **Boufassa F, Bachmeyer C, Carre N.** Influence of neurologic manifestations of primary human immunodeficiency virus infection on disease progression. *J Infect Dis.* 1995;171:1190–5.

108. **Sinicco A, Fora R, Sciandra M, et al.** Risk of developing AIDS after primary acute HIV-1 infection. *J Acquir Immune Defic Syndr Hum Retrovirol.* 1993;6: 575–81.

109. **Pantaleo G, Demarest JF, Schacker T, et al.** The qualitative nature of the primary immune response to HIV infection is a prognosticator of disease progression independent of the initial level of plasma viremia. *Proc Natl Acad Sci U S A.* 1997;94:254–8.

110. **Rosenberg ES, Billingsley JM, Caliendo AM, et al.** Vigorous HIV-1-specific CD4+ T cell responses associated with control of viremia. *Science.* 1997;278: 1447–50.

111. **Cates W, Chesney MA, Cohen MS.** Primary HIV infection: A public health opportunity. *Am J Public Health.* 1997;87:1928–30.

112. **Koopman JS, Jacquez JA, Welch GW, et al.** The role of early HIV infection in the spread of HIV through populations. *J Acquir Immune Defic Syndr Hum Retrovirol.* 1997;14:249–58.

113. **Jolles S, Kinloch de Loes S, Johnson MA, Janossy G.** Primary HIV-1 infection: a new medical emergency? *BMJ.* 1996;312:1243–4.

114. **Jacquez JA, Koopman JS, Simon CP, Longini IM.** Role of the primary infection in epidemics of HIV infection in gay cohorts. *J Acquir Immune Defic Syndr Hum Retrovirol.* 1994;7:1169–84.

115. **Rutherford GW, Lifson AR, Hessol NA, et al.** Course of HIV-1 infection in a cohort of homosexual and bisexual men: an 11-year follow-up study. *BMJ.* 1990; 301:1183–8.

116. **Biggar RJ and the International Registry of Seroconverters.** AIDS incubation in 1891 HIV seroconverters from different exposure groups. *AIDS.* 1990;4: 1059–66.

117. **Ward JW, Bush TJ, Perkins HA, et al.** The natural history of transfusion-associated infection with human immunodeficiency virus: factors influencing the rate of progression to disease. *N Engl J Med.* 1989;321:947–52.

118. **Giesecke J, Scalia-Tomba G, Burglund O, et al.** Incidence of symptoms and

AIDS in 146 Swedish haemophiliacs and blood transfusion recipients infected with human immunodeficiency virus. *BMJ*. 1988;297:99–102.

119. **Donegan E, Stuart M, Niland JC, et al.** Infection with human immunodeficiency virus type 1 (HIV-1) among recipients of antibody-positive blood donations. *Ann Intern Med*. 1990;113:733–9.

120. **Walker B.** *Immune Events in Early HIV Infection*. Session #425, XIIth International AIDS Conference, June 29 to July 2, 1998, Geneva.

121. **Autran B.** *Immune Responses and Reconstitution*. Session #426, XIIth International AIDS Conference, June 29 to July 2, 1998, Geneva.

3

■　■　■

HIV Prevention in Clinical Practice

Robert Garofalo, MD
Harvey J. Makadon, MD

Many challenges remain in the fight against HIV and AIDS. Although significant advances in antiretroviral therapy and the prophylaxis and treatment of opportunistic infections have occurred over the past two decades, a cure or preventive vaccine remains elusive. People continue to become infected with HIV at an alarming rate. In the United States, it has been estimated that over 40,000 new infections are diagnosed each year (1). One quarter of new HIV infections in the United States occurs in people under 22 years of age, and one half occurs in people under 25 (2). In 1995, AIDS ranked as the sixth leading cause of death among those aged 15 to 24 years (3) and is currently the second leading cause of death among those 25 to 44. Preventing new cases of HIV infection is an essential component of efforts to curtail this epidemic.

Most cases of HIV transmission can be linked to specific human behaviors. Epidemiologic and ethnographic studies have shown the effectiveness of community-based programs in targeting specific high-risk behaviors and decreasing HIV transmission. Needle-exchange programs (NEPs) for injection-drug users and widespread educational campaigns to modify the sexual behavior of homosexual men are two such examples (4). A 1997 National Institute of Health (NIH) consensus statement on strategies to prevent HIV risk behaviors concluded that behavioral interventions aimed at reducing the risk for HIV/AIDS are effective and should be disseminated widely (5). However, limitations placed on providing clean needles to drug users and on promoting condom use within public schools have resulted in variable and inconsistent efforts toward behavioral change.

Barriers to Providing HIV Prevention Information in Clinical Practice

Traditionally, our health care system has placed a higher priority on acute care needs of the population than on issues related to disease prevention. A clinician's potential to influence the attitudes and behaviors of patients has gone largely unrealized. Physicians are cited consistently by the public as the most trusted source of health information, and patients often heed their counsel (6). As such, primary care providers have the potential to play an integral role in HIV prevention efforts. However, although physicians are considered valuable sources of information about health issues, one national survey showed that counseling and advice about HIV transmission were given in fewer than 1% of primary care visits (7). Within a clinical setting, four major barriers have been identified as impediments to communicating information about HIV prevention:

1. A narrow conception of health care and the physician's role in prevention efforts

2. Physician attitudes toward HIV-infected people, including the stigma associated with the disease and discomfort discussing sexual and drug-taking behaviors

3. Practical constraints of time and resources

4. Ambiguities in the HIV prevention message, including imprecise information about sexual risk transmission rates associated with various behaviors (6).

In 1992, the Centers for Disease Control and Prevention (CDC) and the Health Resources and Services Administration (HRSA) commissioned a survey of primary care physicians to learn more about practices in the prevention of HIV infection and limitations to those practices. Although most physicians indicated that they "usually" or "always" asked new adult patients about cigarette smoking, inquiries about sexually transmitted diseases (STDs), condom use, sexual orientation, and number of sexual partners were far less frequent (8). One quarter of physicians surveyed believed that their patients would be offended by questions about their sexual behavior, whereas a corresponding survey of patients indicated that nearly all would not object to discussing AIDS (9). These results highlight missed opportunities for HIV prevention counseling during patient encounters and indicate an increased need for focused skills-based training of clinicians in areas such as sexual history taking and HIV risk assessment.

What Is HIV Prevention?

The American Medical Association (AMA) has recommended that a discussion of HIV infection and HIV prevention be part of routine health care maintenance for all patients (10). Clinicians see patients in a variety of settings, and these often dictate the nature and scope of issues that can be addressed. Primary care practitioners should be able to identify which patients are at high risk for HIV infection and to focus prevention efforts on them. Accurate estimates of risk cannot be made solely by appearance or self-reported behaviors. An astute clinician should inquire about sexual and other high-risk behaviors in a manner that is both sensitive and comprehensive (Table 3.1).

Once a patient's risk has been assessed, clinical prevention entails providing information that will help to modify high-risk behaviors. Clinicians should view HIV prevention as health education, not as a specific

---

Table 3.1   Sample HIV Risk-Assessment Instrument for Men and Women

Men
- Did you receive a transfusion of blood or blood products between 1978 and 1985?

- Have you ever, even once, used any kind of injected drug?

- Have you ever had a disease that you contracted through sexual contact?

- Have you ever, even once, had sex with a man?

- Have you ever, even once, had sex with a prostitute or with someone who has used injected drugs?

- Do you have any other reason to suspect you might be at risk for AIDS or HIV?

Women
- Did you receive a transfusion of blood or blood products between 1978 and 1985?

- Have you ever, even once, used any kind of injected drug?

- Have you ever had a disease that you contracted through sexual contact?

- Are you sexually active with men?

- Have you ever, even once, had sex with a bisexual man or someone who has used injected drugs?

- Do you have any other reason to suspect you might be at risk for AIDS or HIV?

Adapted with permission from Libman H, Witzburg RA (eds). *HIV Infection: A Primary Care Manual.* Boston: Little, Brown; 1996.

psychological intervention requiring extensive assessment and counseling skills. Physicians should engage their patients in open discussions about their health and behavioral risk, with careful consideration of their culture and values (Tables 3.2 and 3.3). Although permanent behavioral change is difficult to achieve and no intervention strategy will be completely effective, successful prevention efforts involve the clinician and patient as part of a system of care. That system may include community-based prevention services that emphasize harm reduction, mental health and substance abuse counseling, and educational efforts directed at change in sexual behavior.

Populations at Risk

Approximately one million U.S. citizens are believed to be infected with HIV (11). Since the beginning of the epidemic, high-risk behaviors (e.g., male-to-male sexual contact, injection-drug use [IDU]) have and continue to account for the vast majority of reported AIDS cases. According to statistics from the CDC, individuals with these two risk behaviors accounted for over 75% of reported AIDS cases in 1995 (12). Racial and ethnic minorities also are represented disproportionately in all risk categories, accounting for 55% of adult AIDS cases and 84% of pediatric cases reported in 1995. These groups deserve continued and focused prevention efforts.

However, as the AIDS epidemic grows, its demographics are changing. Women are now one of the fastest growing populations being infected with HIV. It has been estimated that the number of AIDS cases among women is doubling every 1 to 2 years (13). From 1985 through 1996, the proportion of adolescent/adult women reported to the CDC with AIDS increased steadily, from 7% to 20% of cases (14). Heterosexual transmission is the most rapidly increasing transmission category among women. In 1996, 40% of women with AIDS acquired HIV through heterosexual contact with at-risk partners (15). Particularly among women, ethnic and racial minorities are affected disproportionately. Although black and Hispanic women comprise less than one fourth of all women in the United States, they account for more than three fourths of AIDS cases (14).

AIDS is quickly becoming a disease of the young in the United States. Although the rate of new AIDS cases reported among people born before 1960 seems to be reaching a plateau, the rate among younger Americans born after 1960 continues to escalate (16). More than in any other risk group, HIV is spread sexually in young people. Two groups of youths account for roughly three quarters of the adolescent epidemic: men who have sex with men and women who are infected through heterosexual contact (17).

Prevention of Sexual Transmission

HIV is transmitted sexually by exposure of the mucous membranes of the penis, vagina, anus, and rectum to infected semen, pre-ejaculate, vaginal secretions, or blood. Sexual transmission of HIV is relatively inefficient and unpredictable. One person can be infected by a single sexual encounter, whereas others can have multiple exposures and never become infected. Many factors seem to contribute to the sexual risk of HIV transmission. Mucosal factors shown to facilitate transmission include abrasion or tears from mechanical trauma and genital ulcerations from co-existing infections. Viral factors include the particular strain of HIV and its concentration in infected bodily fluids (18). Behavioral factors implicated in HIV transmission include engaging in sexual activity while under the influence of drugs and using condoms inconsistently or inappropriately.

High-Risk Sexual Activities

The per-episode risk associated with a specific sexual act is variable and difficult to quantify. Unprotected receptive anal intercourse is felt to be the highest-risk sexual activity followed by unprotected receptive vaginal intercourse. Few data exist about the estimate of risk associated with insertive anal or vaginal intercourse (19). In general, male-to-male and male-to-female transmission are considered more efficient than female-to-male or fe-

---

Table 3.2   Sexual Risk-Reduction Topics for Discussion with Patients

---

- The importance of taking care of oneself and others by reducing risk for HIV transmission

- The role of "safer sex" in the patient's life with all relevant partners—whether regular, occasional, and/or paid

- The importance of limiting the number of sexual partners

- The importance of knowing the serostatus of sexual partners and frankly discussing risk behaviors with them

- The risk of unplanned or unprotected sexual contact when using drugs or alcohol

- The risk of HIV transmission during pregnancy

- The use of condoms in male–female and male–male sexual activity, including identification of obstacles and strategies to overcome them

---

Adapted with permission from Libman H, Witzburg RA (eds). *HIV Infection: A Primary Care Manual.* Boston: Little, Brown; 1996.

male-to-female transmission (19). Seroconversion as a result of oral sex has been documented (20), and recent data suggest that there is a tangible risk associated with this activity. The correct and consistent use of latex condoms can reduce significantly the risk of transmission during anal, vaginal, and oral sex (21).

Clinicians should provide patients with information about the relative risk of sexual behaviors when educating them about options, including abstinence, for decreasing HIV transmission. However, simply advising abstinence is an unrealistic foundation on which to build an effective HIV prevention strategy, particularly among adolescents and young adults. Sexual activity is a normal experimental step in the human developmental process, a step that is first taken most often during adolescence (17). Most people will choose to have sex, and they should be provided with instructions on safer sex behaviors. Sexually active individuals may be reached more effectively with nonjudgmental messages that emphasize the importance of having satisfying intimate experiences, improving interpersonal communication, maintaining control over their sexual behavior, and taking the responsibility to protect themselves from HIV.

Over the years, safer sex guidelines have emphasized the importance of limiting the number of sexual partners and avoiding those who may be at risk for HIV (22). This message also should include using condoms consistently and limiting oneself to low-risk sexual activities. Individuals should be encouraged to discuss openly their serostatus before engaging in sexual activity, because evidence suggests that high-risk behaviors (e.g., unprotected anal intercourse between homosexual men) are more likely to occur within the context of an ongoing relationship than in anonymous sexual encounters (23). Among individuals infected with HIV, clinicians must continue to advise safer sexual practices and consistent condom use. HIV-infected people remain potentially infectious to others even if antiretroviral therapy has reduced viral load to "undetectable" levels. In general, prevention messages must be designed with a knowledge of the individuals at whom they are targeted and then presented in an easily understood manner.

Treatment of Sexually Transmitted Diseases

Among people who are sexually active, a compelling body of evidence has shown that STD prevention and treatment are an important component to a successful HIV prevention strategy, particularly for young women who are vulnerable to heterosexual transmission. The rise in heterosexual HIV transmission among women closely parallels the rise of other STD epidemics (24). In addition to the common behavioral risk factors between HIV and other STDs, evidence suggests that on a biologic level, STDs facilitate the sexual acquisition of HIV (25). These include ulcerative STDs (e.g., syphilis, herpes, chancroid) and nonulcerative (e.g., chlamydia, gonorrhea, trichomoniasis). In addition, an HIV-infected person with another STD may be more infectious and may transmit the virus to an uninfected partner more easily (25,26). Studies from Africa have shown that treating STDs reduces both how much and how often the HIV virus is shed in genital secretions and lesions (26). A randomized trial in Tanzania demonstrated a 42% decrease in new heterosexually transmitted HIV cases in communities with improved treatment of STDs compared with communities with minimal STD services (27).

Unfortunately, comprehensive STD clinical services are not readily available in all parts of the United States. In fact, only one half of local public health departments provide STD services in comparison to other services such as immunizations, which are provided by 97%. Within the private sector in one state in which health maintenance organization enrollees have more annual preventive care visits than the national average, only an estimated 21% of sexually active teenage women are screened routinely for STDs (28). Expanding STD surveillance programs and improving STD detection and treatment services for individuals who have or who are at risk for STDs should be part of any comprehensive HIV prevention strategy.

Appropriate Use of Condoms

In addition to STD management, consistent use of latex condoms during sexual activity is essential to clinical HIV prevention efforts. Physicians must be able to provide patients with specific instructions about the appropriate use of condoms, because improper use can lead to slippage, breakage, and unnecessary HIV exposure. Instructions for correct latex condom use include (18):

1. Using a new condom for each act of intercourse
2. Checking the expiration date on the package
3. Carefully handling condom to avoid damaging it with sharp objects (e.g., using teeth to open the package)
4. Ensuring that a condom is placed on an erect penis before any genital contact with a partner
5. Ensuring that no air is trapped in the tip of the condom
6. Ensuring adequate lubrication during intercourse with only water-based lubricants
7. Holding the condom at the base of the erect penis during withdrawal to prevent slippage.

Individuals who are allergic to latex should use polyurethane condoms, although their clinical effectiveness in HIV prevention has not been well established. The female condom was introduced as a method that woman can control for preventing pregnancy and STDs. Although the female condom is impenetrable to HIV, its efficacy in preventing HIV infection also has not been established (29). Dental dams (small squares of latex) or, alternatively, nonmicrowaveable plastic wrap is recommended as a barrier during cunnilingus and anilingus. Data on the effectiveness and safety of topical products, such as nonoxynol-9, that might act as an HIV microbicide have been inconclusive (14).

Prevention of Transmission by Injection-Drug Use

Approximately one third of all AIDS cases have been associated with IDU (30). These statistics do not include those individuals who contracted HIV through high-risk behaviors associated with the use of noninjected drugs, such as alcohol and crack cocaine. Data from a CDC study of young adults aged 18 to 29 years showed a high prevalence of HIV among women who recently had had unprotected sex in exchange for crack cocaine or money. In fact, these women were as likely to be HIV infected as men who had sex with men (15). Therefore, in addition to sharing needles, engaging in high-risk sexual activity while under the influence of drugs (either injection or noninjection) and exchanging sex for drugs or money can contribute significantly to HIV transmission in the substance-using population.

Needles and syringes are the primary drug equipment involved in transferring HIV-infected blood between drug injectors (31). Providing non-judgmental advice, counseling, and medical care is the first and perhaps most important component of a clinician's HIV prevention strategy in a substance-using patient. Establishing trust with an individual is critical to the goals of referral to drug treatment programs and abstinence from drug use. Unfortunately, these are not always attainable because patients may be unwilling to accept treatment or access to appropriate substance abuse treatment programs may be limited. In this scenario, the clinician needs to

---

Table 3.3   Drug-Use Risk-Reduction Topics for Discussion with Patients

- The importance of using bleach to clean drug paraphernalia

- The avoidance of "shooting galleries" or trading sex for drugs

- The importance of drug treatment and rehabilitation

- The opportunity to discuss harm-reduction topics and/or offer referral to community-based educational services

---

Adapted with permission from Libman H, Witzburg RA (eds). *HIV Infection: A Primary Care Manual.* Boston: Little, Brown; 1996.

set more realistic goals, emphasizing harm reduction rather than absolute risk elimination. A harm-reduction model accepts that drug use exists but attempts to minimize the adverse consequences of the behavior (32). For the active injection-drug user, clinicians can advise that the most effective way to reduce HIV transmission risk is by not sharing needles or by disinfecting syringes and drug apparatus in bleach (31).

Physicians should advise injection-drug users to use sterile needles for each injection and to avoid sharing needles at all times. Users who share needles should disinfect their injection equipment with bleach, although this practice is not as safe as always using a sterile needle and syringe (31). To kill the HIV virus effectively, the drug apparatus must first be flushed with clean water. It then must soak in full-strength bleach for at least 1 minute, followed by another thorough rinse with clean water (33).

As rates of HIV infection related to drug use continue to rise, there is growing pressure to identify effective prevention strategies. Despite existing controversy and a current lack of federal funding support, in some areas of the United States, physicians can refer injection-drug users to NEPs. Proponents for needle exchange cite an emerging body of scientific evidence supporting its efficacy in reducing HIV transmission among injection-drug users (34–37). In contrast, opponents fear that NEPs may serve as deterrents for individuals to seek drug treatment and send the wrong message to young people who could misinterpret needle exchange as supporting drug use. However, studies have shown consistently that needle exchange is not associated with an increase in injection- or non–injection-drug use (35). Some data even suggest that needle exchange actually may serve as a vehicle for patients to seek ongoing treatment for substance use (38). Along with continuing counseling, support, and education aimed at decreasing rates of high-risk behaviors such as IDU, NEPs should remain a focal point of HIV preventive intervention in this hard-to-reach population.

Prevention of Perinatal Transmission

Perinatal (vertical) transmission of HIV from mother to infant accounts for approximately 90% of pediatric AIDS cases. Epidemiologic studies in the early 1990s in the United States indicated that approximately 7000 infants were born to HIV-infected women each year, with 1000 to 2000 of those infants being infected with HIV. It was estimated that in the absence of antiretroviral therapy, HIV infection is transmitted during pregnancy or labor in 15% to 35% of cases (39). Maternal viral load is an independent predictor (39a).

Although still under active investigation, most vertical HIV transmission is believed to occur during labor and delivery, although it also can occur during gestation and in the postpartum period through breast feeding (40).

Risk factors for perinatal transmission of HIV are listed in Table 3.4. Natural history data suggest that the duration of ruptured membranes is an important obstetric predictor of HIV transmission risk. The mode of delivery also has been examined, with studies demonstrating a benefit with cesarean section over vaginal birth (41). Physicians can decrease the risk of perinatal HIV transmission by avoiding invasive procedures or trauma to the infant, such as fetal scalp monitoring, amniocentesis, and episiotomy. Other obstetrical risk factors for HIV transmission include breaks in the placenta, premature birth, and blood or meconium in the amniotic fluid (42). After delivery, breast feeding increases the risk of transmission of HIV from mother to infant by approximately 10% to 19% (41). In the United States, where safe alternatives to breast milk are available, HIV-infected women are advised against breast feeding.

Primary care physicians have an opportunity to reduce perinatal HIV transmission rates by offering HIV testing and counseling to all women of child-bearing age. For women infected with HIV, physicians must provide counseling about the risks of perinatal transmission as well as explain a variety of options, including the use of contraception to avoid pregnancy, termination of pregnancy, and the use of antiretroviral therapy (*see* Chapter 5). In 1994, the results of the Pediatric AIDS Clinical Trials Group (ACTG) protocol 076 dramatically changed the clinical strategy for reducing perinatal HIV transmission. In this protocol, HIV-infected women were randomized to receive either zidovudine (ZDV) or placebo during pregnancy, labor, and delivery. ZDV also was administered to the infant in the newborn period. HIV transmission was reduced in the ZDV arm of the study to 8% compared with 25% in the placebo arm (39). These results led to recommendations by the Public Health Service advising clinicians to counsel all pregnant women about the benefits of HIV testing and offering voluntary testing (43). Women found to be infected with HIV should be presented with the benefits and potential risks of ZDV treatment so that they may understand their options better. The discussion of treatment recom-

---

Table 3.4   Risk Factors for Perinatal Transmission of HIV

- Maternal viral load

- Placenta rupture or break

- Premature delivery

- Blood or meconium in the amniotic fluid

- Invasive obstetric procedures (e.g., fetal scalp monitoring, amniocentesis, episiotomy, forceps, vacuum extractor, fetal-blood scalp sampling)

- Breast feeding

---

mendations should be noncoercive, and the final decision about antiretroviral therapy is the responsibility of the woman. There are limited data about the safety and efficacy of using antiretroviral medications other than ZDV in pregnancy, but generally it is prescribed in combination with other agents to maximize viral suppression (44).

HIV Postexposure Prophylaxis

Until recently, patients had little motivation to seek medical care soon after exposure to HIV. However, a retrospective study of health care workers found that treatment with ZDV after needle-stick exposure to HIV-infected blood reduced the odds of HIV infection by approximately 80% (45). Although this observation has not been confirmed in a randomized controlled trial, the findings of this study and other data led the CDC to recommend postexposure prophylaxis (PEP) for health care workers who were exposed accidentally to HIV-infected bodily fluids (*see* Chapter 10). Since PEP is now recommended for health care workers, it was logical that it be considered for people exposed to HIV through sexual contact or IDU, because these are more common routes of transmission. The theoretical basis for the use of PEP is that antiretroviral therapy used immediately following exposure to HIV may prevent initial cellular infection, inhibit initial viral replication, and allow host immune defenses to eradicate the virus (46,47). For seronegative individuals who are exposed to HIV, there may be a window of opportunity in the first few hours or days following exposure in which antiretroviral therapy may help prevent infection. Although no direct evidence exists about the efficacy of PEP following sexual contact, it remains biologically plausible given the benefit of treatment following occupational exposure and the immune response similarities between transcutaneous and transmucosal exposure (46,47).

Recently, the CDC published recommendations about PEP following sexual or exposure via IDU but did not offer specific guidelines because of a lack of data (48). Many physicians and clinics across the United States offer PEP in varying forms. Patients should be counseled about PEP if they are candidates for treatment, but deciding whether an individual is appropriate for PEP is often difficult and requires a careful assessment of the following:

1. **Type of Sexual Exposure.** The quantitative HIV risk associated with a specific sexual exposure is difficult to measure. Limited data suggest that the probability of transmission through a single episode of unprotected rectal or vaginal intercourse with someone known to be infected with HIV is similar in magnitude to the probability of transmission associated with occupational needle punctures (~0.003). The probability is highest for unprotected re-

ceptive anal intercourse (49). Unprotected receptive vaginal intercourse seems to be of higher risk than unprotected insertive vaginal intercourse (50–52). Per-episode risk estimates for other types of sexual exposure (e.g., receptive oral sex with ejaculation, insertive anal intercourse) are not available; however, both of these behaviors are thought to transmit HIV (53–55).

2. **HIV Status of the Patient and Sexual Partner.** PEP is given with the assumption that a patient is not already infected with HIV. As such, baseline HIV testing should be available for those who have not been tested recently. For patients who report multiple exposures in the recent past, an HIV viral load should be performed to detect primary HIV infection. However, clinicians should not wait for the results of HIV testing to initiate PEP. The HIV status of the sexual partner may or may not be known. If the partner is known to be infected with HIV, additional information (e.g., stage of illness, results of recent viral load tests) can affect treatment decisions. If the partner's HIV status is unknown and the partner is willing to be tested, treatment can be started and then stopped if the partner tests negative. If the partner is unavailable or unwilling to be tested, the decision to initiate PEP is based on the type of exposure and knowledge of the partner's risk behaviors. In cases of rape in which the perpetrator is unknown, PEP always should be considered (56).

3. **Patient's Attitude Toward Safer Sex.** Patients present with various histories for HIV based on sexual risk. Some individuals diligently practice safer sex but are exposed accidentally to HIV when a condom breaks. Others have isolated episodes of unsafe sex while "high" on substances. Still others have many unsafe sexual exposures with a variety of partners of unknown HIV status. PEP is not appropriate for individuals who intend to continue high-risk behaviors, because it is unlikely to be effective. However, in ambiguous cases, clinicians may choose to offer prophylactic treatment and to emphasize the importance of condom use and safer sexual practices in the future (47). For some exposed individuals, the PEP treatment encounter actually may help motivate behavioral change and ultimately may serve to decrease their long-term behavioral risk.

4. **Length of Time Since Exposure.** The timing of the risk behavior is an important component of the PEP evaluation. Few data exist on which to base a precise cutoff time after exposure, but animal models suggest that delaying therapy more than 24 to 36 hours dramatically decreases the likelihood of effectiveness (57). Although immediate treatment is optimal, PEP should be initi-

ated within 72 hours of exposure. Katz and Gerberding (47) recommend that PEP be offered to individuals who have had recent (<72 hours) unprotected anal or vaginal intercourse (receptive or insertive) or receptive oral sex with ejaculation with a person known to be infected with HIV or in a group at high risk for HIV (e.g., an injection-drug user). Such people should be committed to practicing safer behaviors in the future.

Until further data are available, the treatment regimen for PEP most likely should be modeled after that used for occupational exposures (58,59). Although ZDV is the only drug for which efficacy data are available in the setting of postexposure treatment, a 4-week regimen of ZDV (300 mg bid) and lamivudine (3TC) (150 mg bid) generally is recommended. The addition of a protease inhibitor (e.g., nelfinavir or indinavir) should be considered if the source patient has advanced HIV disease, has been treated previously with one or both of the nucleoside analogues in the two-drug regimen, or is known to have a high HIV viral load (>50,000 copies/mL). People with sexual exposure to HIV also should be screened for other STDs (e.g., syphilis, gonorrhea, chlamydia, and hepatitis B).

Although we do not know whether PEP following sexual encounters or IDU is effective, it provides clinicians in primary care practice, emergency rooms, and STD clinics a valuable opportunity to reach individuals at high risk of HIV seroconversion and to provide them with evaluation, treatment, counseling, and ongoing medical care. In addition, it is unclear whether PEP may motivate individuals to resume unsafe sexual practices because they expect postexposure treatment to be protective. As such, we must be careful not to undermine existing HIV prevention efforts by exaggerating the protective benefits of PEP. Emphasis of condom use, safer sexual practices, and an avoidance of high-risk behaviors must remain the "gold standard."

■   ■   ■

Key Points

- Primary care physicians have the opportunity to play an integral role in HIV prevention. Clinical prevention of HIV infection entails assessing patient risk and providing health education tailored to help modify high-risk behaviors.

- Clinicians should emphasize the importance of safer sexual behaviors, particularly the consistent and appropriate use of condoms. Sexual behaviors can be stratified by their relative risk.

- Because STDs are associated with an increased risk of HIV acquisition, the prevention and treatment of these infections play an important role in HIV prevention.

- Primary care physicians should advise injection-drug users to use sterile needles for each injection and to avoid sharing paraphernalia. Despite political controversies, NEPs appear to be effective at reducing the risk of HIV transmission.

- All pregnant women should undergo an HIV risk assessment and be counseled about HIV antibody testing.

- Postexposure antiretroviral therapy prophylaxis should be considered in people presenting within 72 hours of HIV exposure through sexual contact or IDU, although data are lacking that demonstrate its effectiveness.

■   ■   ■

Resources

Organizations

AIDS Project LA (APLA): 1313 N. Vine Street, Los Angeles, CA 90028; 323-993-1600; www.apla.org

Gay Men's Health Crisis: 119 West 24th Street, New York, NY 10011; 1-800-AIDS-NYC; 212-807-6655; www.gmhc.org

Center for AIDS Prevention Studies (CAPS): University of California, San Francisco, 74 New Montgomery Street, Suite 600, San Francisco, CA 94105; 415-597-9100; www.epibiostat.ucsf.edu/capsweb

Guides and Manuals

The American Medical Association: *A Physician Guide to HIV Prevention 1996*

The Centers for Disease Control and Prevention: *HIV/AIDS Prevention Guide 1994*

Web Sites

The Body: An AIDS and HIV Information Source: www.thebody.com

The Centers for Disease Control and Prevention: www.cdc.gov

▦   ▦   ▦

REFERENCES

1. **Holmberg SD.** The estimated prevalence and incidence of HIV in 96 large US metropolitan areas. *Am J Public Health.* 1996; 86:642–54.

2. **Rosenberg PS, Bigger RJ, Goedert JJ.** Declining age at HIV infection in the United States (Letter). *N Engl J Med.* 1994;330:789–90.

3. **Centers for Disease Control and Prevention.** *Adolescents and HIV/AIDS* [Fact sheet]. Dec 1995.

4. **Coats TJ, Choi KH.** Prevention of HIV infection. *AIDS.* 1994;8:1371–89.

5. **National Institutes of Health.** Consensus Statement: interventions to prevent HIV risk behaviors. 1997;15:1–41.

6. **Makadon HJ, Silin JG.** Prevention of HIV infection in primary care: current practices, future possibilities. *Ann Intern Med.* 1995;123:715–9.

7. **Schappert SM.** *The National Ambulatory Medical Care Survey: 1990 Summary.* Hyattsville, MD: U.S. Department of Health and Human Services, Public Health Service, Centers for Disease Control and Prevention, National Center for Health Statistics; 1992.

8. **Centers for Disease Control and Prevention.** HIV prevention practices of primary care physicians: United States, 1992. *MMWR Morb Mortal Wkly Rep.* 1994;42: 988–92.

9. **Gerbert B, Maguire BT, Coats TJ.** Are patients talking to their physicians about AIDS? *Am J Public Health.* 1990;80:467–9.

10. **Anonymous.** *A Physician Guide to HIV Prevention.* Chicago: American Medical Association; 1996.

11. **Wheeler DA.** Human immunodeficiency virus in the health care setting. *Occup Med.* 1997;12:741–56.

12. **Centers for Disease Control and Prevention.** *AIDS Case Report 1996.*

13. **Ickovics JR, Rodin J.** Women and AIDS in the United States: epidemiology, natural history, and mediating mechanisms. *Health Psychol.* 1992;11:1–16.

14. **Centers for Disease Control and Prevention.** *HIV/AIDS and Women in the United States: Excerpts from the HIV/AIDS Surveillance Report* [Fact sheet]. Jul 1997.

15. **Centers for Disease Control and Prevention.** *Strategies for Preventing HIV in Women* [Fact sheet]. Jul 1997.

16. **Rosenberg P.** Scope of the AIDS epidemic in the United States. *Science.* 1995; 270:1372–5.

17. **Collins C.** *Dangerous Inhibitions: How America Is Letting AIDS Become an Epidemic of the Young.* San Francisco, CA: Center for AIDS Prevention Studies at UCSF; 1997.

18. **Reyes EM, Legg JJ.** Prevention of HIV transmission. *Prim Care.* 1997;24:469–77.

19. **Holmberg SD.** Risk factors for sexual transmission of the human immunodeficiency virus. In *AIDS: Biology, Diagnosis, Treatment, and Prevention,* ed. 4. Philadelphia: J.B. Lippincott-Raven; 1997:569–75.

20. **Lifson AR, O'Malley PM, Hessol NA, et al.** HIV seroconversion in two homosexual men after receptive oral intercourse with ejaculation: implications for counseling safe sexual practices. *Am J Public Health.* 1990;80:1509–11.

21. **Cates W Jr, Stone KM.** Family planning, sexually transmitted diseases, and contraceptive choice. Part 1: A literature update. *Fam Plann Perspect.* 1992;24:75–84.

22. **Hearst N, Hulley SB.** Preventing the heterosexual spread of AIDS: Are we giving our patients the best advice? *JAMA.* 1988;259:2428–32.

23. **King E.** *Safety in Numbers: Safer Sex and Gay Men.* New York: Cassell; 1993.

24. **Centers for Disease Control and Prevention.** *HIV/AID Prevention* [Fact sheet]. Jul 1997.

25. **Wasserheit JN.** Epidemiologic synergy: interrelationships between human immunodeficiency virus infection and other sexually transmitted diseases. *Sex Transm Dis.* 1992;19:61–77.

26. **Cohen MS, Zaidi AA, Peterman TA, et al.** Reduction of concentration of HIV-1 in semen after treatment of urethritis: implications for prevention of sexual transmission of HIV-1. *Lancet.* 1997;349:1868–73.

27. **Grosskurth H, Mosha F, Todd J, et al.** Impact of improved treatment of sexually transmitted diseases on HIV infection in rural Tanzania: randomised controlled trial. *Lancet.* 1995;346:530–6.

28. **Centers for Disease Control and Prevention.** *HIV/AIDS Prevention: The Role of STD Testing and Treatment in HIV Prevention* [Fact sheet]. Jul 1997.

29. **Anonymous.** The female condom. *Med Lett Drugs Ther.* 1993;35:123–4.

30. **Centers for Disease Control and Prevention.** AIDS associated with injecting drug use: United States, 1995. *MMWR Morb Mortal Wkly Rep.* 1996;45:392–8.

31. **Centers for Disease Control and Prevention.** *Drug Use and HIV/AIDS* [Fact sheet]. Jul 1997.

32. **Des Jarlais DC.** Harm reduction: a framework for incorporating science into drug policy. *Am J Public Health.* 1995;83:10–2.

33. **Centers for Disease Control and Prevention.** Use of bleach for disinfection of drug injection equipment. *MMWR Morb Mortal Wkly Rep.* 1993;42:418–9.

34. **Lee FR.** Data show needle exchange curbs HIV among addicts. *The New York Times.* 24 Nov 1994, sec. 1, p. 9.

35. **Loue S, Lurie P, Lloyd LS.** Ethical issues raised by needle exchange programs. *J Law Med Ethics.* 1995;23:382–8.

36. **Hurley SF, Jolley DJ, Kaldor JM.** Effectiveness of needle-exchange programmes for prevention of HIV infection. *Lancet.* 1997;349:1797–800.

37. **Lurie P, Drucker E.** An opportunity lost: HIV infection associated with lack of a national needle-exchange pregramme in the USA. *Lancet.* 1997;349:604–8.

38. **Seattle-King County Department of Public Health.** *Update of the Seattle-King County Needle-Exchange Program.* Mar 1992.

39. **Connor EM, Sperling RS, Gelber R, et al.** Reduction of maternal-infant transmission of human immunodeficiency virus type 1 with zidovudine treatment. *N Engl J Med.* 1994;331:1173–80.

39a. **Garcia PM, et al.** Maternal levels of plasma human immunodeficiency virus type 1 RNA and the risk of perinatal transmission. *N Engl J Med.* 1999;341:394–402.

40. **Zorilla CD.** Obstetric factors and mother-to-infant transmission of HIV-1. *Infect Dis Clin North Am.* 1997;11:109–18.

41. **Hoyt L.** HIV infection in women and children: special concerns in prevention and care. *Postgrad Med.* 1997;102:165–176.

42. **Bryson YJ.** Perinatal HIV-1 transmission: recent advances and therapeutic interventions. *AIDS.* 1996;10(Suppl 3):33–42.

43. **Centers for Disease Control and Prevention.** United States Public Health Service recommendations for human immunodeficiency virus counseling and voluntary testing of pregnant women. *MMWR Morb Mortal Wkly Rep.* 1995;44:1–15.

44. **Mofenson LM.** The role of antiretroviral therapy in the management of HIV infection in women. *Clin Obstet Gynecol.* 1996;39:374–6.

45. **Centers for Disease Control and Prevention.** Case-control study of HIV seroconversion in health care workers after percutaneous exposures to HIV-infected blood: France, United Kingdom, and United States, January 1988 to August 1994. *MMWR Morb Mortal Wkly Rep.* 1995;44:929–33.

46. **Pinto LA, Landay AL, Berzofsky JA, et al.** Immune response to human immunodeficiency virus (HIV) in health care workers occupationally exposed to HIV-contaminated blood. *Am J Med.* 1997;102(Suppl 5B):21–4.

47. **Katz MH, Gerberding JL.** The care of persons with recent sexual exposure to HIV. *Ann Intern Med.* 1998;128:306–12.

48. **Centers for Disease Control and Prevention.** Management of possible sexual, injecting-drug-use, or other nonoccupational exposure to HIV, including considerations related to antiretroviral therapy. *MMWR Morb Mortal Wkly Rep.* 1998;47(RR-17):1–14.

49. **De Gruttola V, Seage GR III, Mayer KH, Horsburgh CR Jr.** Infectiousness of HIV between male homosexual partners. *J Clin Epidemiol.* 1989;42:849–56.

50. **Wiley JA, Herskorn SJ, Padian NS.** Heterogeneity in the probability of HIV transmission per sexual contact: the case of male-to-female transmission in penile-vaginal intercourse. *Stat Med.* 1989;8:93–102.

51. **Peterman TA, Stoneburner RL, Allen JR, et al.** Risk of human immunodeficiency virus transmission from heterosexual adults with transfusion-associated infections. *JAMA.* 1988;259:55–8.

52. **Downs AM, DeVincenzi I.** Probability of heterosexual transmission of HIV: relationship to the number of unprotected sexual contacts. *J Acquir Immune Defic Syndr Hum Retrovirol.* 1996;11:388–95.

53. **Samuel MC, Mohr MS, Speed TP, Winkelstein W.** Infectivity of HIV by anal and oral intercourse among homosexual men. In Kaplan EH, Brandeau ML (eds). *Modeling the AIDS Epidemic: Planning, Policy, and Prediction.* New York: Raven Press, 1994:423–38.

54. **Rozenbaum W, Gharakhanian S, Cardon B, et al.** HIV transmission by oral sex. *Lancet.* 1988;1:1395.

55. **Lane HC, Holmberg SD, Jaffe HW.** HIV seroconversion and oral intercourse. *Am J Public Health.* 1991;81:658.

56. **Gostin LO, Lazzarini Z, Alexander D, et al.** HIV testing, counseling, and prophylaxis after sexual assault. *JAMA.* 1994;271:1436–44.

57. **Geberding JL.** Prophylaxis of occupational exposure to HIV. *Ann Intern Med.* 1996;25:497–501.

58. **Anonymous.** Update: provisional Public Health Service recommendations for chemoprophylaxis after occupational exposure to HIV. *MMWR Morb Mortal Wkly Rep.* 1996;45:468–80.

59. **Centers for Disease Control and Prevention.** Public Health Service guidelines for the management of health care worker exposures to HIV and recommendations for postexposure prophylaxis. *MMWR Morb Mortal Wkly Rep.* 1998;47(RR-7): 1–29.

4

■ ■ ■

Primary Care of HIV Disease

Howard Libman, MD

Raymond Powrie, MD

Michael Stein, MD

The management of HIV-infected patients has undergone dramatic change over the past few years with the advent of combination antiretroviral therapy and the introduction of viral load testing in clinical practice. Patients are diagnosed less frequently with opportunistic infections and are living longer. However, with this encouraging news have come important challenges. For patients, they include difficulties in adhering to a complex medical regimen and the uncertainty of predicting future health. For primary care clinicians, they include keeping up with a rapidly changing but incomplete knowledge base and addressing the needs of complicated outpatients within time constraints.

Competence in HIV care requires adequate clinical experience in the field rather than specific subspecialty training. Also essential are nursing support and access to social services, subspecialty consultations, mental health and additional professionals, and clinical trials. A multidisciplinary approach generally works best for patients and clinicians.

This chapter reviews the major issues related to outpatient HIV care, including antibody testing, clinical evaluation, laboratory studies, management, health care maintenance issues, other health issues, and considerations in women and pregnancy.

HIV Antibody Testing

HIV antibody testing should be recommended to patients at historical risk for HIV infection or with suggestive clinical findings (Table 4.1). Twenty-

Table 4.1   Indications for HIV Antibody Testing

Historical	*Clinical*
• Men who have sex with men	• Tuberculosis
• People with multiple sexual partners	• Syphilis
• Current or past injection drug users	• Recurrent shingles
• Recipients of blood products between 1978 and 1985	• Constitutional symptoms
• People with current or past sexually transmitted diseases	• Generalized adenopathy
• Prostitutes and their sexual partners	• Chronic diarrhea or wasting
• Pregnant women or those of childbearing age who are at risk through drug use, prostitution, or unprotected sex	• Encephalopathy
	• Thrombocytopenia
• Children born to HIV-infected mothers	• Thrush or chronic/recurrent vaginal candidiasis
• Sexual partners of those at risk for HIV infection	• Other HIV-associated opportunistic diseases (e.g., *Pneumocystis carinii* pneumonia and Kaposi's sarcoma)
• People who consider themselves at risk or request testing	
• Donors of blood products, semen, or organs	

five million people in the United States are tested annually for HIV infection. Both confidential and anonymous testing sites exist in most urban centers, and home testing kits are also now available. Knowledge of HIV serostatus has many potential individual health benefits, including the initiation of antiretroviral therapy and prophylaxis for opportunistic infections, screening and prophylaxis for tuberculosis (TB), screening for and treatment of sexually transmitted diseases (STDs), administration of appropriate vaccinations, and institution of other health care maintenance measures. Potential risks of HIV antibody testing include a false-positive test result, a false-negative test result, adverse psychological reactions, breach of confidentiality, and social discrimination.

Pretest and Posttest Counseling

The personal benefits of learning that one is positive for HIV antibodies include the capacity to receive appropriate medical care, including early institution of antiretroviral therapy, and to modify behaviors that may result in transmission to others (Table 4.2). However, testing also is associated with certain risks. Receiving a positive result can have adverse personal and social consequences. HIV seropositivity may compromise eligibility for life insurance, health insurance, employment, and housing. Patients who undergo HIV antibody testing should have a full understanding of its ramifications through pretest and posttest counseling (Table 4.3). Antibody testing is contraindicated in patients who 1) cannot provide informed consent; 2) are unable to understand the implications of test results; 3) are psychotic, suicidal, or emotionally disturbed; or 4) lack adequate personal support systems to cope with the stress of receiving a positive test result.

Characteristics of Test

HIV antibody testing is performed by an enzyme-linked immunosorbent assay (ELISA), which is highly sensitive. Seroconversion, which is the development of antibodies, normally occurs 6 to 8 weeks after infection. If the ELISA is negative, the HIV antibody test is reported as being negative; if it is positive, the test is repeated. If the repeat ELISA is positive, a Western blot (WB) assay, which is more specific, is performed for confirmation. If the WB assay result is positive, the HIV antibody test is reported as being positive. These sequential testing modalities are 99.5% sensitive and over 99% specific. WB results occasionally are described as indeterminate; in these instances, repeat or supplemental testing may be recommended.

It is important to note that the "window period"—the time between infection and first detectable sign of antibody positivity—may last up to 3 months after a high-risk behavior. In people with suspected acute HIV syndrome, an HIV antibody test should be obtained at baseline, but viral load or other supplemental testing is necessary for early diagnosis. Low-titer false-positive HIV viral load assays have been reported in patients with acute non–HIV-related illness, so caution is advised in its interpretation.

Table 4.2   Topics for Discussion in Risk-Reduction Counseling

---

- Reducing or limiting the number of sexual partners

- Using latex condoms and spermicide for all sexual activity

- For injection-drug users, appropriate use and cleaning of needles (e.g., do not share needles; if drug use is continued, use new sterile needles or only one set of works and clean them with diluted chlorine bleach every time)

- Do not share personal items (e.g., razors and toothbrushes)

Table 4.3   Features of Pretest and Posttest Counseling

Pretest Counseling

- Distinction between anonymous and confidential testing and the availability of home testing

- Review of natural history of HIV infection

- Review of reasons for testing and expectations

- Review of individual risk behaviors and risk reduction measures

- Discussion of meaning of positive and negative results

- Assessment of personal and social supports

Posttest Counseling

- Review meaning of test results and implications

- If test result is positive:

    Assess patient's reaction and ability to cope

    Anticipate need for immediate support and close follow-up plan for medical evaluation

- If test result is negative:

    Restate possibility of seroconversion if patient is involved in high-risk activities

    Dispel any false beliefs regarding invulnerability or immunity to HIV infection

Rapid tests to detect HIV antibody within 10 minutes also have been developed. These enable clinicians to provide definitive negative and preliminary positive results immediately. By eliminating the need for follow-up visits, patients seen in settings in which there is a low return-visit rate (e.g., at anonymous test sites and STD clinics) may be served better. Positive rapid HIV tests are confirmed with the ELISA/WB sequence to identify false-positive results.

A low CD4 cell count is not diagnostic of HIV disease and should never be used in lieu of HIV antibody testing. HIV antibody testing does not detect HIV-2 reliably, which is common in West Africa; if this virus is suspected by history, a specific ELISA can be requested.

Clinical Evaluation

The clinical evaluation of HIV-infected patients should include a careful history, review of systems, physical examination, and attention to psychosocial and educational concerns. In newly diagnosed patients, understanding their emotional state and knowledge of HIV disease takes precedence. Denial, anxiety, and depression are often seen in this setting, and mental health concerns should be addressed before dealing with nonurgent medical issues. Patients show great variability in their knowledge of HIV disease despite the widespread availability of information in the press and on the Internet. Comprehension of its natural history, how it is spread, and how it is treated is essential. Information should be provided in the patient's primary language and should be appropriate to his or her level of education.

History

Taking a history from an HIV-infected patient serves to establish rapport, gather clinical data, and facilitate self-care counseling (Table 4.4). Confirmation of HIV antibody status is recommended if documentation is not available. The first visit often provides insight into a patient's understanding of HIV disease. It also serves as an opportunity to discuss psychological factors, social supports, and financial resources, which likely will prove critical to patient use of and adherence to recommended therapies.

The initial medical history should include the items listed in Table 4.4. Particular aspects of the medical history are important in managing HIV-in-

---

Table 4.4   History-Taking in Patients with HIV Infection

Medical History
- Previous medical, surgical, and psychiatric care
- Opportunistic diseases
- CD4 cell count results (nadir and recent) and viral load titer (highest and recent) results
- Exposure to tuberculosis, viral hepatitis, syphilis and other sexually transmitted diseases
- Gynecologic and obstetric history
- Alcohol or drug use
- Travel history
- Immunizations
- Previous use of antiretroviral drugs
- Current medications
- Drug allergies

Psychosocial
- HIV risk behaviors
- Knowledge of HIV infection
- Emotional response
- Family/social situation
- Employment/insurance status

---

fected patients. It is important to inquire about a history of syphilis, because atypical manifestations and responses to treatment have been described in some patients. A history of genital or anal warts or abnormal Pap smears also should be sought because of the association of advanced immunodeficiency with cervical and anal dysplasia/carcinoma in patients co-infected with human papillomavirus (HPV). Inquiry should be made into any history of viral hepatitis. Hepatitis A exposure is common in men who have sex with men (MSM), hepatitis B is frequent in both MSM and injection-drug users, and hepatitis C often occurs in injection-drug users. A history of TB exposure or positive reaction to purified protein derivative (PPD) in HIV-infected patients indicates a significantly increased risk of developing active disease in the absence of antimicrobial prophylaxis.

Review of medications should include all forms of treatment. The use of over-the-counter drugs and complementary therapies is common. An HIV medication poster or chart often is helpful to review timing and doses of specific medications by sight rather than relying on names. Discussion of the nature and severity of any medication side effects also should take place.

Psychosocial issues are important at all stages of HIV disease. Psychological trauma is common in the lives of HIV-infected people. Some face rejection by family and friends and discrimination, which may result in loss of personal supports and income. Disclosure of HIV serostatus to sexual partners is a matter of personal responsibility (although many state health departments now have partner-notification programs); disclosure to family, friends, and children often requires time and support. Many HIV-infected people have concerns related to insurance and housing at some time in the course of their disease, which requires the expertise of case managers or social workers familiar with community resources.

Finally, each visit should include a discussion of current health habits. It is important to ask explicitly about new sexual partners and practices. This allows the opportunity to counsel patients about protecting themselves and their partners by using barrier methods. A discussion of any on-going substance abuse is also critical. For patients who continue to inject drugs, harm-reduction strategies (e.g., cleaning skin with alcohol, using clean needles, and not sharing injection equipment) may be helpful in self-protection and in assessing their readiness to enter formal drug treatment. Heavy alcohol use may contribute to drug use and sexual risk taking and has its own adverse health effects.

Physical Examination

Because HIV infection and its complications may involve nearly every organ system, a comprehensive review of systems and physical examination should be performed, with special focus on the skin, mouth, anogenital re-

Table 4.5   Review of Systems and Physical Examination in Patients with HIV Infection

Constitutional Symptoms
- Fever
- Chills
- Night sweats
- Weight loss

Integumentary
- Seborrhea
- Psoriasis
- Onychomycosis
- Herpes simplex virus
- Varicella zoster virus
- Kaposi's sarcoma
- Generalized adenopathy

Head, ears, eyes, nose, and throat
- Altered vision
- Dysphagia
- Cytomegalovirus retinitis
- Thrush
- Oral hairy leukoplakia
- Periodontal disease

Pulmonary
- Cough
- Dyspnea
- Adventitious breath sounds

Gastrointestinal
- Odynophagia
- Diarrhea
- Organomegaly

Genitourinary
- Vaginitis
- Pelvic inflammatory disease
- Human papillomavirus infection
- Cervical dysplasia
- Anal carcinoma

Neurologic
- Headache
- Problems with memory
- Change in behavior or personality
- Focal findings

gion, and central nervous system (Table 4.5).

Weight loss often suggests undiagnosed opportunistic infections, progressive HIV disease, depression, or substance abuse. As one of the earliest and most meaningful signs of deteriorating clinical status, the patient's weight should be measured at each visit.

The skin may be involved early in the course of HIV disease. HIV-infected patients are at increased risk for a variety of infectious and inflammatory skin conditions. Bacterial agents may cause folliculitis, impetigo, and bacillary angiomatosis. People actively injecting drugs may have infected tracks, skin abscesses, or cellulitis. Superficial fungal infections and warts are common. Molluscum contagiosum, pearly papules most often on the genitalia and face, also may be seen. Herpes simplex or zoster may be the initial presentation of HIV disease and are often more severe than in immunocompetent hosts. Inflammatory disorders, such as seborrheic dermatitis and psoriasis, are often difficult to treat. Kaposi's sarcoma (KS) presents as purplish nodules and plaques, often on the trunk, legs, or oral mucosa.

Most HIV-infected people have palpable lymph nodes at some point during the course of their disease. Such nodes, which may involve multiple sites, do not predict disease progression but often cause discomfort and distress. Patients should be reassured that nodes are common and often spontaneously increase and decrease in size. To exclude an opportunistic disease, lymph node biopsy should be considered if gland enlargement is rapid or continuous or if adenopathy is associated with constitutional symptoms or cytopenia.

Direct ophthalmoscopy with dilatation of the pupils should be performed regularly (if they are asymptomatic) in patients whose CD4 counts are fewer than 100 cells/mm^3 and should be performed urgently if any eye complaint arises. Cytomegalovirus (CMV) retinitis presents with hemorrhagic exudates and can progress quickly to blindness by affecting the macula or by leading to retinal detachment.

Oral lesions may cause discomfort and affect nutrition negatively. Candidiasis, also known as thrush, appears as white plaques on the buccal mucosa and tonsillar areas. Without treatment, thrush may spread throughout the mouth; in people with advanced HIV disease, candidiasis can involve the esophagus, which leads to severe odynophagia. Angular cheilitis is caused commonly by mucosal candidiasis. Oral hairy leukoplakia (OHL), which is caused by Epstein–Barr virus, presents as a white plaque on the side of the tongue. Rough in texture, OHL may cause difficulty chewing but often regresses spontaneously. Ulcerations also are frequent in HIV-infected patients. Those lesions appearing on keratinized epithelium—the lips, tongue, and hard palate—are likely herpetic, whereas those on the buccal mucosa are often aphthous. Periodontal disease can be aggressive in people with HIV disease and, if untreated, can lead to necrotizing gingivitis and tooth loss.

HIV-infected patients who have a history of receptive anal intercourse are at increased risk for HPV-related anal squamous cell cancer. The clinician should be alert also for anal warts, herpetic ulcers, hemorrhoids, fissures, and traumatic tears. Patients with HIV disease are at risk for other STDs, such as syphilis, chlamydia, gonorrhea, herpes simplex virus (HSV), and chancroid. HIV-infected women may develop cervical dysplasia or cancer. A Pap test should be performed every 6 months, and histologic abnormalities should be evaluated with colposcopy. Bacterial vaginosis, candidal vaginitis, and trichomoniasis are common in women with HIV disease. These infections often are recurrent and sometimes are difficult to manage with conventional courses of antibiotic therapy.

A brief, structured cognitive examination using the "mini-mental status" instrument should be performed at regular intervals on all patients. The clinician should screen for affective disorders and alcohol or drug abuse when evaluating complaints of memory difficulty. The other essential part of the neurologic examination involves looking for evidence of peripheral neuropathy, a condition that may be a manifestation of HIV disease but that is often medication related.

Laboratory Studies

Baseline laboratory evaluation of the HIV-infected patient is important to screen for occult systemic disease, to identify latent infections that may reactivate, and to monitor for drug toxicity (Table 4.6).

A complete blood and differential count should be performed on all patients. Cytopenia may occur without symptoms and should prompt appropriate evaluation. Anemia, thrombocytopenia, and/or leukopenia may result from HIV-induced marrow suppression, toxicity from antiviral therapy, or infiltration of the marrow by infection or tumor; thrombocytopenia

---

Table 4.6   Baseline Laboratory Studies in Patients with HIV Infection

- Complete blood and differential counts

- BUN/creatinine, liver function tests, glucose, lipid profile

- CD4 cell count

- HIV viral load titer

- RPR or VDRL

- Hepatitis B core antibody (HBsAb if prior immunization)

- Hepatitis C serology

- Toxoplasmosis serology

- PPD test

- Pap smear in women

- G6PD qualitative, urinalysis, and CMV serology may be indicated in some clinical settings

---

BUN = blood urea nitrogen; CMV = cytomegalovirus; G6PD = glucose-6-phosphate dehydrogenase; HBsAb = hepatitis B surface antibody; PPD = purified protein derivative of tuberculin; RPR = rapid plasma reagin test; VDRL = Venereal Disease Research Laboratory test for syphilis.

and leukopenia also may be mediated by autoantibody production.

Because hepatitis A, B, and C are known to occur with increased frequency among some patients with HIV infection, liver function and serologic tests for these viruses are recommended as part of the initial evaluation. These studies help to identify susceptible individuals who would benefit from hepatitis A and B immunizations and to alert the clinician to the presence of chronic hepatitis B or C virus infections. An isolated increased serum alkaline phosphatase may prompt evaluation for infiltrative diseases of the liver.

Syphilis may progress more rapidly and may be more resistant to standard therapies, more prone to reactivation, and more difficult to detect by serologic tests in HIV-infected people. Baseline screening for syphilis and periodic retesting in those at continued risk are warranted.

In that HIV is a potent activator of latent TB, baseline and follow-up skin testing is important in identifying patients in whom antimicrobial prophylaxis is indicated. Because skin testing depends on intact cell-mediated immunity, lack of reactivity to antigens is more common with advanced immunodeficiency, which leads to a false-negative test. A positive PPD is an indication for prophylactic antimicrobial therapy in the previously untreated individual regardless of age and timing of PPD conversion.

Toxoplasma antibody titers should be obtained as part of the baseline evaluation. This information may have value in selecting patients for antimicrobial prophylaxis and in identifying patients at risk for developing active disease. CMV serology has been advocated by some authorities as a screening test to determine which patients with advanced HIV disease are at increased risk for developing symptomatic infection. It also may be useful in patients who require a blood transfusion to identify those who should be given white blood cell–poor products. Serum cryptococcal antigen screening of asymptomatic individuals has little clinical use.

CD4 Cell Count

The CD4 cell count correlates highly with the progression of HIV disease and is the main surrogate marker for immunologic function (*see* Figure 2.4). Its clinical uses are to monitor antiretroviral therapy, to determine risk for opportunistic diseases and need for antimicrobial prophylaxis, and to assess prognosis. Without effective antiretroviral therapy, the average decline per year in CD4 count is 75–100 cells/mm^3, but there is a great deal of variability among patients and in a given patient over time. A normal CD4 count is generally greater than 500 cells/mm^3 in healthy people, but it may be as few as 350 cells/mm^3. Although opportunistic infections usually do not occur with CD4 counts of greater than 500 cells/mm^3, conventional bacterial infections, HSV, varicella-zoster virus, thrush, TB, KS, generalized lymphadenopathy, and chronic skin conditions may be seen as the count declines. A CD4 count of fewer than 200 cells/mm^3 indicates significant immunodeficiency with increased risk for serious opportunistic infections, such as *Pneumocystis carinii* pneumonia (PCP), toxoplasmosis, and cryptococcal meningitis. Patients with a count of fewer than 50 cells/mm^3 are also at risk for CMV and *Mycobacterium avium* complex (MAC) infection and for lymphoma. The highest risk for death in HIV-infected patients is in those with a CD4 count fewer than 50 cells/mm^3.

Some investigators have suggested that the percentage of total lymphocytes that are CD4 cells may provide a more reliable indication of immune function than the absolute CD4 cell count, but use of this parameter has not gained widespread acceptance. Other proposed surrogate markers, such as beta-2-microglobulin and neopterin levels also are not used routinely. CD4 cell count results may not always be reliable. Because CD4 counts have a diurnal variation, samples should be obtained at the same time of day if possible. Intercurrent illnesses, especially herpesvirus infections, may cause transient CD4 cell count decline. Because inter- and intralaboratory variation in test results may occur, it is wise to confirm the initial CD4 count and any subsequent values that are grossly different from the preceding one, especially if such results would lead to new therapeutic interventions.

Viral Load Titer

The ability to measure HIV viral level in blood has revolutionized disease management. Its clinical uses are to monitor antiretroviral therapy and to assess prognosis. Viral load titer results provide complementary information to the CD4 cell count. Its level correlates with CD4 count decline and clinical disease progression. Measurement of HIV viral RNA in blood is performed using polymerase chain reaction (PCR) or branched-chain DNA (bDNA) techniques. The lower threshold for detection of newer assays is between 50 and 20 copies/mL. The level of HIV in blood correlates well with tissue levels, CD4 cell count decline, and disease progression. There is a variability of 0.3 log (three- to fivefold) in the assay, meaning that differences between sequential values must exceed this standard to be considered significant. Intercurrent illnesses and immunizations may affect HIV viral load results transiently, and the use of the assay in this context is discouraged.

Management

General Approach

Specific management issues in HIV-infected patients include initiation and maintenance of antiretroviral therapy, prophylaxis against PCP and other

---

Table 4.7   Management of HIV Disease Stratified by CD4 Cell Count

---

>500 cells/mm³
- Initiate antiretroviral therapy if patient is symptomatic or has viral load >10,000 copies/mL (bDNA) or >20,000 copies/mL (PCR)

- If the above criteria are not met, either initiate therapy or monitor patient off therapy

- Give attention to health care maintenance issues and immunizations

200-500 cells/mm³
- Initiate or maintain antiretroviral therapy with modification of regimen as necessary

50-200 cells/mm³
- Initiate or maintain antiretroviral therapy with modification of regimen as necessary

- Initiate prophylaxis for *Pneumocystis carinii* pneumonia.*

<50 cells/mm³
- Initiate or maintain antiretroviral therapy with modification of regimen as necessary

- Maintain prophylaxis for *P. carinii* pneumonia.

- Initiate prophylaxis for *Mycobacterium avium* complex.

---

bDNA = branched-chain DNA; PCR = polymerase chain reaction.
*Alternative prophylaxis for toxoplasmosis should be initiated in the patient with CD4 count <100 cells/mm³ and positive toxoplasmosis serology who is not receiving TMP-SMX for *P. carinii* pneumonia prophylaxis.

---

opportunistic infections, and health care maintenance issues. Patients are stratified based on their CD4 cell count (Table 4.7). In general, antiretroviral therapy is initiated if the patient is symptomatic, has a CD4 count of fewer than 500 cells/mm³, or has a significant detectable viral load titer. Prophylaxis against PCP is started in patients with a CD4 count of fewer than 200 cells/mm³ and against toxoplasmosis if the CD4 count is fewer than 100 cells/mm³. Preventive therapy against MAC is begun in patients with a CD4 count of fewer than 50 cells/mm³.

Medical visits should be scheduled with appropriate frequency to monitor for disease progression and complications and to monitor drug therapies. In general, patients with advanced HIV disease require more frequent visits than those with earlier stages.

The initial evaluation generally is accomplished in two appointments. At the first visit, a history and physical examination are performed and baseline laboratory studies are obtained. At the second visit, results of evaluation are reviewed and a management plan is discussed. Before starting antiretroviral medications, factors that could have a negative impact on ad-

Table 4.8   Factors Having Negative Impact on Adherence to Treatment

- Lack of education about HIV disease
- Denial, anxiety, or depression
- Alcohol or drug use
- Poor social situation
- Inadequate health insurance
- Number of medications/pills
- Frequency of dosing
- Stringent dosing requirements
- Presence of side effects

herence should be reviewed (Table 4.8). Frequently missed doses will render a drug regimen ineffective by leading to the development of viral resistance. Every effort should be made to address active substance abuse, alcoholism, or significant psychological problems, all of which may interfere with a patient's ability to take medications reliably. Clear therapeutic goals should be established before starting therapy, and a plan should be in place to facilitate adherence and to monitor for drug toxicity.

If antiretroviral therapy is initiated, a follow-up visit is arranged in 4 weeks to assess the tolerability of the medical regimen and to repeat laboratory parameters used to determine its effectiveness. Once a patient is on a stable treatment regimen, visits every 3 to 4 months are recommended unless intercurrent problems necessitate more frequent appointments. Follow-up laboratory studies should include complete blood and differential counts, BUN/creatinine, liver function tests, glucose and lipid profile, CD4 cell count, and viral load titer. In patients not on antiretroviral therapy, only a CD4 cell count and viral load titer are necessary.

Antiretroviral Therapy

All patients with HIV infection, including those with advanced disease, potentially may benefit from antiretroviral therapy. Because of the rapidly changing nature of clinical practice in this area, expertise should be sought when initiating or changing drug regimens. The following recommendations are based on our current understanding of the pathophysiology of HIV disease and the results of clinical trials. They reflect guidelines of U.S. Department of Health and Human Services (DHHS) and the International AIDS Society USA Panel (*see* Chapter 5).

Contrary to earlier understanding, viral replication occurs throughout the course of HIV infection at astonishing rates. It is estimated that 10 billion viral particles are produced each day. The patient's immune system keeps pace with this activity during the clinical latency period. However, in the absence of effective antiretroviral treatment, the immune system ultimately reaches a "point of exhaustion," at which viral replication exceeds its ability to produce CD4 cells. This leads to a decline in immunologic function and the development of clinical disease manifestations, including opportunistic infections and neoplasms. The rate of viral replication is thought to stabilize after primary infection at a particular level or "set point." This level may be maintained within a 10-fold range over months and possibly years. The viral load titer is highly correlated with the rate of CD4 count decline, disease progression, and mortality.

The primary goal of antiretroviral therapy should be "to keep the viral load as low as possible for as long as possible." Maximal suppression of the virus makes it more difficult for resistance to develop. Partial suppression results in the emergence of "quasi-species," which are pre-existing, resistant, mutant strains in the viral population. These arise because of the rapid turnover of HIV and the many random errors made during replication.

Approximately two thirds of patients started on combination antiretroviral therapy have an undetectable virus 3 years into treatment. Patient adherence to medical therapy is key. Second and subsequent attempts at viral suppression are less often successful. Current antiretroviral drugs are not thought to be curative because of persistence of HIV in latent CD4 lymphocytes (which seem to have a long life span) and in "sanctuary sites" (regions of the body [e.g., central nervous system, gonads] in which some agents may not penetrate well).

Combination antiretroviral therapy now is considered the standard of care for HIV infection. Monotherapy and less potent combination regimens lead to the development of viral resistance within weeks to months. To date, fourteen antiretroviral agents have been approved by the Food and Drug Administration. They are classified by their mode of action against the virus into the following categories: 1) nucleoside reverse-transcriptase inhibitors (NRTIs); 2) nonnucleoside reverse-transcriptase inhibitors (NNRTIs); and 3) protease inhibitors (PIs) (see Tables 5.2, 5.3, and 5.4 and Appendix). Antiretroviral agents vary considerably in dosing and frequency, side-effect profiles, interactions with other drugs, and in how they should be administered (with food or when fasting).

Specific Guidelines
WHEN SHOULD ANTIRETROVIRAL THERAPY BE INITIATED?
Antiretroviral therapy is recommended in HIV-infected patients who meet any of the criteria listed in Table 4.9. Baseline laboratory testing, includ-

Table 4.9   Indications for Antiretroviral Therapy

- Symptomatic disease regardless of CD4 count or viral load titer

- CD4 count >500 cells/mm^3 and viral load titer >10,000 copies/mL (bDNA) or >20,000 copies/mL (PCR)*

- CD4 count <500 cells/mm^3 regardless of viral titer[†]

- Pregnancy

bDNA = branched-chain DNA; PCR = polymerase chain reaction.
* There is some debate about what the viral load threshold should be to initiate therapy in this setting.
[†] Some experts would delay therapy with CD4 count between 350–500 cells/mm^3 in the context of low viral load titer.

ing CD4 cell count and viral load measurement, should be performed before initiating therapy. Because of variability in test results, it may be prudent to obtain repeat CD4 count and viral load titer over a 2- to 4-week period.

WHAT AGENTS SHOULD BE USED?
Combination therapy using three drugs is recommended as the initial therapy in most patients. This should include two NRTI agents given in conjunction with a PI or NNRTI. Three NRTIs also have been used by some clinicians in this setting, although supporting data are limited. The use of all monotherapies, d4T with ZDV, or ddC with ddI, d4T, or 3TC is not recommended. Specific reverse-transcriptase inhibitor and PI combinations may necessitate dose adjustments. PIs have many potential drug interactions (see Tables 5.5 and 5.6). Medication lists should be reviewed carefully before beginning therapy with these agents to determine if there are potential drug–drug interactions.

HOW SHOULD ANTIRETROVIRAL THERAPY BE MONITORED?
Patients started on antiretroviral therapy should return in 4 weeks to assess toxicity of the regimen and to repeat the CD4 cell count and viral load titer. If the drug regimen is well tolerated, CD4 count is rising, and viral load titer is maximally suppressed, therapy is continued and repeat laboratory parameters are obtained in 3 to 4 months.

WHEN SHOULD AN ANTIRETROVIRAL DRUG REGIMEN BE MODIFIED?
Indications for modification of a drug regimen include the inability to tolerate drug(s), rising viral load titer, declining CD4 cell count, or clinical disease progression. A rising viral load is often the first evidence of resistance and tests for this should be repeated before changing a regimen. This finding also should necessitate inquiry into the patient's medication adherence.

IF A MODIFIED ANTIRETROVIRAL REGIMEN IS NECESSARY, HOW SHOULD NEW DRUGS BE CHOSEN?

If the regimen is being changed because of development of viral resistance, an entirely new combination that does not share cross-resistance with current drugs is recommended. A careful history of previous antiretroviral drugs is important in selecting new agents, and HIV genotypic or phenotypic testing may be useful in this setting. However, the clinical role of these studies is still under investigation. This genotype test provides a genetic "blueprint" of the predominant viral strain, and the phenotype test offers a drug-sensitivity profile. Both tests identify medications to which the virus is resistant, but they may be of limited help in selecting an effective new regimen. Expert consultation is recommended for clinicians with limited experience in this area. If the regimen is being modified because of toxicity to one drug, a single agent may be substituted for it.

LIPODYSTROPHY SYNDROME

In addition to specific toxicities listed for individual drugs, lipodystrophy syndrome has been reported in some patients on combination antiretroviral therapy. This syndrome consists of body morphology changes (e.g., deposition of fat in abdomen, breasts, and neck; loss of fat in face and extremities), metabolic changes (e.g., hyperlipidemia, glucose intolerance, diabetes mellitus), or both. It is unclear whether all of these findings are related pathophysiologically. The epidemiology of lipodystrophy syndrome is not understood fully, and its optimal management is unknown.

UNRESOLVED QUESTIONS

There are many questions about antiretroviral therapy that are still unanswered and that are the subject of ongoing research. These include the following:

1. How should patients with low but detectable viral load titers be managed?
2. What is the significance of metabolic complications and body morphology changes?
3. How durable is antiretroviral therapy, and what are the long-term toxicities?
4. How should patients with suboptimal virologic responses be managed?
5. What is the role of genotypic and phenotypic testing in clinical practice?

Prophylaxis of Opportunistic Infections

Pneumocystis carinii *Pneumonia*

Despite recent advances in the management of HIV disease, PCP remains an important complication and cause of significant morbidity. PCP prophylaxis is effective and has been demonstrated to prolong life. The risk of developing PCP becomes significant when the patient's CD4 count falls to approximately 200 cells/mm³ and increases progressively as it gets lower.

An algorithmic approach to PCP prophylaxis is presented in Figure 4.1. Effective agents for PCP prevention include trimethoprim–sulfamethoxazole (TMP-SMX), dapsone, and aerosol pentamidine (AP). Atovaquone also has been shown to be useful but is expensive. All HIV-infected patients who have a previous history of PCP or whose CD4 count is fewer than 200 cells/mm³ should receive prophylaxis. Consideration should be given to starting prophylaxis in patients with higher CD4 counts who have a history of thrush or persistent unexplained fever. Recent data indicate that patients receiving primary prophylaxis can discontinue their medication safely if their CD4 count is greater than 200 cells/mm³ for 3 to 6 months on combination antiretroviral therapy. Until more information becomes available, secondary prophylaxis should be maintained in patients with a previous history of PCP.

The drug of choice for PCP prophylaxis is TMP-SMX. The recommended dosage is one double-strength (DS) tablet per day, although there

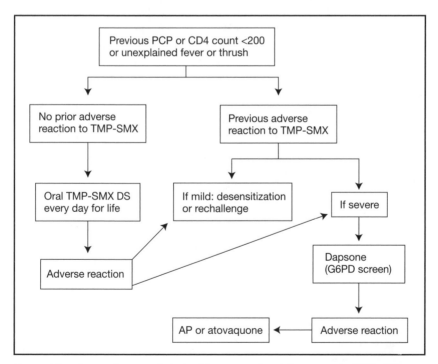

Figure 4.1 Approach to prophylaxis of *Pneumocystis carinii* pneumonia (PCP). AP = aerosol pentamidine; DS = double strength; G6PD = glucose-6-phosphate dehydrogenase; TMP-SMX = trimethoprim-sulfamethoxazole.

is evidence supporting the use of reduced-dose regimens (single-strength [SS] per day or DS three times per week). TMP-SMX is preferred to dapsone because of increased efficacy and protection against conventional bacterial infections. It is preferred to AP because of increased efficacy, lower cost, protection against toxoplasmosis and conventional bacterial infections, and lower risk of extrapulmonary pneumocystosis (Table 4.10). Twenty-five to fifty percent of patients with HIV infection have toxicity to TMP-SMX. The most common side effects include fever, rash, and leukopenia. Strategies for managing mild reactions include discontinuation of the drug, resuming at the same or lower dose at a later date or using a desensitization protocol with gradually increasing doses administered over several days (see Table 6.2). For symptom management of mild drug reactions, many patients can be treated with acetaminophen, an antihistamine, or both.

Dapsone, 100 mg/d taken orally, is recommended as the alternative agent in patients who cannot tolerate TMP-SMX. Side effects of dapsone include fever, rash, and hemolytic anemia. A G6PD qualitative assay should be performed before starting dapsone therapy. For patients who cannot tolerate dapsone, AP is recommended (300 mg/mo by Respirgard II jet nebulizer using 6 mL of sterile water delivered at 6 L/min from a 50-psi compressed-air source until the reservoir is dry, usually over 45 minutes). Active TB should be ruled out with PPD, chest radiograph, and other studies if necessary before initiating AP. Appropriate measures should be in place to prevent TB transmission in people receiving AP. These include use of individual rooms or booths with negative-pressure ventilation, air exhaust to the outside, scheduling to permit air exchange before use by an-

Table 4.10   Comparison of PCP Prophylaxis Regimens

Issue	TMP-SMX	Dapsone	AP	Atovaquone
Efficacy	High	Moderate	Moderate	Moderate
Toxicity	Moderate	Low to moderate	Low	Low
Cost	Low	Low	High	Very high
Toxoplasmosis protection	Yes	Yes*	No	?
Bacterial infection protection	Yes	?	No	No
Risk of extrapulmonary pneumocystosis	No	No	Yes	No

AP = aerosol pentamidine; TMP-SMX = trimethoprim–sulfamethoxazole.
* In conjunction with weekly pyrimethamine.

other patient, use of particulate respirators by workers administering the drug, and restriction of patients from returning to waiting areas until their coughing subsides.

Mycobacterium avium *Complex*

Mycobacterium avium complex is a slow-growing bacterium that is an important cause of disseminated infection in patients with advanced HIV disease. The risk of developing MAC infection becomes significant when the patient's CD4 count falls to approximately 50 cells/mm^3 and increases progressively as it gets lower. Prophylactic therapy has been shown to be effective in preventing MAC infection, with the risk reduced by one half in most studies.

MAC infection presents subacutely with nonspecific symptoms; physical examination shows few, if any, findings. Usually, diagnosis is made by isolator blood cultures, although the organism often can be cultured from body tissues as well. Treatment requires a combination of antimycobacterial agents that generally need to be continued indefinitely.

Prophylaxis is recommended in all patients with CD4 count of fewer than 50 cells/mm^3. Effective agents include rifabutin and the macrolides clarithromycin and azithromycin; their usual oral dosages are 300 mg/d, 500 mg twice daily, and 1200 mg/wk, respectively.

Clarithromycin and azithromycin are more effective than rifabutin. In addition, unlike rifabutin, both can be administered with PIs; in this setting, rifabutin either needs to be dose adjusted or is contraindicated. Furthermore, both macrolides have the advantage of conferring protection against infection with bacterial respiratory pathogens, such as pneumococcus. Clarithromycin is more costly than azithromycin, and their toxicities, which are primarily gastrointestinal, seem to be similar. Although azithromycin in combination with rifabutin provides greater protection against MAC infection than either agent alone, there is also a larger risk of drug toxicity. Clarithromycin with rifabutin is not recommended for MAC prophylaxis. Before MAC prophylaxis is started, assessment to rule out disseminated infection is recommended. If clinically warranted, an isolator blood culture should be obtained.

Recent data indicate that discontinuation of primary MAC prophylaxis is safe in patients whose CD4 cell count has risen to greater than 100 cells/mm^3 for at least 3 to 6 months on combination antiretroviral therapy.

Other Pathogens

Primary prophylaxis is recommended for toxoplasmosis in patients with a positive serology and CD4 count of fewer than 100 cells/mm^3. Either TMP-SMX or dapsone in conjunction with weekly pyrimethamine is useful for toxoplasmosis prophylaxis. Oral ganciclovir has been demonstrated effective for primary prophylaxis of CMV infection but has not come into widespread use because of concerns about toxicity and cost. Secondary prophylaxis is always indicated for TB and is often necessary in advanced HIV disease for relapsing candidiasis and HSV (Table 4.11).

Health Care Maintenance Issues

Immunizations

Patients with HIV disease are at increased risk for a variety of infections that potentially can be prevented by using available vaccine preparations. Immunizations should be given as early in the course of HIV disease as possible for optimal effect. Patients with relatively preserved immune function are more likely to have a favorable response to vaccine challenge than those who are significantly immunocompromised. Initiation of combination antiretroviral therapy in patients with advanced HIV disease may improve the immunologic response to vaccine preparations.

In general, live pathogen vaccines (e.g., measles, mumps, rubella [MMR]; oral polio [OPV]) are contraindicated in HIV-infected patients. However, killed or inactivated vaccines are considered safe in this population. Influenza and other vaccine preparations have been shown to stimulate

Table 4.11   Opportunistic Infection Prophylaxis Stratified by CD4 Cell Count

Infection	CD4 Cell Count		
	>200	*50-200*	*<50*
Tuberculosis*	Isoniazid	Same	Same
PCP	None	TMP-SMX	Same
Toxoplasmosis[†]	None	TMP-SMX	Same
Fungal[‡]	None	Fluconazole	Same
HSV[‡]	None	Acyclovir	Same
MAC	None	None	Macrolide
CMV	None	None	(Oral GCV)

CMV = cytomegalovirus; GCV = ganciclovir; HSV = herpes simplex virus; MAC = *Mycobacterium avium* complex; PCP = *Pneumocystis carinii* pneumonia; PPD = purified protein derivative of tuberculin; TMP-SMX = trimethoprim–sulfamethoxazole.
* In patients with positive PPD
[†] Prophylaxis indicated in patients with CD4 count <100 cells/mm³ and positive serology; alternative therapy is dapsone and pyrimethamine
[‡] Secondary prophylaxis only

HIV replication transiently and increase viral load titer. This phenomenon does not seem to have an impact on overall disease progression.

Specific immunization recommendations are presented in Table 4.12. Pneumococcal vaccine should be administered to all HIV-infected patients. Some experts recommend a booster dose 5 years after immunization. Hepatitis B immunization series should be administered to patients who have a negative screening serologic test for this infection. Hepatitis A vaccine should be given to homosexual and bisexual men and to patients with chronic hepatitis C infection. It also should be considered in injection-drug users, in whom outbreaks have been described. The decision about whether to administer influenza vaccine should be based on an individual's historical risk factors for exposure to the virus and the presence of conditions associated with increased morbidity from influenza infection. Routine use of *Haemophilus* B vaccine is not recommended, but asplenic patients and those with history of recurrent *Haemophilus* infection should be immunized.

Cervical Cancer Screening

HIV disease is associated with an increased risk of cervical dysplasia and cancer in women. Most patients who develop these conditions have a prior history of HPV infection, which is a sexually transmitted pathogen that causes genital warts. The risk of developing cervical disease is greatest in women with advanced HIV disease. Pap smear has been demonstrated to be a useful screening test for cervical dysplasia. Its routine use in populations at risk decreases morbidity and mortality from cervical neoplasia.

A pelvic examination and Pap smear should be performed as part of the initial evaluation of all HIV-infected women; it should be repeated 6 months later and, if normal, repeated at 12-month intervals thereafter. Colposcopy is not recommended as a screening test in this population. More frequent Pap smear evaluations (every 4–6 months) are recommended 1) if endocervical component is absent, 2) if there is a history of HPV infection, or 3) after treatment for any cervical lesion. Women with abnormal Pap smear results showing cellular atypia or any degree of cervical dysplasia should be referred to a gynecologist for further diagnostic evaluation. In general, colposcopy and biopsy are performed.

Tuberculosis: Screening and Prophylaxis

Tuberculosis is a significant cause of morbidity and mortality in HIV-infected patients. The risk of developing active TB in patients with HIV disease if infected with *Mycobacterium tuberculosis* is approximately 10% each year compared with a 10% lifetime risk in immunocompetent hosts. Antimicrobial prophylaxis is effective in HIV-infected patients with a positive PPD, and treatment is effective in those with active TB. TB may pre-

Table 4.12   Immunizations in HIV-Infected Adults

Vaccine	Status	Dose/Regimen	Comments
Pneumococcal vaccine	Recommended	0.5 mL IM	Consider revaccination 5 years after initial dose
Hepatitis B vaccine	Recommended in selected settings; *see* comments	Engerix B, 20 µg, *or* Recombivax HB, 10 µg IM given at 0, 1, and 6 months	Administer to patients without serologic evidence of past or present hepatitis B infection; vaccinated patients should be tested for HBsAb response after the third dose; nonresponding patients should receive booster injections.
Hepatitis A vaccine	Recommended in selected settings; *see* comments	1 mL IM with revaccination in 6–12 months	Administer to homosexual or bisexual men and to patients with chronic hepatitis C infection; serologic testing prior to vaccination is not necessary
Haemophilus influenzae type B vaccine	Consider in selected settings; *see* comments	0.5 mL IM	Administer to asplenic patients and those with history of recurrent *Haemophilus* infection
Influenza vaccine	Recommended in selected settings; *see* comments	0.5 mL IM annually	Administer to patients at high risk for exposure to or morbidity from influenza; there is evidence that the vaccine may promote HIV replication transiently
Td toxoid	Same as for patient without HIV infection	Td 0.5 mL IM	Td booster is recommended every 10 years
Polio vaccine	OPV contraindicated; eIPV if indicated	0.5 mL SC; three doses over 6–12 months for primary immunization	OPV has not proven harmful when given to asymptomatic HIV-infected patients, but eIPV is preferred

eIPV = enhanced inactivated polio vaccine; HBsAb = hepatitis B surface antibody; IM = intramuscularly; OPV = oral polio vaccine; SC = subcutaneously; Td = tetanus–diphtheria toxoid.

sent with extrapulmonary manifestations in advanced HIV disease, and lack of reactivity to skin tests is more common in this context. Diagnosis may be delayed because of these characteristics.

Screening for TB should be part of the initial assessment of HIV-infected patients and repeated annually in high-risk individuals if the test result is negative. Testing is performed with a PPD (intermediate strength, 5TU) administered intracutaneously and read at 48 to 72 hours. The routine use of control agents (e.g., *Candida*, tetanus toxoid, and mumps) is no longer recommended because of their lack of standardization. A positive test in an HIV-infected patient is defined as 5 mm or more of induration.

Prophylactic antimicrobial therapy is recommended for HIV-infected patients regardless of age with any of the following: 1) positive PPD, 2) history of a positive PPD and no documentation of a standard course of prophylaxis, or 3) exposure to active pulmonary TB. Prophylaxis is no longer recommended in HIV-infected patients with anergy who have historical risk factors for TB exposure, such as injection-drug use, alcoholism, homelessness, incarceration, having lived in shelter or institution, and having originated from a country endemic for TB. A chest radiograph should be obtained for all patients with a positive PPD to rule out active pulmonary TB before initiating antimicrobial prophylaxis. If extrapulmonary disease is suspected clinically, the appropriate additional diagnostic evaluation also should be completed.

The standard prophylactic regimen consists of oral isoniazid (INH; 300 mg/d) given with oral pyridoxine (50 mg/d) (in those with history of alcoholism or nutritional deficiency) or directly observed treatment (DOT) of INH 900 mg plus pyridoxine 100 mg, both twice weekly. Treatment is continued for 9 months. Hepatotoxicity to INH increases is uncommon in patients aged under than 35 years but increases with advancing age. Other common side effects include fever and rash. The drug should be discontinued if clinical stigmata of hepatitis develop or if liver transaminases increase to greater than five times baseline. Alternative prophylactic regimens include oral rifampin (RIF; 600 mg/d) for 4–12 months and RIF (600 mg/d) plus pyrazinamide (PZA; 20 mg/kg/d) for 2 months. Infectious disease consultation is recommended in the prophylaxis of multi–drug-resistant (MDR) TB strains.

Sexually Transmitted Diseases

Patients with HIV infection should be screened for other STDs at intake and periodically thereafter if they remain at risk. Emphasis should be placed on prevention. Genital ulcer diseases, such as syphilis and HSV, predispose to transmission of HIV infection. Treatment of pelvic inflammatory disease (PID) may be problematic.

Other Conditions

Age-appropriate screening for other conditions (e.g., breast, colon, and prostate cancers) should be performed in patients with HIV disease. Baseline mammography generally is performed in women between 35 and 40 years of age and repeated annually thereafter. Sigmoidoscopy is recommended every 5 years to patients over 45 years of age, with hemoccult testing of stool in interval years. Digital rectal examination is performed annually in men over 45 years of age. The role of prostate-specific–antigen (PSA) testing to screen for prostate cancer remains controversial.

Psychiatric Disorders

The most common psychiatric diagnoses in patients with HIV disease are adjustment disorder, major depression, anxiety disorder, and substance abuse. Because of the possibility of organic brain disease in this population, a syndrome that manifests itself primarily as a psychiatric disorder merits careful evaluation. Psychological symptoms may be part of an organic syndrome warranting medical intervention. Sometimes, a clinical distinction can be made between early HIV-associated neurocognitive disorder (associated with withdrawal, apathy, avoidance of complex tasks, and mental slowing) and psychological depression (associated with low self-esteem, irrational guilt, and other signs). Neuropsychological testing or an empiric trial of antidepressant therapy may be necessary in more subtle instances.

Adjustment disorder with depressed or anxious mood—considered to be a reaction to the illness—is frequent and may be severe enough to warrant psychotherapeutic or pharmacologic treatment. Stressors may include the following:

1. All of the psychological issues associated with a potentially life-threatening illness

2. The stigmatization that threatens the patient's status in society

3. Uncertainty about the course of illness

4. Difficulty in obtaining adequate health care or financial resources.

Informing patients about support groups and AIDS service organizations available within the community is another important aspect of primary care. "Buddies" available through service organizations can provide long-term emotional support that may otherwise be unavailable to patients who have been estranged from family or friends.

Considerations in Women and Pregnancy

Epidemiology and Transmission

AIDS is presently one of the leading causes of death in women of reproductive age in the United States. The incidence of HIV infection among women in the United States has increased 20-fold since 1981, and the prevalence of HIV disease in this population is estimated to be 0.1%. Approximately 75% of HIV-infected women in the United States are black or Hispanic. Generally, the seroprevalence rate is highest in urban areas and in the Northeast. Initially, injection-drug use was responsible for most cases of HIV disease in women, but since 1993 heterosexual intercourse has been an equally common mode of transmission. The importance of the growing epidemic among women is compounded when one considers that mother-to-infant transmission accounts for nearly all cases of HIV infection among children.

Seronegative women who have sex with HIV-infected men are at higher risk of acquiring HIV infection than are seronegative men who have sex with HIV-infected women. Factors that may increase the risk of HIV transmission to a woman who has sexual contact include intercourse during the menses, anal intercourse, traumatic intercourse, cervical ectopia, and the presence of other STDs in either the man or woman. Transmission of HIV infection through sexual contact between two women, although probably uncommon, also has been reported.

Clinical Manifestations

Despite differences in access to health care, it does not seem that gender significantly affects the course of HIV disease. Reports suggest that women with HIV infection are more likely than men to present with HSV, esophageal candidiasis, and wasting syndrome and are less likely than men to develop KS. Vaginal candidiasis, syphilis, aphthous genital ulcers, HSV infection, and PID often are common and more difficult to manage in HIV-infected women. The incidence of cervical dysplasia, cervical cancer, and vulvar cancer also is increased significantly.

Pregnancy

Reproductive decisions in HIV-infected women seem to be no different than those in age-matched HIV-negative patients. Although sexual transmission of HIV and maternal fetal transmission of the virus are important public health concerns, the clinician should focus on educating the prospective mother about the potential benefits and risks of pregnancy and answering questions she may have.

Management of pregnancy in HIV-infected women includes general prenatal care, maximizing antiretroviral and prophylactic therapies in the mother, and observation for evidence of disease progression. This is best accomplished with a multidisciplinary approach involving an obstetrician, internist, nutritionist, and social worker.

Although pregnancy is associated with a transient 20% decrease in CD4 cell count, it does not seem to have a negative impact on the long-term prognosis of HIV infection. HIV viral load titers are unaffected by pregnancy. Asymptomatic HIV-positive women do not have a significantly greater risk of obstetric complications.

In the absence of effective antiretroviral treatment in the mother, there is a 25% to 30% risk of transmission to the newborn. Evidence exists that maternal–fetal transmission of the HIV virus can occur at any stage in gestation, during labor and delivery, and in the postpartum period through breast feeding. However, presently it is believed that the majority of HIV transmission from mother to infant occurs during labor and delivery. Direct contact of the infant with maternal blood and cervical secretions is the likely mechanism of transmission in this setting. This opinion is supported by the findings that prolonged rupture of membranes is associated with an increased risk of transmission and that the first born of twins, which spends more time in direct contact with maternal bodily fluids, is at higher risk of acquiring the HIV infection than the second born. High maternal HIV viral load, high p24 antigenemia, low CD4 cell count, illicit drug use during pregnancy, and low infant birth weight also are associated with an increased risk of transmission. Recent data about the impact of cesarean section in HIV-infected women show a compelling reduction in the risk of transmission to the newborn.

Table 4.13   Use of Zidovudine During Pregnancy

Maternal Prescription During Second and Third Trimesters
• Administer oral zidovudine, 500–600 mg/d

Intrapartum Prescription
• During labor and delivery, administer intravenous zidovudine, 2 mg/kg loading dose over 30 minutes to 1 hour followed by continuous infusion of 1 mg/kg/h until delivery

Newborn Prescription
• Within 8–12 hours of birth, administer oral zidovudine (syrup), 2 mg/kg 4 times daily for 6 weeks; if infant cannot be given oral medication, then administer intravenous zidovudine, 1.5 mg/kg over 30 minutes every 6 hours

---

Regimens for the use of zidovudine (ZDV) during pregnancy are shown in Table 4.13. Use of ZDV in the mother during pregnancy and in the neonate postpartum has been shown to decrease the rate of vertical transmission of HIV by two thirds. ZDV does not seem to have any adverse fetal effects. How ZDV decreases vertical transmission is not known, but at least part of its benefit is likely due to a postexposure prophylaxis effect. Because of the dramatic effect of ZDV in decreasing neonatal infection, one of the most significant impacts that the primary care clinician can have on the HIV epidemic is to encourage all women of child-bearing age who are pregnant or considering a family to have an HIV antibody test performed. Although no state presently requires testing for HIV infection during pregnancy, many states require physicians to counsel all pregnant women to be tested for HIV antibodies at the beginning of their pregnancy and to inform them of the potential benefits of ZDV in decreasing maternal fetal transmission. Unfortunately, routine voluntary testing for HIV infection has not been implemented successfully in many areas of the country. In addition, even when HIV infection is diagnosed antenatally, as many as 25% of these women decline ZDV therapy.

Despite our understanding of the safety and benefits of ZDV use in pregnancy, there remains little reliable information on the use of other antiretroviral agents in pregnancy. All of the approved agents are listed as pregnancy category B (no evidence of teratogenicity in humans) or C (risk cannot be excluded). A national registry for antiretroviral therapy in pregnancy exists (Antiretroviral Pregnancy Registry; 1-800-258-4263); however, some general principles about drug use in pregnancy are worth reviewing.

First, when considering the use of any medication, it is more helpful to think less in terms of whether a drug is "safe" or "not safe" and more in terms of whether a particular drug's use is justified in the setting of pregnancy based on both what is known about its potential maternal and fetal benefits and toxicity. Second, it is important for the internist to keep in mind that the needs of the mother and the fetus often coincide when it comes to use of medications during pregnancy (i.e., fetal well-being is dependent on that of the mother, so maintenance of maternal health is very much in the interest of the fetus). Furthermore, any medical regimen that can reduce maternal viral load has the theoretical benefit of possibly decreasing vertical transmission. Third, a careful discussion with the patient that emphasizes potential fetal benefits and risks by reviewing what is known and not known about a particular drug regimen is essential. However, the mother's right to make the final decision about use of any medication in pregnancy must be respected. Fourth, organogenesis and therefore teratogenesis occurs in the first trimester of pregnancy. Therefore, use of medications for which there are inadequate pregnancy data should be avoided if possible during the first trimester.

For previously untreated women with HIV infection, many clinicians begin three agents, including ZDV, after completion of the first trimester. The combination of ZDV, 3TC, and nevirapine is well tolerated and a popular initial option. For women already on an effective established antiretroviral regimen, clinicians should counsel them to consider remaining on their medications throughout gestation because stopping the drugs even for the brief period of organogenesis may result in a substantial increase in viral load. If a regimen is stopped during the first trimester, it is important that all agents be stopped and reinstated simultaneously to minimize the likelihood of development of viral resistance. The addition of ZDV during the second and third trimesters to a non–ZDV-containing regimen should be strongly considered.

Recommendations for initiation and maintenance of prophylaxis of opportunistic infections in the pregnant women are standard. TMP-SMX, despite theoretical concerns about its use in pregnancy, has an excellent safety profile in doses used for prophylaxis of PCP and toxoplasmosis. Isoniazid, azithromycin, and clarithromycin have human data supporting their use during pregnancy. Influenza, pneumococcal, and hepatitis B immunizations can all be administered safely.

The optimal mode of delivery for the HIV-infected woman is a matter of some controversy. A recent meta-analysis suggests that cesarean section is associated with less vertical transmission of HIV than vaginal delivery and even confers additional protection to infants of mothers receiving ZDV. Whether cesarean section offers benefit to women on suppressive combination antiretroviral therapy presently is not known. Use of intravenous ZDV intrapartum clearly is warranted and other antiretroviral agents should be continued throughout parturition. Avoidance of fetal scalp monitors and artificial rupture of membranes and the use of forceps or vacuum extractor and fetal blood scalp sampling are important in decreasing the risk of vertical transmission. Following delivery, HIV-infected mothers must be observed carefully for any symptoms or signs of infection, because there may be an increased risk of postpartum endometritis. Infant bonding should be encouraged, although contact with maternal body fluids should be avoided. Patients also should be counseled extensively about options for contraception. Arrangements for medical follow-up should be made before patients are discharged. Finally, many patients are at risk for depression and social isolation and may have few resources for support. They should be made aware of community services that are available to them during this period of significant adjustment.

In the United States, breast feeding is contraindicated in HIV-infected women because of the increased risk of transmission. Seronegative women with a history of high-risk behaviors also may be counseled against breast feeding in the event that they may not have developed HIV antibody to recent infection. However, bottle feeding is often not practical in developing countries in which acceptable alternatives to breast milk are not available because of poor sanitation, high rates of infectious disease, and economic limitations.

Neonates

Testing neonates for HIV infection is complicated by the fact that maternal HIV antibodies readily cross the placenta and may be found in the infant's serum for up to 18 months after delivery. Neonates are considered HIV-infected if two separate blood specimens test positive for HIV by nucleic acid, p24 antigen, or viral culture. Ideally, to allow early intervention in the HIV-infected neonate, DNA PCR testing should be performed at birth and weekly for the first month of life. Careful follow-up of both positive and negative newborn test results, with repeat studies that include viral culture for confirmation, will increase the accuracy of diagnosis of HIV infection in the newborn.

Other Health Issues

Complementary Medical Therapies

Complementary or alternative medical therapies are commonly used by HIV-infected patients, often in conjunction with conventional treatments. Individuals may not volunteer such information unless it is requested specifically. The safety and efficacy of alternative medical therapies for HIV disease are not well established but are in the process of investigation.

Clinical Trials

Participation in clinical trials should be encouraged for HIV-infected patients in therapeutic areas in which optimal management is not known. For example, what is the best therapeutic approach in an individual who has received several different antiretroviral regimens but continues to have a detectable viral load? Good communication between research staff and the primary care clinician is important to ensure coordination of care.

Substance Abuse

Some HIV-infected patients have a history of substance abuse involving alcohol, cocaine, crack, or opiates. Clinicians should recognize that the stress of being seropositive or developing symptomatic disease may lead to substance abuse relapse. Fostering sobriety is an important component of care. In some situations, substance abuse treatment may be a higher priority than treatment for HIV infection because the latter may be impossible in the context of active drug use.

Personal Finances

Assessment of the patient's financial situation and insurance status also should be part of the intake process with attention given to ascertaining eligibility for health care, general relief, disability, and housing programs.

Legal Issues

A variety of legal issues can take on dramatic significance for those with HIV disease, especially if the patient is involved in a long-term homosexual relationship. Patients may need to anticipate transfer in custody of their children and should be encouraged to arrange for others to make medical judgments on their behalf in case of severe illness by executing an advance directive for health care, a durable power of attorney, or both. Many AIDS service organizations assist patients in executing legal instruments and re-solving custody issues.

Food Safety and Other Concerns

Caution in food preparation and handling is important given the vulnera-bility to infections that accompanies immunodeficiency. Using plastic or glass rather than wooden cutting boards may decrease the chance of bac-terial contamination. Microwaved foods should be allowed to stand for a few minutes after cooking to ensure that heat is evenly distributed. Be-cause of the risk of salmonellosis, raw egg products should not be con-sumed. Raw seafood (e.g., sashimi, sushi, oysters), poultry, or meat (e.g., steak tartar) should be avoided because of the potential transmission of bacteria and protozoa. All produce should be washed before eating it. Practical measures to limit exposure to other pathogens are described in Table 4.14.

Table 4.14   Measures to Limit Exposure to Pathogens

- Wash hands after bathroom use or contact with animals or soil
- Do not drink water from an untested source
- Use care in selecting and handling of animals
- Discuss travel plans with knowledgeable health care professional
- Follow safer sex and drug use recommendations

■ ■ ■

Key Points

- All people at risk for HIV infection or in whom it is suspected should be counseled about HIV antibody testing.
- The clinical evaluation of HIV-infected patients should include not only history taking, physical examination, and laboratory testing but also attention to psychosocial and educational needs.
- Baseline laboratory studies are performed to identify occult systemic disease and latent infections and to determine the HIV disease stage.
- Management of HIV-infected patients includes addressing the issues of antiretroviral therapy, prophylaxis against opportunistic infections, health care maintenance, and treatment of diseases acquired as their immunologic function diminishes.
- Use of ZDV during pregnancy and in the postpartum infant significantly decreases the risk of HIV transmission.

■ ■ ■

Resources

Web Sites

The Johns Hopkins AIDS Service: www.hopkins-aids.edu
HIV Information Network: www.hivline.com
HIV InSite (University of California/San Francisco General Hospital): hivinsite.ucsf.edu
DHHS HIV/AIDS Treatment Information Service: www.hivatis.org
National AIDS Treatment Information Project (patient education materials): www.natip.org

■ ■ ■

SUGGESTED READINGS

Bartlett JG (ed). *Hopkins HIV Report.* Baltimore, MD: Johns Hopkins University AIDS Service [Published bimonthly].

Carpenter CCJ, et al. Antiretroviral therapy in adults: updated recommendations of the International AIDS Society, USA Panel. *JAMA.* 2000;283:381–90.

Centers for Disease Control and Prevention. CDC guidelines for national human immunodeficiency virus case surveillance, including monitoring for human immunodeficiency virus infection and acquired immunodeficiency syndrome. *MMWR Morb Mortal Wkly Rep.* 1999;48(RR-13):1-31.

Centers for Disease Control and Prevention. Report of the NIH panel to define principles of therapy of HIV infection and guidelines for the use of antiretroviral agents in HIV-infected adults and adolescents. *MMWR Morb Mortal Wkly Rep.* 1998; 47:1-82. (Available as "living document" an DHHS HIV/AIDS Treatment Information Service Web site at http://www.hivatis.org).

Centers for Disease Control and Prevention. Public Health Service Task Force recommendations for the use of antiretroviral drugs in pregnant women infected with HIV-1 for maternal health and for reducing perinatal HIV-1 transmission in the United States. *MMWR Morb Mortal Wkly Rep.* 1998;47:1-30.

Cotton DJ (ed). *AIDS Clinical Care.* Waltham, MA: Massachusetts Medical Society [Published monthly].

Drugs for HIV infection. *Med Lett Drugs Ther.* 2000;42:1-6.

Hirsch MS, et al. Antiretroviral drug resistance testing in adults with HIV infection: implications for clinical management. *JAMA.* 1998;279:1984-91.

Mellors JW, et al. Plasma viral load and CD4 lymphocytes as prognostic markers of HIV-1 infection. *Ann Intern Med.* 1997;126:946-54.

O'Brien WA, et al. Changes in plasma HIV RNA levels and CD4+ lymphocyte counts predict both response to antiretroviral therapy and therapeutic failure. *Ann Intern Med.* 1997;127:939-45.

Powderly WG, Landay A, Lederman MM. Recovery of the immune system with antiretroviral therapy: the end of opportunism? *JAMA.* 1998;280:72-77.

United States Public Health Service, Infectious Disease Society of America. 1999 guidelines for the prevention of opportunistic infections in persons infected with HIV. *MMWR Morb Mortal Wkly Rep.* 1999;48:1-66.

5

■ ■ ■

Antiretroviral Therapy

Colm Bergin, MD

Timothy Cooley, MD

he first antiretroviral drug, zidovudine (ZDV), was introduced in 1987. Since that time, fourteen agents have been approved by the Food and Drug Administration (FDA) for the treatment of HIV disease. The use of these drugs in combination has had a dramatic impact on the course of HIV disease. AIDS mortality declined from 43,000 in 1995 to 17,000 in 1997. In addition, hospitalizations and the incidence of opportunistic infections also have decreased significantly. An improved understanding of the pathogenesis of HIV infection and the development of reliable assays to quantify plasma viral RNA have paralleled the increased number of therapeutic options. Data from the Multicenter AIDS Cohort Study (MACS) and others demonstrate the association of higher HIV viral loads and lower CD4 counts with progression to AIDS. The primary goal of antiretroviral therapy is to suppress HIV viral load to an undetectable level.

The topic of antiretroviral therapy is both complex and evolving. The focus of this chapter is to review drugs currently prescribed for the treatment of HIV disease and to present guidelines for the clinical management of adult patients. Although starting treatment in HIV-infected patients with advanced disease is the standard of care, there are both potential benefits and risks to initiating therapy in patients with early disease (Table 5.1), and treatment decisions must be individualized.

Goal of Antiretroviral Therapy

The monitoring of viral RNA is an important determinant in deciding when to initiate antiretroviral therapy and when to consider changing regimens that are failing. The specific goals of treatment are to decrease the HIV viral load by at least 1 log in the first 4 weeks after starting therapy and to the undetectable range using the most sensitive assay (20–50 copies/mL) by 3 to 6 months. The achievement of complete viral suppression depends on the baseline viral load and CD4 count, the potency of the regimen used, patient adherence, and previous exposure to antiretroviral drugs. The nadir of viral load response and the time to achieve an undetectable level strongly predict the durability of response to treatment.

In clinical trials, approximately 80% of subjects have complete viral suppression on their first antiretroviral drug regimen, and most of these remain suppressed for at least 3 years. In clinical practice, the response rate range is between 50% and 80%, depending on adherence of the patient population. Subsequent antiretroviral regimens are generally less successful at achieving viral suppression.

Drug Failure and Adherence

Drug failure does not always equal viral resistance and may be caused by a number of other factors, including suboptimal choice of regimen, pharmacokinetic variability, drug–drug interactions, or a combination of these factors.

Genotypic and phenotypic testing of viral isolates is becoming more common in clinical practice and will serve an increasingly important role in the management of HIV-infected patients over time. The genotype test

Table 5.1   Risks and Benefits of Antiretroviral Therapy in Asymptomatic HIV-infected Patients

Potential Benefits	*Potential Risks*
• Control of viral replication and mutation	• Drug toxicities
• Reduction of viral burden	• Drug–drug interactions
• Control of disease progression	• Excessive medication burden
• Maintenance of immunologic function	• Early drug resistance
• Decreased risk of HIV transmission	• Cross-resistance
	• Transmission of drug-resistant virus

detects specific viral mutations associated with drug resistance based on polymerase chain reaction (PCR) technique. It is relatively simple and is less expensive than the phenotypic assay. The phenotype test measures the 50% or 90% inhibitory concentrations of a drug against the virus. It may be of use when evaluating complex cases of heavily pretreated patients or in cases in which the genetic basis of resistance to a particular drug is unknown.

The association between genotype, phenotype, and clinical outcome is not well defined. HIV resistance assays may provide data on which drugs will *not* be successful rather than on which drugs will. This is because small populations of resistant virus undetected by the assay may be present and may predominate under selective pressure when a specific drug is used.

Adherence is clearly an important factor in determining the likelihood of success of an antiretroviral regimen. Studies of other chronic medical conditions have identified a number of factors associated with nonadherence (*see* Table 4.8). Alcoholism and psychiatric disease (particularly affective disorders) are associated with poor adherence, but socioeconomic characteristics are not predictive. The issue of prescribing antiretroviral therapy to patients actively using illicit drugs remains controversial, and decisions need to be made on an individual basis.

Interventions that may improve adherence include patient education before starting treatment and adaptation of a drug regimen to an individual's lifestyle. Unfortunately, methods of monitoring adherence, including patient self-report and pill counts, are not always reliable.

Antiretroviral Drugs

Antiretroviral drugs are classified into three categories: nucleoside reverse-transcriptase inhibitors (NRTIs), nonnucleoside reverse-transcriptase inhibitors (NNRTIs), and protease inhibitors (PIs). Their characteristics are described in Tables 5.2, 5.3, and 5.4. Fourteen drugs and sixteen formulations have been approved by the FDA. Tenofovir, a nucleotide agent, and ABT-378/ritonavir (lopinavir), a PI, are now available through pharamceutical company expanded-access programs. Antiretroviral drugs vary greatly in their dosaging, toxicity, and interactions with other drugs. Because of the effect of NNRTIs and PIs on hepatic metabolism, certain medications cannot be co-administered with these agents (Table 5.5), and others may require dosage adjustment or careful monitoring. NNRTI and PI dosing also may need to be modified when these drugs are given concurrently (Table 5.6). Patients on antiretroviral therapy should contact their HIV care provider before starting any new medications.

Table 5.2   Characteristics of Nucleoside Reverse-Transcriptase Inhibitors

Generic Name Trade Name	Dosage	Oral Bioavailability	Serum Half-life	Intracellular Half-life	Elimination	Toxicity
Zidovudine (AZT, ZDV) *Retrovir*	300 mg bid, or with 3TC as Combivir 1 bid	60%	1.1 hours	3 hours	Metabolized to AZT glucuronide (GAZT) Renal excretion of GAZT	GI intolerance, headaches, insomnia, asthenia, anemia, neutropenia, lactic acidosis (rare)
Didanosine (ddI)* *Videx*	Tablet: 200 mg bid or 400 mg qd in patients weighing ≥60 kg; 125 mg bid or 250 mg qd in <60 kg Powder: 250 mg bid in patients weighing ≥60 kg; 167 mg bid in <60 kg Take 30 minutes before or 2 hours after meal	Tablet: 40% Powder: 30%	1.6 hours	25–40 hours	Renal excretion 50%	Pancreatitis, peripheral neuropathy, GI intolerance, lactic acidosis (rare)
Zalcitabine (ddC) *HIVID*	0.75 mg tid	85%	1.2 hours	3 hours	Renal excretion 70%	Peripheral neuropathy, stomatitis, lactic acidosis (rare)
Stavudine (d4T)* *Zerit*	40 mg bid in patients weighing ≥60 kg; 30 mg bid in <60 kg	86%	1.0 hour	3.5 hours	Renal excretion 50%	Peripheral neuropathy, lactic acidosis (rare)
Lamivudine (3TC) *Epivir*	150 mg bid or with ZDV as combivir 1 bid	86%	3–6 hours	12 hours	Renal excretion unchanged	Minor, lactic acidosis (rare)
Abacavir (ABC) *Ziagen*	300 mg bid	83%	1.5 hours	3.3 hours	Renal excretion of metabolites 82%	Hypersensitivity reaction[†] (fever, rash, nausea, vomiting, malaise, fatigue, respiratory symptoms), lactic acidosis (rare)

GI = gastrointestinal.

* Hydroxyurea sometimes is prescribed in conjunction with these agents to enhance their antiviral activity.

[†] Patients who develop symptoms or signs of hypersensitivity reaction should discontinue abacavir; the drug should not be restarted because of risk of severe toxicity or death. Adapted from Centers for Disease Control and Prevention. Report of the NIH panel to define principles of therapy of HIV infection and guidelines for the use of antiretroviral agents in HIV-infected adults and adolescents. *MMWR Morb Mortal Wkly Rep.* 1998;47:1–82. (Available as "living document" on DHHS HIV/AIDS Treatment Information Service Web site at www.hivatis.org).

Table 5.3   Characteristics of Nonnucleoside Reverse-Transcriptase Inhibitors

Generic Name Trade Name	Dosage	Oral Bioavailability	Serum Half-life	Elimination	Toxicity
Nevirapine *Viramune*	200 mg/d every 14 days, then 200 mg bid	>90%	25–30 hours	Metabolized by cytochrome p450; 80% excreted in urine (glucuronidated metabolites, <5% unchanged), 10% in stool	Rash, hepatitis, increased transaminases
Delavirdine *Rescriptor*	400 mg tid (two 200-mg tablets in ≥3 oz water to produce slurry) Separate dosing with ddI or antacids by 1 hour	85%	5.8 hours	Metabolized by cytochrome p450; 51% excreted in urine (<5% unchanged), 44% in stool	Rash, increased transaminases, headaches
Efavirenz *Sustiva*	600 mg qhs Avoid taking after high-fat meal	Data not available	40–55 hours	Metabolized by cytochrome p450; 14%–34% excreted in urine, 16%–61% in stool	Neurocognitive dysfunction (e.g., confusion, somnolence, difficulty concentrating, depersonalization, insomnia, altered dreams), rash, increased transaminases

Adapted from Centers for Disease Control and Prevention. Report of the NIH panel to define principles of therapy of HIV infection and guidelines for the use of antiretroviral agents in HIV-infected adults and adolescents. *MMWR Morb Mortal Wkly Rep.* 1998;47:1–82. (Available as "living document" on DHHS HIV/AIDS Treatment Information Service Web site at www.hivatis.org).

Nucleoside Reverse-Transcriptase Inhibitors

Nucleoside reverse-transcriptase inhibitors serve as the foundation of most antiretroviral drug regimens and are often prescribed in combination with an NNRTI or PI. These drugs include ZDV, didanosine (ddI), zalcitabine (ddC), stavudine (d4T), lamivudine (3TC), and abacavir (ABC). NRTIs are incorporated into the HIV deoxyribonucleic acid-ase (DNAase), and after

Table 5.4   Characteristics of Protease Inhibitors

Generic Name / Trade Name	Form	Dosage	Oral Bioavailability	Serum Half-life	Route of Metabolism	Storage	Toxicity
Saquinavir / *Invirase, Fortovase*	200-mg capsule	Invirase: 400 mg when given with ritonavir. Fortovase: 1200 mg tid. Take with food	Invirase: 4% Fortovase: 13%	1–2 hours	p450 cytochrome 3A4	Room temperature	GI intolerance, headaches, increased transaminases, hyperglycemia, fat redistribution, lipid abnormalities
Ritonavir / *Norvir*	100-mg capsule 600-mg/ 7.5-mL solution	600 mg every 12 hours* Take with food. Separate dosing with ddI by 2 hours	NA	3–5 hours	p450 cytochrome 3A4 >2D6	Refrigerate capsules; do not refrigerate solution	GI intolerance; circumoral and extremity paresthesias; asthenia; taste perversion; increased transaminases, CPK, and uric acid; hyperglycemia; fat redistribution; lipid abnormalities
Indinavir / *Crixivan*	200- and 400-mg capsule	800 mg every 8 hours. Take 1 hour before or after meals; may take with skim milk or low-fat meal. Separate dosing with ddI by 1 hour	65%	1.5–2.0 hours	p450 cytochrome 3A4	Room temperature	Nephrolithiasis, GI intolerance, headaches, asthenia, blurred vision, dizziness, rash, metallic taste, indirect hyperbilirubinemia, thrombocytopenia, hyperglycemia, fat redistribution, lipid abnormalities
Nelfinavir / *Viracept*	250-mg tablet 50-mg/g oral powder	750 mg tid. Take with food	20%–80%	3.5–5.0 hours	p450 cytochrome 3A4	Room temperature	Diarrhea, hyperglycemia, fat redistribution, lipid abnormalities
Amprenavir / *Agenerase*	150-mg tablet	1200 mg bid	63%	NA	p450 cytochrome 3A4	Room temperature	GI intolerance, rash, headaches

CPK = creatine phosphokinase; GI = gastrointestinal; NA = data not available.

* Dose escalation for ritonavir: day 1–2: 300 mg bid; day 3–5: 400 mg bid; day 6–13: 500 mg bid; day 14+: 600 mg bid.

Adapted from Centers for Disease Control and Prevention. Report of the NIH panel to define principles of therapy of HIV infection and guidelines for the use of antiretroviral agents in HIV-infected adults and adolescents. *MMWR Morb Mortal Wkly Rep.* 1998;47:1–82. (Available as "living document" on DHHS HIV/AIDS Treatment Information Service Web site at www.hivatis.org).

cell uptake they are converted by cellular kinases to a triphosphate. This form competes with the HIV reverse transcriptase, is incorporated into the DNA strand, and causes premature termination of the DNA intermediate because it lacks the 3-hydroxyl group necessary for deoxyribonucleotide linkage. Reverse-transcriptase enzyme is not present in human cells.

In addition to convenience, the choice of which NRTI agents to use should be based on efficacy, ability to penetrate the central nervous system, and interactions with other NRTIs. Many studies have found no significant differences in the effectiveness of various NRTI combinations; ZDV/3TC, ZDV/ddI, ddI/d4T and d4T/3TC seem similar in terms of their anti-HIV effect. There are fewer studies of ddC-containing regimens.

Resistance to 3TC emerges rapidly, especially in people with detectable viral loads. There is some *in vitro* evidence to suggest that 3TC-resistant virus may be less susceptible to ddI and ddC. Paradoxically, the mutation that confers 3TC resistance may reverse resistance to ZDV by suppressing the effect of ZDV mutations at codons 215 and 70. However, this benefit may be transient with the emergence of other mutations. The response to d4T in patients previously treated with ZDV may be impaired because continual ZDV therapy renders cells less efficient in phosphorylating other NRTIs. Resistance to ddI/d4T is unusual, making this combination a possible alternative to ZDV/3TC as the initial choice of NRTIs. The frequency of neuropathy with ddI/d4T is no greater than that described with either drug alone.

Zidovudine

Zidovudine (ZDV) is a thymidine analog. The antiviral effect of ZDV monotherapy has been shown to be transient because of the development of multiple mutations in HIV reverse transcriptase that renders the virus progressively less susceptible to the drug. The first mutation is usually Lys-70-Arg followed by Thr-215-Tyr. Highly resistant virus generally arises after three to four mutations. Increased resistance to ZDV correlates with decreased susceptibility to other NRTIs. Common toxicities of ZDV include nausea, headaches, anemia, and neutropenia.

Didanosine

Didanosine (ddI) is a purine analog. The CD4 response, viral load decrease, and toxicity profile of once-daily dosing seems similar to twice-daily administration. ddI may soon be available as "enteric-coated" 400-mg pills. Resistance develops slowly during monotherapy. The most common mutation is Leu-74-Val and confers a four- to tenfold increase in IC_{50}. Gastrointestinal intolerance, including lack of palatability, nausea, and diarrhea are the most common side effects. Pancreatitis and peripheral neuropathy occur less frequently.

Table 5.5   Drugs Contraindicated for Use with Antiretroviral Agents*

Drug	Cardiac Agents	Lipid-Lowering Agents	Antimyco-bacterial Agents	Calcium-Channel Blockers
Delavirdine	None	Simvastatin Lovastatin	Rifampin Rifabutin	None
Efavirenz	None	None	None	None
Saquinavir	None	Simvastatin Lovastatin	Rifampin Rifabutin	None
Ritonavir	Amiodarone Flecainide Propafenone Quinidine	Simvastatin Lovastatin	None	Bepridil
Indinavir	None	Simvastatin Lovastatin	Rifampin	None
Nelfinavir	None	Simvastatin Lovastatin	Rifampin	None
Amprenavir	None	Simvastatin Lovastatin	Rifampin	Bepridil

Zalcitabine

Zalcitabine (ddC) is a cytidine analog. Resistance develops slowly, with Lys-65-Arg and Thr-69-Asp being the usual mutations. ddC appears to be the least effective NRTI and is not prescribed frequently. The most common toxicity is peripheral neuropathy. Oral ulcers and pancreatitis also may occur.

Stavudine

Stavudine (d4T) is also a thymidine analog with similar clinical efficacy to ZDV. The most common side effect is peripheral neuropathy, which may

Table 5.5   *Continued*

Antihistamines	Gastro-intestinal Drugs	Neuroleptics	Psychotropics	Ergot Alkaloids
Astemizole Terfenadine	Cisapride H$_2$-blockers Proton-pump inhibitors	None	Midazolam Triazolam	Dihydro-ergotamine Ergotamine
Astemizole Terfenadine	Cisapride	None	Midazolam Triazolam	Dihydro-ergotamine Ergotamine
Astemizole Terfenadine	Cisapride	None	Midazolam Triazolam	Dihydro-ergotamine Ergotamine
Astemizole Terfenadine	Cisapride	Clozapine Pimozide	Midazolam Triazolam	Dihydro-ergotamine Ergotamine
Astemizole Terfenadine	Cisapride	None	Midazolam Triazolam	Dihydro-ergotamine Ergotamine
Astemizole Terfenadine	Cisapride	None	Midazolam Triazolam	Dihydro-ergotamine Ergotamine
Astemizole	Cisapride	None	Midazolam Triazolam	Dihydro-ergotamine Ergotamine

* Other medications coadministered with NNRTIs and PIs may require dosage adjustment or careful monitoring (*see* package insert or *Physicians Desk Reference* for details).
Adapted from Centers for Disease Control and Prevention. Report of the NIH panel to define principles of therapy of HIV infection and guidelines for the use of antiretroviral agents in HIV-infected adults and adolescents. *MMWR Morb Mortal Wkly Rep.* 1998;47:1–82. (Available as "living document" on DHHS HIV/AIDS Treatment Information Service Web site at www.hivatis.org).

improve with dose reduction. Pancreatitis also has been described rarely when the drug is co-administered with ddI.

Lamivudine

Lamivudine (3TC), another cytidine analog, is associated with the rapid development of resistance (Met-184-Val) if used as monotherapy. This mutation also may affect susceptibility to ABC. Toxicity from 3TC is uncommon. 3TC also has activity against hepatitis B. FTC, a fluorinated form of 3TC,

Table 5.6   Nonnucleoside Reverse-Transcriptase Inhibitor and Protease Inhibitor Drug Interactions*

Drug Affected	Nevirapine	Delavirdine	Efavirenz	Saquinavir	Ritonavir	Indinavir	Nelfinavir	Amprenavir
Nevirapine	—	NR	NR	No data	Standard dose	Standard dose	Standard dose	No data
Delavirdine	NR	—	NR	Standard dose	Standard dose	Standard dose	No data	No data
Efavirenz	NR	NR	—	NR	Standard dose	Standard dose	Standard dose	Standard dose
Saquinavir	No data	Fortovase 800 mg tid	NR	—	Fortovase 400 mg bid	No data	Fortovase 800 mg tid	No data
Ritonavir	Standard dose	No data	Standard dose	400 mg bid	—	400 mg bid	400 mg bid	200 mg bid
Indinavir	1000 mg q8h	600 mg q8h	1000 mg q8h	No data	400 mg bid	—	1200 mg bid	Standard dose
Nelfinavir	Standard dose	No data	Standard dose	Standard dose	500–750 mg bid	1250 mg bid	—	1250 mg bid
Amprenavir	No data	No data	1200 mg tid or 1200 mg bid with RTV 200 mg bid	No data	600 mg bid	Standard dose	750 mg bid	—

*Drug doses refer to bold agents at beginning of each row.

NR = not recommended for coadministration; RTV = ritonavir.

Adapted from Centers for Disease Control and Prevention. Report of the NIH panel to define principles of therapy of HIV infection and guidelines for the use of antiretroviral agents in HIV-infected adults and adolescents. *MMWR Morb Mortal Wkly Rep.* 1998;47:1–82. (Available as "living document" on DHHS HIV/AIDS Treatment Information Service Web site at www.hivatis.org).

currently is being studied, with its prolonged half-life making once-daily dosaging possible.

Abacavir

Abacavir (ABC) is a guanosine analog. Initial studies with this drug as monotherapy showed viral load drops of 1.5 to 2.0 logs over 4 weeks. Trials comparing ZDV/3TC/ABC to ZDV/3TC/indinavir and combinations of ABC with PIs are ongoing. Patient response to ABC seems to be lessened in the presence of three or more mutations to nucleoside analogues. Resistance mutations are found at codons 184, 74, and 115. The 184 mutation associated with 3TC resistance decreases susceptibility to ABC twofold; however, at least three mutations are required to result in a 10-fold change in viral susceptibility. More than 90% of isolates resistant to ZDV, 3TC, or ZDV/3TC remain susceptible to ABC. Although usually well tolerated, it is imperative that physicians and patients be aware of the occurrence of a hypersensitivity reaction to ABC in 3% of patients (see Table 5.2). If hypersensitivity develops, ABC should be discontinued permanently as serious toxicity and death have been reported on rechallenge of the drug.

Tenofovir

Tenofovir is an experimental nucleotide reverse-transcriptase inhibitor that is available through an expanded-access program from Gilead Pharmaceuticals (1-800-GILEAD-5). It is also active against hepatitis B. Tenofovir does not appear to be as nephrotoxic as adefovir. Toxicities to date have included increased serum creatine phosphokinase and transaminase levels.

Combivir

The introduction of Combivir (ZDV/3TC) reduced the pill burden for patients taking ZDV and 3TC. Pharmacokinetic studies showed that combining these drugs does not affect their absorption, toxicity profile, or anti-HIV effect.

Nonnucleoside Reverse-Transcriptase Inhibitors

Nonnucleoside reverse-transcriptase inhibitors bind directly and noncompetively to reverse transcriptase downstream from the active catalytic site to inhibit production of viral DNA. They act at different sites than NRTIs and do not require phosphorylation for activation. NNRTIs and NRTIs have different viral resistance patterns. However, resistance to this class of drugs can develop easily from a single mutation. In vitro mutation sites include codon 103 (common to all), 106, 108, 181, 190, and 236 (which seems unique to delavirdine).

Nevirapine

Nevirapine was the first licensed NNRTI. In the INCAS trial, treatment-naive subjects with CD4 counts of 200-600/mm^3 and a mean HIV RNA of 25,000 copies/mL were randomized to ZDV/ddI, ZDV/nevirapine, or ZDV/ddI/nevirapine; 55% of subjects on triple therapy had undetectable viral load at 52 weeks compared with none in the other arms. Data from AIDS Clinical Trials Group (ACTG) study 241 show diminished efficacy in pretreated subjects. Other studies have suggested decreased benefit in patients with high baseline viral loads. Common toxicities include rash, which rarely may be severe, and increased liver function test (LFT) levels.

Delavirdine

Delavirdine has not been studied as much as nevirapine but seems similar in effectiveness. Unlike nevirapine and efavirenz, it inhibits p450 cytochrome and, therefore, may increase levels of drugs metabolized in the liver, including indinavir and nelfinavir. Rash and increased LFT levels may occur but are less common with nevirapine.

Efavirenz

Studies comparing ZDV/3TC/indinavir to ZDV/3TC/efavirenz and indinavir/efavirenz have demonstrated that the rates of complete viral suppression are greater in the groups receiving efavirenz, including a subset of subjects with high baseline viral loads. High-level resistance to the drug occurs more slowly than with the other NNRTIs, and at least two mutations are necessary to cause phenotypic resistance. Resistance is associated most commonly with K103N, which also confers resistance to the other NNRTIs. Multiple mutations are required for high-level resistance. Neuropsychiatric side effects are common with efavirenz. They tend to occur in the first few weeks of therapy and are reduced when the drug is given at night. Rash is not as frequent as with the other NNRTIs. Because of concerns about teratogenicity, efavirenz is not recommended for pregnant women or those of child-bearing age who do not use barrier-contraceptive methods.

Protease Inhibitors

Protease inhibitors are the most potent antiretroviral agents available, with viral replication suppressed by 2 logs or more. PIs prevent HIV from being assembled and released from the CD4 lymphocyte by inhibiting the viral enzyme that cleaves large viral polyproteins into small functional units. Despite the potent antiviral effect of PIs, problems with their use include bioavailability, difficult dosage requirements, side effects, and drug–drug interactions. Whether these drugs should be used as first-line agents or reserved for patients whose viral load is not suppressed on a PI-sparing regimen is currently under investigation.

Saquinavir (Invirase)

The Invirase preparation of saquinavir was the first PI to be evaluated in clinical trials. Its bioavailability is only 4%, with most of the drug undergoing first-pass hepatic metabolism. Invirase should only be used in combination with other PIs that increase its plasma level and antiviral effect. The most common toxicities of saquinavir are nausea and diarrhea.

Saquinavir (Fortovase)

The Fortovase preparation of saquinavir contains lipids that facilitate absorption of the drug and reduces the effect of hepatic enzymatic metabolism. Data from the CHEESE study confirm its efficacy in treatment-naive subjects.

Ritonavir

Ritonavir is a potent antiretroviral drug when used in combination with other agents; however, concerns about pill burden, toxicity, and drug interactions have limited its use as a single PI. However, it is prescribed commonly in reduced dosage as part of a dual-PI regimen (see Dual-Protease Inhibitor Therapy below).

Indinavir

Indinavir is also a potent PI when combined with other antiretroviral agents. However, its dosage schedule (three times per day), dietary restrictions, and fluid requirements (to decrease the risk of nephrolithiasis) may make administration difficult. Twice-daily dosing of indinavir is not recommended based on a study of treatment-naive subjects taking ZDV/3TC with indinavir either every 8 hours or 12 hours. There were fewer than 400 copies/mL of HIV RNA in 91% of subjects on every-8-hour indinavir compared with only 64% of those on every-12-hour indinavir. Similar dosage-related outcomes were seen in the ACTG study 368. Viral resistance to indinavir is often associated with cross-resistance to saquinavir and ritonavir.

Nelfinavir

Nelfinavir has similar antiviral activity to ritonavir and indinavir. Its most common side effect is diarrhea, which occurs in up to 30% of patients and may require treatment with antidiarrheal agents or pancreatic enzyme supplement. Results from the Agouron study 542 comparing every-12-hour and every-8-hour dosing showed similar results in both arms. Nelfinavir has a different resistance pattern compared with the other PIs exhibiting the primary mutation of D30N.

Amprenavir

Amprenavir is the newest PI to be approved by the FDA. The ACTG study 347 assessed efficacy in PI-naive and 3TC-naive subjects. In combination with ZDV and 3TC, 63% of subjects treated with amprenavir had undetectable viral load at 24 weeks. Data are being collected on its use in combination with other PIs. Amprenavir selects for a unique resistance pattern (I50V) *in vitro*, suggesting that it may be of benefit for patients who have relapsed on other PIs or as a first-line PI, which enables the other agents to be used for salvage therapy. Common toxicities of amprenavir include diarrhea, rash, and headaches.

ABT-378/Ritonavir (Lopinavir)

ABT-378 is an experimental PI that is available through an expanded-access program from Abbott Laboratories (1-888-711-7193). It is combined with ritonavir to enhance the oral bioavailability. ABT-378 may be active against HIV strains that are resistant to other PIs. Toxicities to date have included gastrointestinal intolerance, rash, and lipodystrophy syndrome.

Dual-Protease Inhibitor Therapy

The use of ritonavir to inhibit hepatic metabolism of other PIs has prompted the use of dual-PI regimens for both initial and salvage treatment. This approach was first used in studies of saquinavir and ritonavir. Administration of twice-daily ritonavir at 400 mg results in a 20-fold increase in saquinavir levels, permitting change of the saquinavir dosaging schedule from three times per day to two. This effect significantly reduces both the number of pills taken and the toxicity from ritonavir. Ninety percent of subjects in one study had a viral load of fewer than 200 copies/mL after 72 weeks of treatment. Similar effects have been reported with the combination of indinavir and ritonavir, both at 400 mg twice daily without dietary restrictions. Various other PI combinations currently are being evaluated. Benefits of dual-PI regimens include improved pharmacokinetics, less variability in drug levels, decreased pill burden, and more convenient dosage schedule.

Hydroxyurea

Hydroxyurea is not an antiretroviral agent but has been used to augment the effectiveness of ddI and d4T. It inhibits ribonucleotide reductase, which reduces the availability of intracellular deoxyribonucleotides. Depletion of this pool favors incorporation of antiviral nucleoside analogs into viral DNA. There is disproportionate depletion of deoxyadenosine triphosphate (dATP) by hydroxyurea *in vitro*, possibly explaining the specific hydroxyurea-associated antiviral effect seen with ddI. Cells exposed to d4T show a three- to four-fold increase in d4T phosphorylation in the presence of hydroxyurea regardless of previous NRTI exposure. By targeting cellular rather than viral enzymes, hydroxyurea can be used in treatment-experienced patients. Toxicities include myelosuppression, blunted CD4 count response, nausea, rash, proteinuria, and hepatitis. Cases of severe pancreatitis recently have been reported in patients receiving ddI with hydroxyurea. Women should be advised to avoid becoming pregnant.

Lipodystrophy Syndrome

Adverse long-term reactions to combination antiretroviral therapy, especially regimens containing PIs, have become the focus of much debate. In one study of 486 subjects on a PI for a mean of 18 months, 78% of subjects had evidence of lipodystrophy syndrome. Its clinical features include increased breast size and abdominal girth, loss of subcutaneous fat in the extremities, facial wasting, and development of a dorsocervical fat pad. These body morphology changes may be associated with glucose intolerance (rarely diabetes mellitus) and significant hyperlipidemia. It has been reported recently that PIs may cross-react with enzymes necessary for lipid metabolism, including lipoprotein-receptor-like protein (LRP) and *cis*-retinoic acid-binding protein type 1 (CRABP-1). However, the epidemiology, pathophysiology, and management of this condition remain the subject of active investigation.

Clinical Guidelines

Initiation of Antiretroviral Therapy

Indications for initiating antiretroviral therapy include:
1. Symptomatic HIV disease
2. CD4 cell count of fewer than 500 copies/mm^3 *or* viral load of more than 10,000 copies/mL by branched-chain DNA (bDNA) or more than 20,000 copies/mL by PCR
3. Acute retroviral syndrome or being within 6 months of documented HIV seroconversion (*see* Chapter 2)
4. Prevention of perinatal transmission (*see* Chapter 4)
5. Postexposure prophylaxis (*see* Chapters 3 and 10)

Preferred initial regimens consist of a combination of two NRTIs with either a PI or an NNRTI. NRTI combinations to avoid include ZDV/d4T because of drug antagonism and ddI/ddC because of the concern for increased risk of peripheral neuropathy. An alternative initial regimen is ABC with two other NRTIs *or* two NRTIs with hydroxyurea, with the potential benefits including a simple dosaging schedule, reduced pill burden, and lack of dietary restrictions. PI-containing regimens have been well studied and shown to be associated with potent and sustained viral response. Dual-PI therapy with saquinavir and ritonavir seems to be successful in suppressing viral RNA to undetectable levels but is not yet recommended as an initial regimen given the lack of direct comparison data. Because resistance to 3TC and NNRTIs develops rapidly, it is advised that these agents be used only as part of regimens in which maximal viral suppression is likely. In the future, HIV genotypic testing may become more common in newly diagnosed patients to help choose a drug regimen because of concern about transmission of resistant viral strains.

Antiretroviral treatment should not be interrupted during an intercurrent illness unless there is concern about drug toxicity, intolerance, or interactions. If therapy needs to be discontinued, it is advisable that all drugs be stopped at the same time to reduce the likelihood of development of resistance. In general, "drug holidays" are discouraged, not so much because of concern about viral resistance but rather because of the possible deterioration of immune function.

Modification of Antiretroviral Therapy

Indications for modifying antiretroviral therapy include:

1. Drug failure, defined as inability to decrease viral load by more than 1 log after 2 to 4 weeks of treatment or a failure to obtain undetectable viral load at 3 to 6 months

2. Relapse in detectable viral load from an undetectable level

3. Drug toxicity

4. Nonadherence

It is advisable to base any decision to change therapy on two separate measurements of viral load and CD4 cell count. The precise timing of when to switch an antiretroviral regimen is controversial. When viral load rebounds occur, the virus may not be resistant to all the drugs in that regimen. Genotypic and phenotypic resistance testing may help determine how best to address this situation. The aggressive approach—switching treatment early with low levels of detectable virus—is based on retrospective evidence showing that patients respond better to new regimens; however, for heavily pretreated patients, this option may not be realistic.

The decision to change antiretroviral agents should include knowledge of available treatment options, issues of cross resistance, potential toxicities, and drug-drug interactions. A significant change in viral RNA levels is considered to be a 0.5-log decrease. A significant change in CD4 cell count is a drop of more than 30% for absolute number or greater than 3% in CD4 cell percentage. Discordance between the viral load and CD4 count may occur sometimes.

Lack of patient adherence or altered pharmacokinetics may lead to viral resistance and failure of an antiretroviral regimen. It is essential to distinguish between drug failure and intolerance. In the latter situation, it is necessary to change only the one offending agent rather than the whole regimen. In contrast, a failing regimen requires starting at least two and preferably all new drugs that ideally do not share cross-resistance with the current regimen. However, for patients with advanced disease and a history of exposure to multiple agents, it may not be possible to do so. Furthermore, drug toxicity or nonadherence may limit treatment choices. For patients with detectable virus and for whom a switch of regimen is not possible, maintaining a suboptimal regimen pending the availability of newer drugs may be necessary. Although there is little information available on the effectiveness of re-introducing a previously used drug (so-called "recycling"), this practice is common when there are no other alternatives. General guidelines for modifying a failing antiretroviral regimen are shown in Table 5.7.

The recent availability of ABC, tenofovir, amprenavir, lopinavir, and hydroxyurea provides additional potential options for drug modification. A wider understanding of disease pathogenesis and results from pending clinical trials inevitably will result in changes in therapeutic preferences. Another recent study demonstrated that a brief course of nevirapine also may be effective.

Antiretroviral Therapy in Pregnancy

Guidelines for the use of antiretroviral therapy in pregnancy were published by the Center for Disease Control and Prevention in 1998. ZDV has been demonstrated effective in reducing HIV transmission regardless of maternal viral load. The ACTG study 076, which consisted of antepartum, intrapartum, and postpartum treatment with ZDV, was associated with a reduction of perinatal transmission by 66%. Short courses of antenatal and intrapartum oral ZDV (300 mg twice daily for 4 weeks antepartum then 300 mg every 8 days intrapartum) studied in Thailand showed a 50% reduction of perinatal transmission risk. Although short courses of oral ZDV may be less effective in the prevention of perinatal transmission than that used in ACTG 076, it may be more practical in settings in which medical resources are limited. The PETRA study data show that ZDV/3TC given at 36 weeks and for 1 week postpartum reduced perinatal transmission by 50%; if given at onset of labor and for 1 week postpartum, transmission was reduced by 37%.

Table 5.7   Approach for Changing Antiretroviral Regimen Because of Drug Failure

---

- Criteria include any of the following: suboptimal reduction in viral load after initiation of therapy, significant increase of viremia after suppression, declining CD4 cell count

- Repeat viral load measurement and exclude patient nonadherence to current regimen before considering modification of it

- If early resistance is present, substitute three new drugs for existing regimen or, as an alternative strategy, consider adding one new agent to existing regimen (intensification)

- If late resistance is present, substitute at least three new drugs for existing regimen

- Base decision of which new medications to use on previous antiretroviral drug history, avoiding those agents if possible and others that are cross-resistant to them

- Avoid substituting ritonavir for indinavir or vice versa because high-level cross-resistance is likely

- Avoid substituting one NNRTI for another because high-level cross-resistance is likely

- Consider HIV genotypic or phenotypic testing to help facilitate treatment decision-making

---

NNRTI = nonnucleotide reverse-transcriptase inhibitor.
Adapted from Centers for Disease Control and Prevention. Report of the NIH panel to define principles of therapy of HIV infection and guidelines for the use of antiretroviral agents in HIV-infected adults and adolescents. *MMWR Morb Mortal Wkly Rep.* 1998;47:1–82. (Available as "living document" on DHHS HIV/AIDS Treatment Information Service Web site at www.hivatis.org).

Future Directions

Although significant improvement has been achieved in the management of HIV disease in recent years, a number of important issues remain. Newer drugs with simplified dosaging schedules and requirements, decreased pill burden, minimized cross-resistance, and fewer side effects and drug-drug interactions need to be developed. Trials to determine the ideal initial treatment regimen are ongoing. Currently, the use of triple NRTI therapy, which spares NNRTI and PI agents for salvage regimens, is being evaluated. A recent study has demonstrated that a brief course of nevirapine also may be effective. Also being assessed are the use of "strategic treatment interruption" in patients on a fully suppressive antiretroviral regimen, the role of therapeutic drug monitoring, and strategies for choosing second and subsequent drug combinations in patients with resistant viral strains.

Cross-resistance among the NNRTI and PI agents leaves limited therapeutic options for heavily pretreated patients. Several new drugs in both classes are currently under investigation. Whether they will prove to be less cross-resistant remains to be seen.

Stemming from an improved understanding of the pathogenesis of HIV disease, new therapeutic modalities also are being developed. These include fusion inhibitors (e.g., T-20), cytokine-receptor inhibitors, integrase inhibitors, ribonuclease-H inhibitors, immunotherapy with interleukins 2 and 10, and cytotoxic T lymphocytes directed against HIV gag.

■ ■ ■

Key Points

- Combination antiretroviral therapy has resulted in significant decreases in the incidence of AIDS-related opportunistic infections, hospitalizations, and deaths.

- The goal of therapy is to decrease HIV viral load by at least 1 log during the first 4 weeks of treatment and for the viral load to be undetectable by 3 to 6 months. In clinical practice, between 50% and 80% of patients will achieve a maximally suppressed viral load in response to their initial antiretroviral regimen. However, the success rate decreases with each successive drug combination.

- Lack of adherence to therapy is associated with the development of viral resistance and drug failure.

- NRTIs provide the foundation for most combination regimens. Two NRTIs commonly are administered with a PI or NNRTI.

- NNRTIs have easier dosing schedules than PIs, but drug resistance can develop from a single viral mutation.

- PIs are the most potent of the antiretroviral therapy drug classes, but therapy is difficult for some patients to maintain because of side effects and adverse drug interactions.

- If a change in antiretroviral therapy is indicated, it is usually best to switch drugs early, when levels of detectable virus are still low. If the regimen is being modified because of the development of viral resistance, an entirely new combination that does not share cross-resistance with current drugs is recommended. If the regimen is being modified because of toxicity to one drug, a single agent may be substituted for it.

- HIV genotypic and phenotypic testing is being used increasingly in clinical practice to help select an appropriate drug regimen for treatment-experienced patients.

■ ■ ■

SUGGESTED READINGS

Boden D, et al. HIV-1 drug resistance in newly infected individuals. *JAMA.* 1999; 282:1135–41.

Carpenter CCJ, et al. Antiretroviral therapy in adults: updated recommendations of the International AIDS Society—USA Panel. *JAMA.* 2000;283:381–90.

Carr, et al. Pathogenesis of HIV-1-protease inhibitor-associated peripheral lipodystrophy, hyperlipidemia, and insulin resistance. *Lancet.* 1998;351:1881–3.

Centers for Disease Control and Prevention. Public Health Service recommendations for the management of health-care worker exposures to HIV and recommendations for postexposure prophylaxis. *MMWR Morb Mortal Wkly Rep.* 1998;47(RR-7):1–33.

Center for Disease Control and Prevention. Public Health Service Task Force recommendations for the use of antiretroviral drugs in pregnant females infected with HIV-1 for maternal health and for reducing perinatal HIV-1 transmission in the United States. *MMWR Morb Mortal Wkly Rep.* 1998;47(RR-2):1–30.

Centers for Disease Control and Prevention. Report of the NIH panel to define principles of therapy of HIV infection and guidelines for the use of antiretroviral agents in HIV-infected adults and adolescents. *MMWR Morb Mortal Wkly Rep.* 1998;47:1–82. (Available as "living document" on DHHS HIV/AIDS Treatment Information Service Web site at www.hivatis.org).

Collier A, et al. Treatment of human immunodeficiency virus infection with saquinavir, zidovudine, and zalcitabine: AIDS Clinical Trials Group. *N Engl J Med.* 1996; 334:1011–7.

Condra, et al. *In vivo* emergence of HIV-1 variants resistant to multiple protease inhibitors. *Nature* 1995;374:569–71.

Cooper D. Therapeutic strategies for HIV infection: time to think hard. *N Engl J Med.* 1998;339:1319–21.

Cooper D, et al. Zidovudine in persons with asymptomatic HIV infection and CD4 counts greater than 400 per cubic millimeter. *N Engl J Med.* 1993;329:297–303.

D'Aquila R, et al. Nevirapine, zidovudine, and didanosine compared with zidovudine and didanosine in patients with HIV-1 infection: a randomized, double-blind, placebo-controlled trial. *Ann Intern Med.* 1996;124:1019–30.

Durant J, et al. Drug-resistance genotyping in HIV-1 therapy: the VIRADAPT randomised controlled trial. *Lancet.* 1999;353:2195–9.

Eron J, et al. Treatment with lamivudine, zidovudine, or both in HIV-positive patients with 200 to 500 CD4 cells per cubic millimeter. *N Engl J Med.* 1995;333:1662–9.

Fischl M, et al. The efficacy of azidothymidine in the treatment of patients with AIDS and AIDS-related complex. *N Engl J Med.* 1987;317:185–91.

Fischl M, et al. The safety and efficacy of zidovudine in the treatment of subjects with mildly symptomatic human immunodeficiency virus type 1 infection: a double-blind, placebo-controlled trial. *Ann Intern Med.* 1990;112:727–37.

Flexner C. HIV protease inhibitors. *N Engl J Med.* 1998;338:1281–92.

Gerberding. The care of persons with recent sexual exposure to HIV. *Ann Intern Med.* 1998;128:306–12.

Gulick R, et al. Treatment with indinavir, zidovudine, and lamivudine in adults with human immunodeficiency virus infection and prior antiretroviral therapy. *N Engl J Med.* 1997;337:734–9.

Hammer S, et al. A controlled trial of two nucleoside analogues plus indinavir in persons with human immunodeficiency virus infection and CD4 counts of 200 per cubic millimeter or less. *N Engl J Med.* 1997;337:725–33.

Havlir D, et al. Maintenance antiretroviral therapies in HIV-infected subjects with undetectable plasma HIV RNA after triple-drug therapy. *N Engl J Med.* 1998;339:1261–8.

Henderson. Postexposure chemoprophylaxis for occupational exposures to the human immunodeficiency virus. *JAMA.* 1999;281:931–6.

Henry, et al. Severe premature coronary artery disease with protease inhibitors. *Lancet.* 1998;351:1328.

Ho D. Time to hit HIV early and hard. *N Engl J Med.* 1995;333:450–1.

International AIDS Society Panel. Antiretroviral drug resistance testing in adults with HIV infection: implications for clinical management. *JAMA.* 1998;279:1984–92.

Mellors J, et al. Plasma viral load and CD4 lymphocytes as prognostic markers of HIV-1 infection. *Ann Intern Med.* 1997;126:946–54.

Mellors J, et al. Prognosis in HIV-1 infection predicted by the quantity of virus in plasma. *Science.* 1996;272:1167–70.

Mellors J, et al. Quantitation of HIV-1 RNA in plasma predicts outcome after seroconversion. *Ann Intern Med.* 1995;122:573–9.

Minkoff, et al. Antiretroviral therapy for pregnant women. *Am J Obstet Gynecol.* 1997;176:478–89.

Mirochnick, et al. Pharmocokinetics of nevirapine in HIV type 1-infected pregnant women and their neonates. *J Infect Dis.* 1998;178:368–74.

Mocroft, et al. Changing patterns of mortality across Europe in patients infected with HIV-1. *Lancet.* 1998;352:1725–30.

Montaner J, et al. A randomized, double-blind trial comparing combinations of nevirapine, didanosine, and zidovudine for HIV-infected patients. *JAMA.* 1998;279:930–7.

O'Brien W, et al. Changes in plasma HIV-1 RNA and CD4 lymphocyte counts and the risk of progression to AIDS: Veterans Affairs Co-operative Study Group. *N Engl J Med.* 1996;334:426–31.

O'Brien W, et al. Serum HIV-1 RNA levels and time to development of AIDS in the multicenter Hemophilia Cohort Study. *JAMA.* 1996;276:105–11.

Palella, et al. Declining morbidity and mortality among patients with advanced human immunodeficiency virus infection. *N Engl J Med.* 1998;338:853–60.

Sperling S, et al. Maternal viral load, zidovudine treatment, and the risk of transmission of HIV from mother to infant. *N Engl J Med.* 1996;335:1621–9.

Spooner, et al. Guide to major clinical trials of antiretroviral therapy administered to patients infected with HIV. *Clin Infect Dis.* 1996;23:15–27.

Staszewski S, et al. Efavirenz plus zidovudine and lamivudine, efavirenz plus indinavir, and indinavir plus zidovudine and lamivudine in the treatment of HIV-1 infection in adults. *N Engl J Med.* 1999;341:1865–73.

Stein, et al. CD4 lymphocyte cell enumeration for prediction of clinical course of human immunodeficiency virus disease. *J Infect Dis.* 1992;165:352–63.

Stephenson. HIV drug resistance testing shows promise. *JAMA.* 1999;281:309–10.

Volberding P, et al. Zidovudine in asymptomatic human immunodeficiency virus infection: a controlled trial in persons with fewer than 500 CD4-positive cells per cubic millimeter. *N Engl J Med.* 1990;322:941–9.

6

■ ■ ■

Prevention of Opportunistic Infections

Helen M. Jacoby, MD
Judith S. Currier, MD, MSc

Prevention of opportunistic infections (OIs) is a major goal in the treatment of HIV disease. Rates of AIDS-related mortality and rates of OIs have declined dramatically since 1996 with the advent of potent combination antiretroviral therapy, which includes protease inhibitors (1). The extent to which specific types of OI prophylaxis have contributed to this decline in infection rates has been difficult to determine. This chapter reviews data about the risk of the major OIs, available drugs for use as primary prophylaxis, and current recommendations for the use of these agents. Secondary prophylaxis (maintenance therapy) for established OIs is addressed in Chapter 8.

Although it is clear that antiretroviral therapy is the most important intervention for the prevention of OIs, the extent of immune recovery conferred on patients with HIV disease who achieve a good response to treatment continues to be studied. Currently available data suggest that after the introduction of antiretroviral therapy, CD4 cell reconstitution occurs in several phases. Initially, there is an expansion of existing memory T cells, followed by a reduction in T-cell activation with improved CD4 cell reactivity to recall antigens, and then a rise in naive CD4 lymphocytes (2). Thus, it is possible that immune recovery for patients who begin therapy when their CD4 cell count is low may be incomplete or delayed. As our understanding of the critical measures of protection against OIs has improved, published recommendations for the use of prophylaxis have been updated (3). Studies are ongoing to determine when prophylaxis against specific OIs can be discontinued safely in patients whose CD4 cell counts have risen on combination antiretroviral therapy. Recent data suggest that primary prophylaxis for *Pneumocystis carinii* pneumonia (PCP) and *Mycobacterium avium* complex (MAC) infection can be stopped in this setting (4–7).

Unfortunately, some patients respond poorly to antiretroviral medications or have difficulty tolerating them. In addition, some patients who initially respond to combination therapy may develop drug resistance and progressive immunosuppression over time. For patients in these groups, prophylactic therapies remain important in the effort to decrease mortality and improve the quality of life.

Several factors need to be considered when deciding to initiate specific types of OI prophylaxis. These factors include infection risks and consequences, prophylactic agent efficacy (e.g., impact on disease severity, known survival benefit), drug toxicities, drug interactions, regimen complexity, the likelihood of inducing drug resistance, and cost.

Detailed guidelines about all aspects of OI prevention (e.g., primary prophylaxis, secondary prophylaxis, prevention of exposure) have been published by the U.S. Public Health Service in conjunction with the Infectious Disease Society of America (3). Primary prophylaxis is recommended under specific clinical circumstances for PCP, toxoplasmosis, MAC infection, and tuberculosis (TB). It is not routinely advocated for localized or systemic fungal disease or for herpes simplex, varicella-zoster, or cytomegalovirus infections.

Pneumocystis carinii Pneumonia

Incidence

Prophylaxis for PCP is a cornerstone of effective management of patients with AIDS. Patients with a CD4 count of fewer than 200 cells/mm^3 are at significant risk of PCP. Before the widespread use of prophylaxis and potent antiretroviral therapy, the infection was the most common opportunistic disease in this group, affecting 40% to 60% of patients (8,9). The introduction of prophylactic therapies in the late 1980s and early 1990s led to a significant decline in the incidence of PCP as well as decreased mortality (10).

Drug Therapy

Four drugs have been demonstrated to reduce the incidence of PCP in patients at risk: trimethoprim-sulfamethoxazole (TMP-SMX), dapsone, aerosol pentamidine (AP), and atovaquone (11,12) (Table 6.1). Of these, TMP-SMX is clearly the drug of choice, because it is both effective and inexpensive.

Table 6.1   PCP Prophylaxis Regimens

Drug	Recommended Dosage	Annual Cost*	Comments
TMP-SMX	1 DS po qd *or* 1 SS po qd *or* 1 DS po 3 times/wk	$60	Prophylaxis of choice
Dapsone	100 mg/d po	$72	Do not use in G6PD-deficient patient
Aerosol pentamidine	300 mg/mo via Respirgard II nebulizer	$1185	Less desirable than either TMP-SMX or dapsone
Atovaquone suspension	1500 mg/d po	$9363	High cost and limited clinical data to support use

DS = double-strength; G6PD = glucose-6-phosphate dehydrogenase; SS = single-strength; TMP-SMX = trimethoprim-sulfamethoxazole
* Republished with permission from *Drug Topics Red Book.* Montvale, NJ: Medical Economics; 1997.

The failure rate of TMP-SMX in preventing PCP is close to zero in patients who reliably take the drug. TMP-SMX also provides excellent prophylaxis against toxoplasmosis (*see* section below) and reduces the incidence of conventional bacterial infections. Three dosage regimens of TMP-SMX have been shown to be effective in preventing PCP. These include one double-strength (DS) tablet per day, one single-strength (SS) tablet per day, and one DS tablet three times per week.

The incidence of TMP-SMX side effects is between 25% and 50% in HIV-infected patients. Adverse drug reactions include fever, rash, liver function test abnormalities, and leukopenia. Lower-dose regimens seem to be somewhat better tolerated than one DS tablet per day. In addition, a study suggested that the number of adverse effects in the first 12 weeks of TMP-SMX therapy can be reduced by gradually increasing the dose of the drug during the first 2 weeks (13). Patients who have a history of a non–life-threatening adverse reaction to TMP-SMX can often be "desensitized" to the drug. This process involves rechallenging the patient with gradually increasing doses of TMP-SMX over a period ranging from 1 day to 2 weeks. A variety of desensitization regimens have proven successful (14,15). One commonly used protocol is outlined in Table 6.2. Given the many advantages of TMP-SMX over alternative regimens, desensitization should be considered in those patients who cannot tolerate TMP-SMX be-

Table 6.2   TMP-SMX Oral Desensitization Protocol*

Day	Dilution†	Serial Doses‡			
1	1:1,000,000	1 mL	2 mL	4 mL	8 mL
2	1:100,000	1 mL	2 mL	4 mL	8 mL
3	1:10,000	1 mL	2 mL	4 mL	8 mL
4	1:1000	1 mL	2 mL	4 mL	8 mL
5	1:100	1 mL	2 mL	4 mL	8 mL
6	1:10	1 mL	2 mL	4 mL	8 mL
7	1:1	1 mL	2 mL	4 mL	8 mL
8	Full strength	5 mL	10 mL	20 mL	1 DS tab

DS = double-strength
* "Treating through" mild to moderate symptoms should be attempted. Low-grade fevers and myalgias can be managed with acetaminophen, and mild rashes can be treated with an antihistamine.
† Dilutions are made by pharmacist from a standard oral suspension of trimethoprim-sulfamethoxazole (TMP-SMX), which contains 40 mg of TMP and 200 mg of SMX per 5 mL.
‡ Gradually increasing doses of each day's dilution should be taken 4 times per day.
Protocol developed by Marcus Conant, MD, San Francisco, CA. Republished with permission.

cause of fever, rash, or other mild to moderate side effects. It should not be used in patients who have a history of anaphylaxis or Stevens–Johnson syndrome when exposed to the drug.

Dapsone generally is considered the second choice for PCP prophylaxis. Like TMP-SMX, it provides systemic protection against *P. carinii* and is inexpensive. Pyrimethamine can be added to confer protection against toxoplasmosis (*see* section below). Failure of prophylaxis is more common in patients on dapsone than in those taking TMP-SMX. A dosage of 100 mg/d seems to be more effective than 50 mg/d. The incidence of dapsone side effects is nearly as high as with TMP-SMX. These can include rash, fever, liver function test abnormalities, anemia, and leukopenia. In addition, dapsone can cause hemolysis in patients who are deficient in glucose-6-phosphate dehydrogenase (G6PD). A G6PD qualitative assay is recommended before starting a patient on dapsone.

Patients who are unable to take either TMP-SMX or dapsone generally should receive AP as prophylaxis against PCP. AP usually is well tolerated, although bronchospasm may occur during treatment; also, AP prophylaxis is less desirable than either TMP-SMX or dapsone for a number of reasons. AP costs more than ten times as much as either of the other two drugs and provides protection against only pulmonary infection because of its lack of systemic absorption. In addition, AP is less effective in preventing PCP than either TMP-SMX or dapsone, especially in patients with CD4 counts of fewer than 100 cells/mm^3 (11). Based on this information, AP generally is reserved for patients who are unable to tolerate either TMP-SMX or dapsone. The usual dosage of AP is 300 mg/mo administered with a Respirgard II nebulizer.

A recent clinical trial demonstrated that atovaquone suspension at a dosage of 1500 mg/d was as effective as dapsone 100 mg/d in preventing PCP (16). The rate of adverse effects was similar between the two regimens. However, atovaquone is used infrequently for PCP prophylaxis because its cost is over 100 times that of either TMP-SMX or dapsone and data supporting its efficacy are sparse compared with those for the other regimens.

The combination of clindamycin and primaquine—sometimes used for the treatment of PCP—has not been shown to provide adequate PCP prophylaxis when compared with the standard regimens described above and therefore is not recommended.

Recommendations

Prophylaxis for PCP should be given to all HIV-infected patients with a CD4 count of fewer than 200 cells/mm^3 and to those who meet other diagnostic criteria for AIDS (see Chapter 1). HIV-infected patients with thrush or a more than 2-week history of unexplained fever also should receive prophylaxis. TMP-SMX is the drug of choice, with alternative regimens outlined above (see Figure 4.1).

Recent data indicate that primary prophylaxis for PCP can be discontinued safely in patients who are on combination antiretroviral therapy, whose viral load is well suppressed, and whose CD4 count rises to over 200 cells/mm^3 for at least 3 to 6 months and whose viral load is well suppressed (3–6).

Toxoplasmosis

Incidence

Toxoplasmic encephalitis is one of the most common neurologic complications of HIV infection. Nearly all cases result from reactivation of latent *Toxoplasma gondii* infection. Most patients who have had a primary infection with *Toxoplasma* and who therefore are at risk of reactivated disease have detectable serum antibody (IgG) against the organism. The rate of seropositivity varies from country to country, but it has been estimated to be between 10% and 40% in the United States. Without effective antiretroviral therapy and antitoxoplasmosis prophylaxis, approximately one third of patients with *Toxoplasma* antibodies eventually will develop toxoplasmic encephalitis. This infection generally occurs in HIV-infected patients with a CD4 count of fewer than 100 cells/mm^3.

Drug Therapy

The two drug regimens commonly used to prevent toxoplasmosis are TMP-SMX and dapsone plus pyrimethamine. TMP-SMX is the prophylactic agent of choice. Although no prospective randomized trial has examined the role of TMP-SMX in preventing toxoplasmosis, data from numerous studies of TMP-SMX as a PCP prophylaxis show that patients only rarely develop toxoplasmosis while taking the drug. An Australian retrospective study of 155 patients receiving secondary PCP prophylaxis during a 3-year period showed that none of 60 patients on TMP-SMX developed toxoplasmic encephalitis, whereas 13% of 95 patients on AP developed the complication (17). The doses of TMP-SMX typically used for PCP prophylaxis seem adequate for toxoplasmosis prophylaxis.

The combination of daily dapsone and pyrimethamine given once per week also is effective in preventing toxoplasmosis. In a French study comparing AP to the combination of dapsone (50 mg/d) plus pyrimethamine (50 mg/wk) and folinic acid (25 mg/wk), toxoplasmosis developed in 16% (28/176) of patients receiving AP as compared with 3% (5/173) of patients receiving dapsone plus pyrimethamine (18). Pyrimethamine alone does not seem to be as effective as the combination of dapsone plus pyrimethamine. Atovaquone in doses used for PCP prophylaxis also may protect against toxoplasmosis (3).

Recommendations

All HIV-infected patients should have a *Toxoplasma* IgG antibody level checked at baseline. Patients with a positive test result and a CD4 count of fewer than 100 cells/mm^3 should receive prophylaxis as outlined below. Patients without detectable antibody presumably have never been infected with the organism and therefore are not at risk of reactivation but should be counseled about methods to avoid primary infection. Patients should be advised to avoid eating raw or undercooked red meat and to avoid contact with cat feces. Specific recommendations for avoiding exposure to *T. gondii* have been published (3). Patients without *Toxoplasma* antibody on initial presentation should have a repeat test performed if their CD4 count drops below 100 cells/mm^3 to determine if they were newly infected in the interim.

The choice of prophylactic agent for toxoplasmosis depends on what is given for PCP prophylaxis. Patients who are already receiving TMP-SMX or atovaquone need no additional prophylaxis for toxoplasmosis. However, in patients receiving dapsone as PCP prophylaxis, pyrimethamine (50 mg/wk) and folinic acid (25 mg/wk to prevent pyrimethamine-induced bone marrow suppression) should be added if the CD4 count drops below 100 cells/mm^3.

At this time, there are insufficient data to ascertain whether primary prophylaxis for toxoplasmosis can be discontinued safely in patients on combination antiretroviral therapy who have a sustained rise in their CD4 count greater than 100 cells/mm^3 (3). Studies are ongoing to address this question.

Mycobacterium avium Complex Infection

Incidence

The risk of disseminated MAC infection increases as the CD4 cell count falls, with the highest risk occurring when it is fewer than 50 cells/mm^3. Before the advent of combination antiretroviral therapy, 40% to 50% of patients with an AIDS diagnosis could be expected to develop MAC eventually. In one study from 1993, 18% of patients with a CD4 count of fewer than 200/mm^3 who did not take prophylaxis developed MAC after a median follow-up of 38 weeks (19). More recent data show an encouraging decline in the incidence of MAC. The AIDS Clinical Trials Group (ACTG) 320 study, which looked at patients with CD4 count of fewer than 200 cells/mm^3 who were receiving either zidovudine/lamivudine or zidovudine/lamivudine/indinavir showed that the rate of MAC infection was below 2% (20).

It is important to note that these data include some patients who were receiving MAC prophylaxis, so it is difficult to sort out the relative contributions of prophylaxis and of antiretroviral therapy.

Drug Therapy

Rifabutin, clarithromycin, and azithromycin are all approved for use as prophylaxis against MAC (Table 6.3). Randomized trials have shown each of these drugs to be superior to placebo in preventing MAC bacteremia (19,21,22). Clarithromycin prophylaxis also was demonstrated to decrease mortality in a placebo-controlled trial (21).

The California Collaborative Treatment Group (CCTG) compared once-weekly azithromycin (1200 mg) to daily rifabutin (300 mg) and to the combination of these two drugs (23). In an intent-to-treat analysis, the 1-year cumulative incidence of disseminated MAC was 15.3% in the rifabutin group, 7.6% in the azithromycin group, and 2.8% in the combination ther-

Table 6.3   *Mycobacterium avium* Complex Prophylaxis Regimens

Drug	Recommended Dose	Annual Cost*	Comments
Azithromycin	1200 mg/wk po	$1490	Least expensive
Clarithromycin	500 mg po twice daily	$2347	—
Rifabutin	300 mg/d po[†]	$2916	Less effective than macrolides; drug interactions are problematic

* Republished with permission from *Drug Topics Red Book*. Montvale, NJ: Medical Economics; 1997.
[†] The dose of rifabutin is 150 mg/d orally if given with indinavir, nelfinavir, or amprenavir, and is 450 mg/d orally if given with efavirenz. Rifabutin is contraindicated for use in patients on saquinavir, ritonavir, nevirapine, or delavirdine.

apy group. After adjustment for CD4 cell count, the risk of MAC was 72% lower with combination therapy than with rifabutin alone and 47% lower than with azithromycin alone. The risk of MAC infection in patients taking azithromycin was 47% lower than the risk in patients taking rifabutin. Azithromycin- and clarithromycin-resistant MAC was identified in 11% (2/18) of the breakthrough isolates on azithromycin and in none on the combination arm. Dose-limiting toxicity was highest in the combination arm (21%) which was statistically significant compared with the azithromycin arm (13%) and the rifabutin arm (16%).

The ACTG 196/CPCRA 009 study compared clarithromycin (500 mg twice daily) to rifabutin (300 mg/d) and to the combination of these two drugs (24). The cumulative incidence of MAC infection at 1 year in an intent-to-treat analysis was 5% in the clarithromycin recipients, 10% in the rifabutin recipients, and 5% in the combination arm (C. Benson, personal communication). Therefore, in contrast to the CCTG results, the addition of rifabutin added no further protection against MAC, suggesting that maximal efficacy was obtained by clarithromycin alone. Clarithromycin resistance was observed in 28% of the breakthrough isolates.

Currently, no data exist about the direct comparison between clarithromycin and azithromycin for the prevention of MAC. However, both agents seem more effective than rifabutin. Azithromycin has the advantages of once-weekly dosing, fewer drug interactions, and lower cost. Their tolerability is comparable, with gastrointestinal side effects being relatively common. The lowest effective dose of these agents is not known.

An added benefit of both clarithromycin and azithromycin over rifabutin is protection conferred against conventional bacterial infections. In the CCTG MAC prevention study, there were more bacterial infections in the rifabutin arm compared with the azithromycin-containing arms (risk ratio [RR]: 1.58; 95% confidence interval [CI]: 1.10–2.30) (19). In addition, the risk of sinusitis and bacterial pneumonia was reduced by 50% in azithromycin compared with rifabutin recipients. Preliminary data also indicate that patients on macrolide prophylaxis for MAC infection have a lower incidence of PCP than those receiving rifabutin (25).

Recommendations

Prophylaxis against MAC infection using either azithromycin or clarithromycin is recommended for HIV-infected patients with CD4 counts of fewer than 50 cells/mm^3. Rifabutin is less attractive because it is less effective and is difficult to administer with protease inhibitors and nonnucleoside reverse-transcriptase inhibitors. Recent data suggest that primary prophylaxis for MAC infection can be discontinued safely in patients who are on combination antiretroviral therapy, whose viral load is well suppressed, and whose CD4 cell count rises to over 100 cells/mm^3 for at least 3 to 6 months (3,7).

It is worth noting that MAC infection presenting as inflammatory lymphadenitis has been reported shortly after initiating combination antiretroviral therapy with a protease inhibitor (26). All of these cases have occurred in patients with a low CD4 cell count who were not receiving prophylaxis. This suggests that subclinical MAC disease was present and that early immune restoration may have unmasked the infection. These cases highlight the potential benefit of starting MAC prophylaxis before antiretroviral therapy in patients with a very low CD4 count.

Tuberculosis

Incidence

TB is not an OI in the strictest sense, but it does pose a special problem in HIV-infected patients (27). HIV disease is the greatest known risk factor for the development of active TB (28). It has been estimated that an HIV-infected patient with a positive skin test for TB has a 10% risk per year of developing active infection. This is in contrast to the 10% lifetime risk of active TB in an HIV-negative individual. Active tuberculosis can affect patients with any CD4 cell count, but extrapulmonary disease is seen mainly in those with advanced immunodeficiency.

The tuberculin skin test (PPD) remains the best method of assessing a patient's risk of developing active TB. Unfortunately, the test is less sensitive in HIV-infected patients, especially those with lower CD4 cell counts. Because of this observation, the Centers for Disease Control and Prevention (CDC) has defined induration of 5 mm or greater to constitute a positive test in HIV-infected people. Because of problems with standardization, routine anergy testing is no longer recommended (29).

Drug Therapy

Isoniazid (INH) significantly lowers the incidence of active TB in HIV-positive patients with evidence of previous infection. In a randomized trial in Haiti, 12 months of isoniazid given to HIV-infected patients with a positive PPD reduced the risk of active tuberculosis by 83% over a 3-year period (30). The recommended dosage of INH is 300 mg/d. The drug usually is given with pyridoxine (50 mg/d) to decrease the risk of peripheral neuropathy. INH given in a dosage of 900 mg twice per week as directly observed therapy (DOT) in patients with a history of poor medication adherence is also effective. Based on results of other studies, 9 months of therapy is now recommended in HIV-infected patients.

Recent data have shown that the combination of rifampin (600 mg/d) plus pyrazinamide (20 mg/kg/d) given for 2 months was as effective as INH given for 12 months in reducing the incidence of active tuberculosis in HIV-infected, PPD-positive patients (31). This regimen also might be considered when adherence to medications is problematic.

Recommendations

All HIV-positive patients should have a PPD performed when entering care and periodically thereafter. Patients who are thought to be at high risk of exposure to TB should have yearly tests. Induration of ≥ 5 mm indicates previous infection with *M. tuberculosis* and the need for prophylactic therapy. Active tuberculosis should be excluded by clinical assessment and chest radiography before prophylaxis is started. Prophylaxis is recommended for all HIV-infected patients with a history of a positive PPD who do not have medical contraindications, regardless of their age. Prophylactic therapy also should be given to any HIV-infected patient who recently has been in contact with a person who has infectious tuberculosis. If the patient's PPD remains negative 3 months after exposure, clinical considerations should dictate whether the full course of prophylaxis is to be given.

Prophylaxis should consist of INH and pyridoxine (300 mg and 50 mg/d, respectively, *or* 900 mg and 100 mg twice weekly [DOT], respectively) for 9 months. If the patient has been exposed to drug-resistant TB, other regimens may be indicated, and consultation with an infectious disease specialist is advised.

Fungal Infections

Incidence

Fungal infections that occur in the context of HIV disease can be divided into superficial (oropharyngeal and vaginal candidiasis) and invasive (cryptococcal meningitis or fungemia, disseminated histoplasmosis, coccidioidomycosis, and esophageal candidiasis). Oropharyngeal candidiasis is extremely common, eventually affecting over 90% of people with AIDS. Before the advent of combination antiretroviral therapy, esophageal candidiasis was the most common invasive fungal infection, with a lifetime risk of 20% to 30% compared with 5% to 10% for cryptococcosis and 2% to 5% for histoplasmosis (with higher rates in endemic areas). The incidence of fungal infections has declined dramatically since the introduction of protease inhibitors. Data from the French Clinical Epidemiology Study, a prospective study of 60,000 HIV-infected adults, demonstrated a 69% decline in the rate of *Candida* esophagitis from the first 6 months of 1996 through the first 6 months of 1997 (32). In this database, the rates of cryptococcal meningitis fell 70% over the same time period.

Drug Therapy

Preventive therapies for fungal infections include nystatin, clotrimazole, fluconazole, and itraconazole. Randomized trials have demonstrated the benefit of prophylaxis for oropharyngeal candidiasis, vaginal candidiasis, and invasive fungal infections.

The largest study of fungal prophylaxis was ACTG 981, which compared daily fluconazole (200 mg) to oral clotrimazole troches five times daily in patients with a CD4 count of fewer than 200 cells/mm^3 (33). The study demonstrated a statistically significant reduction in overall rates of invasive fungal infections, from 11% in patients receiving clotrimazole troches to 4% in patients receiving fluconazole. This difference was primarily the result of a reduction in the rates of esophageal candidiasis and cryptococcal disease, and benefit was greatest among patients with a CD4 count of fewer than 50 cells/mm^3. No survival benefit was shown. This study also demonstrated a significant reduction in the rate of thrush, from 45% in the clotrimazole group to 15% in the fluconazole group.

Fluconazole (200 mg/wk) also has been compared with placebo for the prevention of vaginal candidiasis in HIV-infected women (34). This study found a 37% decrease in the rate of vaginal candidiasis in the fluconazole group and a decrease in overall rates of mucosal candidiasis. Rates of resistance to fluconazole were not different between study arms among the isolates studied.

Itraconazole, an azole that is superior to fluconazole in treating histoplasmosis, has been studied for its ability to prevent fungal infections in patients residing in histoplasmosis-endemic areas. Results from a study of 295 patients randomized to receive either itraconazole (200 mg/d) or placebo showed that after a median 16 months of follow-up, itraconazole prophylaxis reduced the risk of systemic fungal infections from 11.6% to 4.0% (35). This finding was the result of a reduction in the rate of histoplasmosis from 6.8% in placebo recipients to 2.7% in itraconazole recipients and also a reduction in the rate of cryptococcosis from 5.5% to 0.7%. Surprisingly, there was no reduction in the rate of mucosal candidiasis.

Recommendations

Despite the proven efficacy of fluconazole in preventing both superficial and invasive fungal infections, the use of this agent for primary prophylaxis is not recommended. Long-term use of fluconazole may predispose to the development of azole-resistant *Candida* infections. In addition, the low incidence rates of invasive fungal disease do not make the widespread use of fluconazole prophylaxis a cost-effective strategy. Fluconazole at a dosage of 200 mg/d costs $5018 per year wholesale.

Itraconazole prophylaxis (200 mg/d) may be warranted to prevent histoplasmosis in patients with a CD4 count of fewer than 100 cells/mm^3 who also reside in endemic areas. Issues to consider when deciding about itraconazole prophylaxis include potential drug interactions, the risk of other fungal infections, and the cost of the drug, which is currently $4239 per year wholesale.

Cytomegalovirus Infection

Incidence

Cytomegalovirus (CMV) disease in AIDS is the result of reactivation of latent infection in the vast majority of cases. Between 95% and 98% of homosexual men and injection-drug users have antibody to CMV, which indicates a previous infection and places them at risk of reactivation if severe immunodeficiency occurs.

Before the advent of combination antiretroviral therapy, CMV disease was a common complication of advanced HIV infection, primarily affecting patients with a CD4 count of fewer than 50 cells/mm^3. One study found that 25% of men with CD4 counts of fewer than 100 cells/mm^3 developed CMV retinitis in 4 years of follow-up (36). Autopsy studies showed that up to 75% of patients who died of AIDS showed evidence of CMV infection in one or more organ systems. The use of combination antiretroviral therapy has led to a dramatic decline in the incidence of CMV disease, making it evident that the best way to prevent CMV disease is to administer effective antiretroviral therapy.

Drug Therapy

The only agent proven effective in preventing CMV disease in advanced AIDS patients is oral ganciclovir. In 1996, Spector and coworkers (37) published the results of a double-blind, placebo-controlled trial of oral ganciclovir (1000 mg tid) versus placebo in 725 AIDS patients who had either a CD4 count of fewer than 50 cells/mm^3 or fewer than 100 cells/mm^3 combined with a history of an AIDS-defining OI. The incidence of CMV retinitis after 12 months was 24% in the placebo group compared with 12% in the patients who received ganciclovir. There was no significant difference in mortality between the two groups. Anemia and neutropenia were common and problematic in the patients who received ganciclovir, so much so that 14% of the group received erythropoietin and 24% received granulocyte colony-stimulating factor. Comparative data for the placebo group were 6% and 9%, respectively.

A second study done by the Community Programs for Clinical Research on AIDS (CPCRA 023) did not confirm the efficacy of oral ganciclovir in preventing CMV disease (38); 994 patients with a CD4 count of fewer than 100 cells/mm^3 were randomly assigned to either oral ganciclovir 1000 mg three times per day or placebo. No difference in the incidence of either CMV disease or death was seen between the two groups. Similar to the previous trial, the patients on ganciclovir experienced significantly more neutropenia than those receiving placebo.

Recommendations

Primary prophylaxis against CMV disease generally is not recommended for a number of reasons, including conflicting data about regimen efficacy, large daily pill burdens, potential bone marrow suppression, and cost concerns. One year of oral ganciclovir costs $17,082 wholesale, which is dramatically more than the cost of other prophylactic medications or antiretroviral agents. In addition, a substantial proportion of patients on ganciclovir requires colony-stimulating factors to prevent anemia and neutropenia, adding further to the cost of treatment. Because ganciclovir prophylaxis has not been shown to decrease mortality, most authorities do not believe its potential benefits outweigh its costs. Studies are being performed to better define which AIDS patients are at the greatest risk of CMV disease, so that prophylaxis can be better targeted at those patients who would be most likely to benefit from it.

HIV-infected patients who are not thought to be at high risk of having had primary CMV infection may benefit from being screened for CMV antibody. HIV-positive patients who are CMV antibody–negative and require a blood transfusion should receive only leukocyte-depleted blood to avoid transfusion-associated primary CMV infection.

Summary

Over the past few years, it has become clear that the best way to prevent OIs is to treat HIV infection aggressively, thus delaying the decline in immune function that predisposes to them. However, the importance of prophylaxis against historically common OIs should not be forgotten. The current standard of care is to provide 1) PCP prophylaxis to all patients who have a CD4 count of fewer than 200 cells/mm^3 or another AIDS-defining condition, 2) toxoplasmosis prophylaxis to those with a positive *Toxoplasma* antibody test and a CD4 count of fewer than 100 cells/mm^3, and 3) MAC prophylaxis to those with a CD4 count of fewer than 50 cells/mm^3. In addition, all HIV-infected patients with a positive TB skin test should receive 9 months of INH therapy. Primary prophylaxis against fungal infections, CMV disease, or other OIs is not recommended for most patients, although such prophylaxis may be desirable in selected clinical circumstances.

Based on recent data, primary prophylaxis for PCP and MAC infection can be discontinued safely in patients on combination antiretroviral therapy whose viral load is well suppressed and whose CD4 cell counts rise above the "threshold" for these conditions for at least 3 to 6 months (3).

■   ■   ■

Key Points

- Despite the success of combination antiretroviral therapy, prophylactic treatment for specific OIs remains critically important.

- There are recent data to support the withdrawal of primary PCP and MAC prophylaxis in patients who have shown a significant rise in CD4 cell count in response to antiretroviral therapy.

- Patients with a CD4 count of fewer than 200 cells/mm^3 are at risk of PCP if they do not receive prophylactic treatment; TMP-SMX is the drug of choice. Desensitization may be possible if there is a history of non–life-threatening drug reaction. Dapsone, atovaquone, and aerosol pentamidine can be used as alternative agents if necessary.

- Prophylaxis against toxoplasmosis should be provided in patients with a CD4 count of fewer than 100 cells/mm³ and serologic evidence of previous *Toxoplasma* infection. TMP-SMX is the drug of choice; dapsone along with weekly pyrimethamine is an alternative treatment.

- Prophylaxis against MAC with azithromycin or clarithromycin should be initiated in patients with a CD4 count of fewer than 50 cells/mm³. Rifabutin is also effective but may be problematic to administer because of drug interactions.

- The use of prophylactic fluconazole for fungal infections is not recommended because of its high cost and the risk of development of resistant organisms.

- The use of oral ganciclovir for CMV prophylaxis generally is not recommended because of its high cost and potential toxicity.

■ ■ ■

REFERENCES

1. **Palella FJ, Delaney KM, Moorman AC, et al.** Declining morbidity and mortality among patients with advanced HIV infection. *N Engl J Med.* 1998;338:853–60.

2. **Autran B, Carcelain G, Li TS, et al.** Positive effects of combined antiretroviral therapy on CD4+ T cell homeostasis and function in advanced HIV disease. *Science.* 1997;227:112–16.

3. **US Public Health Service, Infectious Disease Society of America.** 1999 guidelines for the prevention of opportunistic infections in persons infected with human immunodeficiency virus. *Morbid Mortal Wkly Rep MMWR.* 1999;48(RR-10):1–66.

4. **Furrer H, et al.** Discontinuation of primary prophylaxis against *Pneumocystis carinii* pneumonia in HIV-1 infected adults treated with combination antiretroviral therapy. *N Engl J Med.* 1999;340:1301–6.

5. **Schneider MME, et al.** Discontinuation of *Pneumocystis carinii* pneumonia prophylaxis in HIV-1 infected patients treated with highly active antiretroviral therapy. *Lancet.* 1999;353:201–3.

6. **Weverling GJ, et al.** Discontinuation of *Pneumocystis carinii* pneumonia prophylaxis after start of highly active antiretroviral therapy in HIV-1 infection. *Lancet.* 1999;353:1293–8.

7. **Currier JS, et al.** A randomized, placebo-controlled trial of azithromycin prophylaxis for the prevention of *Mycobacterium avium* complex (MAC) in subjects with increases in CD4 cells on antiretroviral therapy. Paper presented at the 39th ICCAC, San Francisco; Abstract no. LB8.

8. **Phair J, Munoz A, Detels R, et al.** The risk of *Pneumocystis carinii* pneumonia among men infected with human immunodeficiency virus type 1. *N Engl J Med.* 1990;233:161–5.

9. **Moore RD, Chaisson RE.** Natural history of opportunistic disease in an HIV-infected urban clinical cohort. *Ann Intern Med.* 1996;124:633–42.

10. **Chaisson RE, Keruly J, Richman DD, Moore RD.** *Pneumocystis* prophylaxis and survival in patients with advanced human immunodeficiency virus infection treated with zidovudine. *Arch Intern Med.* 1992;152:2009–13.

11. **Bozzette SA, Finkelstein DM, Spector SA, et al.** A randomized trial of three antipneumocystis agents in patients with advanced human immunodeficiency virus infection. *N Engl J Med.* 1995;332:693–9.

12. **Ioannidis JPA, Cappelleri JC, Skolnik PR, et al.** A meta-analysis of the relative efficacy and toxicity of *Pneumocystis carinii* prophylactic regimens. *Arch Intern Med.* 1996;145:177–188.

13. **Para MF, Dohn M, Frame P, et al.** ACTG 268 trial: gradual initiation of trimethoprim/sulfamethoxazole as primary prophylaxis for *Pneumocystis carinii* pneumonia. In *Program and Abstracts of the Fourth Conference on Retroviruses and Opportunistic Infections.* Alexandria, VA: Infectious Diseases Society of America; 1997, abstract 2.

14. **Absar N, Daneshvar H, Beall G.** Desensitization to trimethoprim/sulfamethoxazole in HIV-infected patients. *J Allergy Clin Immunol.* 1994;93:1001–5.

15. **Gluckstein D, Ruskin J.** Rapid oral desensitization to trimethoprim-sulfamethoxazole (TMP-SMZ): use in prophylaxis for *Pneumocystis carinii* pneumonia in patients with AIDS who were previously intolerant to TMP-SMZ. *Clin Infect Dis.* 1995;20:849–53.

16. **El-Sadr W, Murphy R, Luskin-Hawk R, et al.** Atovaquone compared with dapsone for the prevention of *P. carinii* pneumonia in patients with HIV infection who cannot tolerate trimethoprim, sulfonamides, or both. *N Engl J Med.* 1998;339:1889–95.

17. **Carr A, Tindall B, Brew BJ, et al.** Low-dose trimethoprim-sulfamethoxazole prophylaxis for toxoplasmic encephalitis in patients with AIDS. *Ann Intern Med.* 1992;117:106–11.

18. **Girard PM, Landman R, Gaudebout C, et al.** Dapsone-pyrimethamine compared with aerosolized pentamidine as primary prophylaxis against *Pneumocystis carinii* pneumonia and toxoplasmosis in HIV infection. *N Engl J Med.* 1993;328:1514–20.

19. **Nightingale SD, Cameron DW, Gordin FM, et al.** Two controlled trials of rifabutin prophylaxis against *Mycobacterium avium* complex infection in AIDS. *N Engl J Med.* 1993;329:828–33.

20. **Currier JS, Williams PL, Becker S, et al.** Incidence rates and risk factors for opportunistic infections in a randomized trial comparing AZT+3TC to the AZT+3TC+Indinavir (ACTG 320). In *Fifth Conference on Retroviruses and Opportunistic Infections.* Chicago: Infectious Diseases Society of America; 1998:abstract 257.

21. **Pierce M, Crampton S, Henry D, et al.** A randomized trial of clarithromycin as prophylaxis against disseminated *Mycobacterium avium* complex infection in patients with advanced acquired immunodeficiency syndrome. *N Engl J Med.* 1996; 335:384–91.

22. **Oldfield EC, Fessel WJ, Dunne MW, et al.** Once weekly azithromycin therapy for prevention of *Mycobacterium avium* complex infection in patients with AIDS: a randomized, double-blind, placebo-controlled multicenter trial. *Clin Infect Dis.* 1998;26:611–9.

23. **Havlir DV, Dube MP, Sattler FR, et al.** Prophylaxis against disseminated *Mycobacterium avium* complex with weekly azithromycin, daily rifabutin, or both. *N Engl J Med.* 1996;335:392–8.

24. **Benson CA, Cohn DL, Williams P, and the ACTG 196/CPCRA 009 Study Team.** A phase III prospective, randomized, double-blind study of the safety and efficacy of clarithromycin (CLA) versus rifabutin (RBT) versus CLA+RBT for prevention of *Mycobacterium avium* complex (MAC) in HIV+ patients with CD4 counts < 100 cells/µl. *Third Conference on Retroviruses and Opportunistic Infections.* Washington, DC: Infectious Diseases Society of America; 1996:abstract 205.

25. **Dunne MW, Havlir D, Dube M, et al.** Efficacy of azithromycin in the prevention of *Pneumocystis carinii* pneumonia: a randomised trial. *Lancet.* 1999;354:891–5.

26. **Race EM, Adelson-Mitty J, Kriegel GR, et al.** Focal mycobacterial lymphadenitis following initiation of protease inhibitor therapy in patients with advanced HIV-1 disease. *Lancet.* 1998;351:252–5.

27. **Markowitz N, Hansen NI, Hopewell PC, et al.** Incidence of tuberculosis in the United States among HIV-infected persons. *Ann Intern Med.* 1997:126:123–32.

28. **Shafer RW, Edlin BR.** Tuberculosis in patients infected with human immunodeficiency virus: perspective on the past decade. *Clin Infect Dis.* 1996;22:683–704.

29. **Centers for Disease Control and Prevention.** Anergy skin testing and preventive therapy for HIV-infected persons:revised recommendations. *Morbid Mortal Wkly Rep MMWR.* 1997;46(RR-15):1–10.

30. **Pape JW, Jean SS, Ho JL, et al.** Effect of isoniazid prophylaxis on incidence of active tuberculosis and progression of HIV infection. *Lancet.* 1993;342:268–72.

31. **Gordin F, Chaisson R, Matts J, et al.** A randomized trial of 2 months of rifampin and pyrazinamide versus 12 months of isoniazid for the prevention of tuberculosis in HIV-positive, PPD-positive patients. *Fifth Conference on Retroviruses and Opportunistic Infections.* Chicago: Infectious Diseases Society of America; 1998: abstract LB5.

32. **Costagliola D.** Trends in incidence of clinical manifestations of HIV infection and antiretroviral prescriptions in French university hospitals. *Fifth Conference on Retroviruses and Opportunistic Infections.* Chicago: Infectious Diseases Society of America; 1998:abstract 182.

33. **Powderly WG, Finkelstein DM, Feinberg J, et al.** A randomized trial comparing fluconazole with clotrimazole troches for the prevention of fungal infections in patients with advanced human immunodeficiency virus infection. *N Engl J Med.* 1995; 332:700–5.

34. **Schuman P, Capps L, Peng G, et al.** Weekly fluconazole for the prevention of mucosal candidiasis in women with HIV infection: a randomized, double-blind, placebo-controlled trial. *Ann Intern Med.* 1997;126:689–96.

35. **McKinsey D, Wheat J, Cloud G, et al.** Itraconazole is effective primary prophylaxis against systemic fungal infections in patients with advanced HIV infection. *34th Interscience Conference on Antimicrobial Agents and Chemotherapy.* New Orleans; 1996:abstract LB-9.

36. **Hoover DR, Peng Y, Saah A, et al.** Occurrence of cytomegalovirus retinitis after human immunodeficiency virus immunosuppression. *Arch Ophthalmol.* 1996;114: 821–7.

37. **Spector SA, McKinley GF, Lalezari JP, et al.** Oral ganciclovir for the prevention of cytomegalovirus disease in persons with AIDS. *N Engl J Med.* 1996;334:1491–7.

38. **Brosgart CL, Craig C, Hillman D, et al.** A randomized, placebo-controlled trial of the safety and efficacy of oral ganciclovir for prophylaxis of CMV disease in HIV-infected individuals. *AIDS.* 1998;12:269–77.

7

■ ■ ■

Diagnostic Approach to Common Clinical Symptoms

Lisa R. Hirschhorn, MD, MPH
Peter J. Piliero, MD

The introduction of combination antiretroviral therapy into clinical practice has altered the natural history and manifestations of HIV disease. Although opportunistic infections (OIs) and malignancies continue to occur, their incidence has declined dramatically (1,2). The utility of previously validated clinical algorithms and approaches must be updated to reflect these changes. This chapter reviews the diagnosis of common clinical syndromes associated with HIV disease. For details on prevention and treatment of these conditions, the reader is referred to other chapters in this text as well as published guidelines (3).

Traditionally, the diagnostic approach to HIV-related complaints has been influenced in large part by the degree of immunosuppression as defined by CD4 cell count. For example, cough and dyspnea in an individual with a CD4 count of greater than 300 cells/mm^3 was evaluated differently from a patient with a CD4 count of fewer than 200 cells/mm^3 who was not on prophylaxis for *Pneumocystis carinii* pneumonia (PCP) (4). More recent data from a number of cohorts have shown that a high plasma viral load, particularly in more immunosuppressed individuals, is also an independent risk factor for OIs (2,5).

Effective antiretroviral therapy results in suppression of viral replication, with improvement of CD4 cell counts over time. In many patients, enhanced clinical immune function also occurs (6). A decline in the risk for OIs has been described 3 to 6 months after initiation of combination antiretroviral therapy (2,5). Rates of other HIV-related bacterial infections and certain HIV-related malignancies also have decreased. For individuals responding to antiretroviral therapy, a CD4 count of greater than 200 cells/mm^3 is now the strongest predictor for OI-free survival, whereas a low plasma viral load is an additional predictor for individuals with CD4 counts of fewer than 200 cells/mm^3. However, it is important to note that atypical presentations of OIs have been described from immune reconstitution associated with initiation of combination antiretroviral therapy in patients with advanced HIV disease (7).

As the frequency of OIs decreases, and as the risk for comorbid conditions increases (because of the aging HIV-infected population), non–HIV-related conditions may account for a greater proportion of clinical complaints. For example, coronary artery disease and chronic obstructive pulmonary disease (COPD) should be considered in the differential diagnosis in an older individual presenting with dyspnea. Complications of combination antiretroviral therapy also need to be considered in the evaluation of new symptoms.

A rational approach to an HIV-infected patient who presents with new symptoms must start with a complete physical examination and a thorough history, including comorbid conditions, medications and other therapies, substance abuse, and travel (Table 7.1). This information is interpreted in the context of the patient's immune status as assessed by his lowest CD4 count, previous OIs, and degree and duration of virologic and CD4-cell-count response if on combination antiretroviral therapy. Once this initial evaluation is completed, diagnostic tests often are required. If these initial studies are not revealing, more extensive testing, empiric treatment, or both are then considered.

A number of advances in diagnostic technology in the past decade have added greatly to our ability to diagnose infections and other complications in individuals with HIV infection. These tools have decreased the need for invasive procedures while also decreasing the time required for making a diagnosis. For example, early in the HIV epidemic, diagnosing PCP required bronchoscopy with bronchoalveolar lavage (BAL) and transbronchial biopsy. The introduction of sputum induction with the use of monoclonal antibodies is a highly sensitive diagnostic tool that has reduced dramatically the number of bronchoscopies necessary in this population. Another example is the diagnosis of intracellular and more fastidious organisms, such as mycobacteria and fungi, using blood cultures with lysis-centrifugation (Isolator) and radiometric systems (8). These blood cultures become positive in a few days to a few weeks, reducing the need for liver and bone marrow biopsies.

The increasing use of polymerase chain reaction (PCR) testing in diagnostic technology also has improved the care of HIV-infected patients. For example, the diagnosis of cytomegalovirus (CMV) central nervous system

Table 7.1   Diagnostic Approach to Common Clinical Syndromes

History

- Current condition (duration, severity, associated symptoms, precipitating factors, prior history)

- Exposures (travel, occupational, similar illness in household and other close contacts)

- Sexual behaviors

- Drug and alcohol use

- Risk factors for cardiopulmonary disease and neoplasia

- Medications (prescribed, over-the-counter, and complementary; adherence to medical therapies)

- Degree of immunosuppression (lowest and current CD4 count, response to antiretroviral therapy)

Physical Examination

- Complete examination with attention to symptomatic areas

Laboratory Studies

- Choice of specific tests guided by symptoms and signs

- Chest radiograph, sputum examination, and culture if pulmonary symptoms are present

- Blood, urine, and other cultures if fever is present

(CNS) infection has improved significantly with the introduction of CMV PCR on spinal fluid (9). Now this technology is being used for the diagnosis of progressive multifocal leukoencephalopathy and the rapid differentiation of tuberculosis (TB) from atypical mycobacteria. Other new diagnostic techniques have facilitated detection of viral pathogens, *Cryptococcus neoformans, Histoplasma capsulatum,* and *Legionella pneumophila* (10,11).

The final area in which tremendous progress has been achieved is in radiologic imaging. The use of magnetic resonance imaging (MRI), improved computed tomography (CT) scans, and other new radiologic and nuclear medicine techniques have enhanced noninvasive diagnosis of many clinical conditions.

Fever

The approach to the HIV-infected patient with fever is determined by the presence and nature of accompanying symptoms; duration, pattern, and degree of fever; and the level of immunodeficiency as measured by CD4 cell count, viral load titer, and duration of response to treatment if on combination antiretroviral therapy. If localized symptoms are present, they should be evaluated as discussed in other sections of this chapter. This section focuses on fever without an evident source.

Studies in the early 1990s that examined fever of unknown origin (FUO) in HIV-positive cohorts reported high rates of mycobacterial disease, including *Mycobacterium avium* complex (MAC), TB, lymphoma, and drug fever, with increased risk for these conditions as the CD4 cell count dropped (12). However, the incidence of many of these infections varied significantly depending on the population. For example, one study of HIV-infected patients hospitalized with fever in a public hospital in the United States documented a source in 87% of cases, with bacterial infections diagnosed in 60% of these (13).

In HIV-infected patients who present with a nonlocalizing fever, TB should always be considered. In advanced HIV disease, extrapulmonary disease is more common, and manifestations may consist of fever, adenopathy, or nonspecific laboratory findings (e.g., anemia, increased serum alkaline phosphatase) (14,15). MAC infection occurs with increasing frequency as the CD4 count falls to fewer than 100 cells/mm^3, presenting with fever and nonspecific symptoms (e.g., weight loss, anemia). In its disseminated form, the organism can be isolated from blood, bone marrow, and lymph nodes. Diagnosis is made in over 90% of cases by blood culture using a lysis-centrifugation or radiometric system (8). CMV infection also occurs in patients with advanced HIV disease, typically as retinitis or gastrointestinal tract disease but may present with fever alone. Other infections, including cryptococcosis, histoplasmosis, and toxoplasma encephalitis, also may initially present with fever and have manifestations related to specific organ systems later in their course. Finally, both community-acquired and nosocomial bacteremia, which is a major cause of morbidity in patients with HIV infection, may present solely with fever.

Limited information exists about the epidemiology and evaluation of patients with FUO in the context of widespread use of antimicrobial prophylaxis and combination antiretroviral therapy. Standard diagnostic approaches for FUO can be used in HIV-infected patients with higher CD4 counts (>200/mm^3) with the proviso that increased rates of TB, bacterial pneumonia, and sinusitis occur in this population (16). HIV-related OIs generally do not occur until the CD4 count drops to 100–200 cells/mm^3. For patients with CD4 counts of fewer than 200 cells/mm^3, the differential diagnosis broadens to include HIV-related OIs and malignant complications including MAC, CMV, disseminated fungal infections, and non-Hodgkin's lymphoma (Table 7.2).

The clinician evaluating a patient with fever should begin with a history of the present illness (including duration, degree, and pattern of the fever), an evaluation of potential exposures (e.g., occupational, geographic region of origin and travel history, animals, sexual practices, injection drug use), and a review of systems. Both recent and past travel are important in approaching patients with fever. For example, a patient from Southeast Asia may present with *Penicillium marneffei* infection, whereas a traveler to Southern California may have acute coccidioidomycosis (10,17). A history of past medical conditions, including TB, bacterial infections, OIs, malignancies, and other potential sources of infection (e.g., intravascular line, surgery, trauma) should be reviewed. A medication history, including any recent changes, should be obtained. Fever associated with immune reconstitution has been described for patients with latent OIs who were recently started on combination antiretroviral therapy (7). For individuals presenting with fever since starting a new medication, drug toxicity even in the absence of a rash should be considered. For example, abacavir can induce a

Table 7.2 Causes of Fever Without Localizing Symptoms or Signs

Etiology	Examples	Comments
Medications	TMP-SMX, dapsone, abacavir, penicillins, and many others	Increased rate of drug reactions in HIV disease
Infections		
Bacterial	Sinusitis, endocarditis, occult abscess, PID, TB, MAC	Atypical manifestations with low CD4 count
Fungal	Histoplasmosis, coccidioido-mycosis, *Penicillium marneffei* infection, cryptococcosis	Diagnosis made by culture, biopsy, or antigen detection
Parasitic	Toxoplasmosis, PCP, malaria, babesiasis, leishmaniasis	Travel exposures important
Viral	CMV	CD4 count $<$ 75–50 cells/mm^3
Neoplasia	Lymphoma	Usually with adenopathy
Endocrine	Hypoadrenalism	Adrenal disease with CMV and mycobacterial infections

CMV = cytomegalovirus; MAC = *Mycobacterium avium* complex; PCP = *Pneumocystis carinii* pneumonia; PID = pelvic inflammatory disease; TB = tuberculosis.

delayed hypersensitivity reaction characterized by fever and generalized symptoms, with no rash evident in 40% of cases (18).

Physical examination with emphasis on the skin, fundi, oral cavity, lymph nodes, sinuses, heart, abdomen, and pelvis should be performed. Initial laboratory tests should include review of recent CD4 cell count, viral load titer, complete blood count (CBC) and differential, urinalysis, and liver function tests (LFTs). Additional studies to consider include a TB skin test (PPD), chest radiography, conventional blood cultures, isolator blood culture for patients with CD4 count of fewer than 100 cells/mm^3, and syphilis and viral hepatitis serologies.

Further evaluation is based on the results of initial laboratory tests. For example, LFT abnormalities may prompt abdominal imaging with CT or ultrasound, whereas an abnormal chest radiograph may be further investigated with CT or bronchoscopy with biopsy as indicated. Other diagnostic studies to consider in patients with normal initial tests include abdominal CT scan looking for adenopathy, MRI or CT scan of the brain for mass lesions, gallium scan for occult infection and malignancy (18a), and examination of the cerebrospinal fluid (CSF) for infection. Bone marrow biopsy may be useful, with a 25% diagnostic yield in patients with fever and neutropenia or anemia (19). Liver biopsy should be considered in patients with advanced HIV disease who have an increased serum alkaline phosphatase level or in whom mycobacterial infection is suspected clinically (20).

The need for hospitalization and empiric antibiotic therapy in an HIV-infected patient with fever is determined by the severity of presentation and probability of a bacterial or fungal infection in which delay may have an impact on outcome.

Pulmonary Symptoms

Pulmonary symptoms, including cough and dyspnea, are common in HIV-infected patients, and the risks of several infectious and noninfectious conditions are increased (Table 7.3). Bacterial pneumonia and TB are frequent early in the course of HIV disease, whereas PCP may occur when the CD4 count falls to fewer than 200 cells/mm^3. Other HIV-related pulmonary conditions include lymphocytic interstitial pneumonitis (LIP), pulmonary hypertension, and Kaposi's sarcoma (KS). In addition, a number of non–HIV-related conditions, including asthma, COPD, and congestive heart failure, also need to be considered as HIV-infected patients grow older.

The most common AIDS-defining OI is PCP, usually presenting subacutely with a nonproductive cough, dyspnea, and interstitial infiltrates on chest radiography. The radiographic findings of PCP may be atypical in individuals receiving aerosol pentamidine prophylaxis with upper lobe disease or pneumothorax. Bacterial infections from encapsulated organisms (*Streptococcus pneumoniae* and *Haemophilus influenzae*) and TB are also a major cause of morbidity and mortality (11,14). As HIV-mediated immuno-deficiency progresses, other pathogens increase in importance. In this population, bacterial etiologies that also should be considered include *Pseudomonas* species, *S. aureus, Rhodococcus equi,* and *Norcardia aster-oides,* the latter two often presenting as cavitary disease (15,21,22). Fungi, including *Cryptococcus* species, *Histoplasma capsulatum,* and *Coccidioides immitis* also can present initially with pulmonary abnormalities. Invasive disease caused by *Aspergillus* species has been described predominantly in patients with advanced HIV disease and coexisting risk factors (e.g., granulocytopenia, exposure to antibiotics or steroids) (10).

Although the differential diagnosis for pulmonary symptoms is broad in HIV disease, a history, physical examination, and the judicious use of laboratory and radiographic studies can narrow the possibilities and provide guidance in the management. History should include duration and nature of symptoms, presence of other complaints, TB exposure, travel, underlying pulmonary or cardiac disease, and current medications. Effective combination antiretroviral therapy and antimicrobial prophylaxis will decrease the risk of PCP, TB, and, in some instances, conventional bacterial infections. Physical examination should include vital signs and should focus on the pharynx, sinuses, heart, lungs, and extremities. Measurement of oxygen saturation is often helpful in assessing severity of the condition. Desaturation with exercise increases the probability of PCP or another interstitial process.

The diagnostic evaluation of an HIV-infected patient with pulmonary symptoms will depend on the results of history and physical examination and the degree of immunodeficiency. Laboratory studies should include a review of recent CD4 cell count, viral load titer, CBC, sputum for Gram stain and culture, and usually chest radiography. If dyspnea is present or if PCP is suspected clinically, an arterial blood gas should be performed.

Chest radiography is often helpful in narrowing differential diagnosis. Diffuse infiltrates are suggestive of PCP, TB, KS, cryptococcosis, histoplasmosis, viruses (e.g., influenza, adenovirus), and LIP. Focal infiltrates usually represent infections with *S. pneumoniae, H. influenzae, Legionella* species, *Mycoplasma* species, or TB. Cavitary lesions should raise the possibility of TB, aspergillosis, nocardial infection, or aspiration pneumonia. A normal chest radiograph may represent early infection or noninfectious processes, such as asthma, COPD, or pulmonary hypertension.

If PCP is suspected clinically, an induced sputum for examination by monoclonal antibodies is highly sensitive, although this may be somewhat lower in patients receiving aerosol pentamidine for prophylaxis. Bronchoscopy with BAL usually is needed only to make the diagnosis for PCP if monoclonal antibody staining is not available. The patient with suspected TB should be evaluated with a PPD and three sputum tests for acid-fast stain and culture. Although acid-fast stain may be negative in up to 70% of patients with advanced immunodeficiency or chest radiograph findings suggestive of primary TB, cultures are positive in 93% of cases and isolator

Table 7.3   Conditions Associated with Pulmonary Symptoms

Condition	Characteristics
Bacterial infections	
Streptococcus pneumoniae, Haemophilus influenzae	Occurs at all stages of HIV disease; acute presentation with fever and purulent sputum production
Gram-negative bacteria	Acute presentation; generally in hospitalized patients
Legionella pneumophila	Acute presentation with constitutional symptoms and variable sputum production
Rhodococcus equii	Subacute presentation with minimal sputum production
Staphylococcus aureus	Acute or subacute presentation with purulent sputum production
Mycobacterium tuberculosis	Acute or subacute presentation, usually with constitutional symptoms
Viral infections	
Influenza	Acute presentation with variable sputum production
CMV, HSV, VZV	Usually seen with involvement of other systems
Fungal infections	
Pneumocystis carinii	Acute or subacute presentation; dry cough and dyspnea common
Cryptococcus neoformans	May be associated with meningitis
Histoplasma capsulatum	Acute to subacute presentation, often with systemic involvement
Coccidioides immitis	Often with meningitis and skin lesions
Noninfectious diseases	
Kaposi's sarcoma	Subacute to chronic presentation with chest pain, dyspnea, and hemoptysis
Lymphocytic interstitial pneumonitis	Chronic progressive dyspnea, usually associated with nonproductive cough; hepatosplenomegaly and parotid enlargement may be present
Lymphoma	Subacute to chronic presentation with constitutional symptoms and adenopathy
Other diseases	
Congestive heart failure	Acute or subacute in presentation; dyspnea often with signs including S3 gallop and rales
Asthma and COPD	Acute or chronic in presentation; cough often associated with wheezing

Table 7.3 *Continued*

Diagnostic Findings	*Comments*
Lobar or bronchopneumonia; diagnosis by sputum gram stain and culture or blood culture	Pneumococcal vaccine indicated for all patients with HIV
Lobar or bronchopneumonia; diagnosis by sputum gram stain and culture or blood culture	*Pseudomonas aeruginosa* seen in patients with neutropenia or low CD4 count
Gram stain is nondiagnostic; urinary antigen test may be useful	
Cavitary lesions common	
Septic emboli, cavitary lesions, lobar pneumonia, and/or pleural effusion; diagnosis by sputum gram stain and culture or blood culture	Usually seen as septic emboli from endocarditis; less commonly after viral pneumonia
Lobar pneumonia, cavitary lesions, hilar adeno-pathy; diagnosis by AFB stain and culture of sputum or isolator blood culture; bronchoscopy with BAL and biopsy may be necessary in some cases	May present with extrapulmonary disease in patients with advanced HIV disease
Interstitial infiltrates; nasopharyngeal washings for viral antigen may be useful	
Reticulonodular or diffuse infiltrates; transbronchial biopsy is necessary for definitive diagnosis	Uncommon, but may be seen in patients with advanced HIV disease (CMV), in intubated patients (HSV), or in pregnant women (VZV)
Interstitial infiltrates; examination may be normal, but oxygen saturation is usually decreased; induced sputum examination by monoclonal antibodies is very sensitive	Desaturation with exercise common; decreased DLCO on PFTs and positive gallium scan.
Focal or diffuse infiltrates; diagnosis by sputum or BAL culture; positive serum cryptococcal antigen	
Focal or nodular infiltrates, hilar adenopathy, and effusions; diagnosis by bronchoscopy, isolator blood culture, or bone marrow biopsy; urinary antigen test may be useful	Seen in patients from or visiting endemic areas including Ohio and Mississippi valleys, parts of Caribbean and South and Central America, Southeast Asia, and Africa
Reticular nodular or focal infiltrates; diagnosis by bronchoscopy, isolator blood culture, or bone marrow biopsy; complement fixation antibody usually positive	Seen in patients from or visiting endemic areas in southwestern U.S. and parts of South and Central America
Nodular or interstitial infiltrates; diagnosis by biopsy of other sites or bronchoscopy	May present with fever due to involvement of internal organs
Interstitial infiltrates; diagnosis by bronchoscopy	Responds to prednisone; may flare with initiation of antiretroviral drugs
Nodular or interstitial infiltrates; diagnosis by biopsy of involved sites	
ECG and echocardiographic abnormalities	May be HIV-related or due to underlying cardiac risk factors. Role of antiretroviral drug-induced hyperlipidemia still unclear
Chest radiograph may show hyperinflation and other characteristic changes; peak flow measurements and PFTs useful	

AFB = acid-fast bacillus; BAL = bronchoalveolar lavage; CMV = cytomegalovirus; COPD = chronic obstructive pulmonary disease; DLCO = carbon monoxide diffusion in the lungs; ECG = electrocardiogram; HSV = herpes simplex virus; PFTs = pulmonary function tests; VZV = varicella-zoster virus.

blood cultures are positive in 20% of cases (14,15). Other diagnostic tests that may be useful in selected clinical instances include *Legionella* urinary antigen and rapid viral culture for influenza and other respiratory viruses.

For patients with acute symptoms in whom infection is suspected, the decision about the need for hospitalization may be difficult. If upper airway infection is suspected and PCP is not a consideration, symptomatic treatment for viral infections or an empiric trial of antibiotics for sinusitis or bronchitis with close follow-up is reasonable. If pneumonia is diagnosed or suspected, most clinicians recommend admission. For patients in whom initial evaluation is nondiagnostic or initial treatment is unsuccessful, bronchoscopy with BAL and transbronchial biopsy should be considered. Specimens should be examined and cultured for bacteria, *Mycobacterium*, *Pneumocystis*, fungi, and viruses, including herpes simplex virus (HSV) and CMV if appropriate. Cryptococcal antigen can be detected in BAL fluid in patients with cryptococcal pneumonia. Biopsy specimens also should be examined for evidence of malignancy and LIP. The role of open-lung biopsy in this population is unclear, but it is generally reserved for instances in which the transbronchial biopsy is nondiagnostic (23).

Diagnostic studies that may be useful in evaluating chronic cough or dyspnea include pulmonary function tests for reactive airway and interstitial disease, bronchoscopy with BAL and transbronchial biopsy, echocardiography, and exercise tolerance test.

Gastrointestinal Symptoms

In HIV disease, gastrointestinal manifestations are common (24). Syndromes include diarrhea, oral and esophageal conditions, viral hepatitis, and wasting syndrome.

Diarrhea

Diarrhea may be the most frequently reported HIV-related symptom. Several series have shown a 0.9% to 14.0% incidence of diarrhea, which is greatest in patients with advanced disease (25). Its etiology is often multifactorial, with opportunistic diseases, medications, and non–HIV-related conditions included in the differential diagnosis.

The most concerning diarrheal syndromes are those caused by OIs, which fortunately have declined in recent years. However, in patients with a CD4 count of fewer than 200 cells/mm^3, MAC infections and pathogens (e.g., *Cryptosporidium*, Microsporidia, and CMV, still need to be considered. For individuals with a higher CD4 count, diarrhea from medications or non–HIV-related disorders (e.g., viral gastroenteritis, bacterial colitis, lactose intolerance, inflammatory bowel disease) are more common. *Clostridium difficile* colitis, which is associated with recent antibiotic use, can occur at any CD4 count. Although salmonellosis was common before 1989, the widespread use of trimethoprim-sulfamethoxazole (TMP-SMX) for PCP prophylaxis has made this condition unusual.

The evaluation of diarrhea in an HIV-infected person is greatly influenced by history. The characteristics of diarrhea to consider include volume (small vs. large), frequency, consistency, duration (acute vs. chronic), and associated symptoms, such as tenesmus, abdominal cramping, nausea, and vomiting (Table 7.4). The patient's level of immunodeficiency also should be considered. Determination of exposures should include recent travel, drinking water supply (reservoir vs. well), sick contacts, sexual activity, and

Table 7.4   Conditions Associated with Diarrhea

Condition	Characteristics	Diagnostic Findings	Comments
Infections			
Cryptosporidium	Subacute course; may be associated with wasting	Stool for cryptosporidium; small bowel biopsy may be necessary	CD4 count < 200 cells/mm³
Microsporidia	Subacute course; may be associated with wasting, cholangiopathy	Stool for microsporidium; small bowel biopsy may be necessary	CD4 count < 200 cells/mm³
Giardia lamblia	Acute or chronic course; upper and/or lower GI symptoms	Stool for ova and parasite (may require more than one specimen) or duodenal aspirate	Any CD4 count; risks include oral–anal sex, travel, and well water
Cytomegalovirus	Acute to subacute course; may be associated with fever or evidence of retinitis	Colonoscopy with biopsy	CD4 count < 75–50 cells/mm³
Enteroviruses	Acute, self-limited course	Diagnosed presumptively	—
Bacterial enteritis	Acute course; watery and/or bloody diarrhea	Stool for enteric pathogens; blood culture if fever present	Increased risk of bacteremia; food history and local epidemiology
Clostridium difficile	Acute course; associated with fever	Stool for toxin	Recent antibiotic therapy or hospitalization
Mycobacterium avium complex	Chronic course; fever and constitutional symptoms; may be associated with wasting	Isolator blood or bone marrow culture; colonoscopy with biopsy sometimes necessary	CD4 count < 75–50 cells/mm³
Medication-related diseases	Usually occurs within 4 weeks of initiation of therapy	May require discontinuation of suspected agent, followed by rechallenge	More common with lower CD4 counts and on initiation of treatment

GI = gastrointestinal.

family history of colitis. In addition, a list of medications may provide clues (Table 7.5). If a medication likely to cause diarrhea has been started, a short trial off this medication or of antimotility drugs may be appropriate.

The physical examination should focus on 1) the oral cavity looking for ulcerations, 2) the abdomen to evaluate for tenderness, masses, or hepatosplenomegaly, and 3) the rectum to check for any external lesions and to assess for occult blood or the presence of mucus in the stool. Laboratory studies should consist of review of recent CD4 cell count, CBC, electrolytes, amylase and lipase (if pancreatitis is suspected), blood cultures (if fever is present), and stool (for leukocytes and specific pathogens). If this approach is nondiagnostic, referral to a gastroenterologist for colonoscopy should be considered.

Hepatitis

Hepatitis, both drug-induced and viral, has become an increasing problem for HIV-infected patients in recent years (Table 7.6). Unfortunately, many patients may have a component of each, which can make diagnosis and treatment complex (25,26). Drug-induced hepatitis is defined as an increase in LFTs associated with the use of a known hepatotoxin. Earlier in the epidemic, zidovudine (ZDV) and other nucleoside reverse-transcriptase inhibitors (NRTIs) were associated with a fulminant hepatitis associated with fatty steatosis and lactic acidosis (27). More recently, nonnucleoside reverse-transcriptase inhibitors (NNRTIs) and protease inhibitors (PIs) also have been shown to cause drug-induced hepatitis, as have other medications used for HIV-related conditions. These include rifabutin, rifampin, isoniazid, and anabolic steroids. Some of these agents are direct hepatotoxins, whereas others also affect the major hepatic metabolic pathways, especially the cytochrome p450 enzyme system.

The viral hepatitides, specifically hepatitis A (HAV), hepatitis B (HBV), and hepatitis C (HCV), frequently occur in HIV-infected individuals. An increase in chronic HBV- and HCV-related morbidity and mortality in recent years has been described (28). Initial assessment of an HIV-infected patient

---

Table 7.5 Medications That Often Cause Diarrhea

• Didanosine	• Azithromycin
• Saquinavir	• Clindamycin
• Ritonavir	• Human growth hormone
• Nelfinavir	• Nutritional supplements
• Clarithromycin	

Table 7.6 Conditions Associated with Abnormal Liver Function Tests

Condition	Characteristics	Diagnostic Findings	Comments
Viral infections			
Hepatitis A	Acute onset of fever, constitutional symptoms, jaundice	Positive HAV IgM	Men who have sex with men at highest risk
Hepatitis B	Acute or chronic (10%)	Positive HBsAg	Sexual or bloodborne transmission
Hepatitis C	Acute or chronic; most have progressive disease; may be asymptomatic until cirrhotic	Positive HCV antibody test with confirmatory RIBA or HCV RNA	Injection drug users at highest risk
Cholangiopathy	Subacute onset of jaundice	Increased serum bilirubin and alkaline phosphatase levels; diagnosis by MRCP or ERCP	CD4 count < 200 cells/mm^3
Medication-related diseases	Acute or subacute onset; NRTI-induced hepatitis can be acute and fulminant	Usually mildly to moderately increased serum transaminases	Any CD4 count
Opportunistic diseases			
Cytomegalovirus	Subacute onset; usually associated with retinitis or GI tract involvement	Liver biopsy may be necessary	CD4 count < 75–50 cells/mm^3
MAC infection	Subacute; associated with fever, GI symptoms, wasting, and/or pancytopenia	Positive isolator blood or bone marrow culture	CD4 count < 75–50 cells/mm^3
Pneumocystis carinii infection	Subacute; may be associated with pulmonary involvement	Liver biopsy	CD4 count < 200 cells/mm^3
Bacillary angiomatosis	Subacute; associated with characteristic skin lesions	Liver biopsy	CD4 count < 100 cells/mm^3
Lymphoma	Subacute; associated with fever, adenopathy, and/or hepatomegaly	Liver biopsy	CD4 count < 200 cells/mm^3

HAV = hepatitis A virus; IgM = immunoglobulin M; HBsAg = hepatitis B surface antigen; GI = gastrointestinal; NRTI = nucleoside reverse-transcriptase inhibitor; RIBA = recombinant immunoblot assay; HCV = hepatitis C virus; MRCP = magnetic resonance cholangiopancreatography; ERCP = endoscopic retrograde cholangiopancreatography.

with LFT abnormalities should include serologies for these three pathogens. For patients who test seronegative for HAV or HBV, the appropriate vaccine series should be administered.

The LFT abnormality pattern and its duration and degree will help define the most likely diagnoses. In an asymptomatic patient, mildly increased transaminases with a normal bilirubin are often caused by drug toxicity, alcohol use, or chronic HBV or HCV infection. A patient presenting with a febrile illness, moderately to severely increased transaminases, and increased bilirubin level will most likely have acute HAV or HBV infection, although an acute drug reaction is also possible. A cholestatic profile raises the possibility of obstruction from stones or malignancy, cryptosporidial or microsporidial infection, or HIV-related cholangiopathy. Abdominal ultrasonography or CT scanning may be useful in this setting.

Odynophagia and Dysphagia

Upper gastrointestinal tract disease associated with HIV infection remains a significant problem (29). The most common mouth lesions are exudative or ulcerative. Oral candidiasis (thrush) is seen in most HIV-infected patients at some time during their illness, usually when the CD4 count is fewer than 300 cells/mm^3. Patients may be asymptomatic and have a white fluffy exudate on their buccal mucosa, palate, tongue, or posterior pharynx. A potassium hydroxide (KOH) preparation will reveal budding yeast and pseudohyphae. This condition is sometimes confused with oral hairy leukoplakia (OHL). In contrast to thrush, OHL is found on the lateral margins of the tongue and appears as vertically-oriented, white, linear plaques that cannot be scraped off. The causative agent is Epstein–Barr virus (EBV), and the diagnosis is made clinically. Ulcerative oral lesions usually come to attention secondary to pain, and patients often have multiple lesions. The three most common causes are aphthous ulcers and HSV and CMV infections (Table 7.7). Syphilis and lymphoma are less frequent causes.

Odynophagia and dysphagia are frequent symptoms in patients with advanced HIV disease, with the cause often being infectious. Most patients with *Candida* esophagitis have thrush. Treatment with a systemic azole, such as fluconazole, is usually effective. In those patients who present with typical esophagitis symptoms but without thrush or who do not respond to empiric therapy, alternative diagnoses (e.g., HSV and CMV infections) must be considered. In addition to odynophagia, these conditions may be associated with fever. Upper endoscopy with biopsy and cultures is needed to establish the diagnosis. Although biopsies of esophageal HSV and CMV show characteristic viral inclusions, no such abnormalities are seen with aphthous esophagitis. In patients with a CD4 count greater than 200 cells/mm^3 who present with esophageal symptoms, reflux disease, stricture, spasm, and other non–HIV-related causes should be considered in the differential diagnosis.

Table 7.7   Conditions Commonly Associated with Oral Ulcers

Condition	Characteristics	Diagnostic Findings	Comments
Herpes simplex virus	Multiple shallow ulcers < 1 cm on buccal mucosa, labia, and/or tongue	Positive culture	Any CD4 count
Cytomegalovirus (CMV)	Several shallow ulcers ≤ 1 cm, usually on buccal mucosa	Positive culture	CD4 count < 75–50 cells/mm^3
Aphthous ulcers	Multiple punched-out ulcers < 0.5 cm with surrounding erythema; on buccal mucosa and/or labia	Diagnosis of exclusion	Any CD4 count

Weight Loss and Change in Body Habitus

The traditional change in body habitus associated with HIV disease has been weight loss. However, lipodystrophy syndrome—characterized by central obesity, loss of subcutaneous fat in the extremities, and metabolic abnormalities (hyperlipidemia, glucose intolerance)—has been reported with increasing frequency in recent years predominantly among individuals on PIs (30). Although advanced HIV infection can cause weight loss and wasting, more often it is caused by an undiagnosed OI. These include MAC infection, cryptosporidiosis or microsporidiosis, disseminated fungal infection, or any of the esophageal diseases that limit oral intake. Wasting syndrome—defined as loss of greater than 10% of baseline body weight associated with chronic diarrhea, weakness, or fever in the absence of a known cause—was one of the earliest recognized manifestations of AIDS. However, lesser degrees of weight loss are clinically significant, and it has now been shown that a 5% reduction is associated with increased risk of OIs and death (31). Other etiologies for weight loss include decreased intake because of limited access to food and increased loss of nutrients from diarrhea or malabsorption.

When a patient presents with weight loss, the history will elucidate possible etiologies and appropriate diagnostic evaluation and management (Table 7.8). Review of weight over time, dietary history, presence of diarrhea, problems with food intake, medications, and illicit drug use is important. The optimal management of lipodystrophy syndrome is undefined at this time. Bioelectric impedance analysis (BIA) has been used to monitor changes in body weight and composition.

Neurologic Symptoms

Neurologic complaints are common at all stages of HIV infection, although significant complications generally occur in patients with advanced immuno-deficiency. The most common symptoms are headache, altered mental status, and painful extremities (Table 7.9).

Headache

In the patient with a CD4 count of 200 cells/mm^3 or greater, non-OI causes of headache (e.g., muscle tension, vascular, and sinus-related) predominate (31a). In the patient with advanced HIV disease, OIs also must be considered in the differential diagnosis of headache. The three most common OIs are cryptococcal meningitis, toxoplasmic encephalitis, and CNS lymphoma; less frequent infections include coccidioidomycosis, histoplasmosis, and TB.

History should include duration, location, and precipitants of headache; associated symptoms; and potential exposures (e.g., travel, TB, drug use). Physical examination should focus on the head and neck, and a detailed neurologic assessment should be performed. For a patient who has a CD4

Table 7.8   Factors Contributing to Weight Loss

Problem	Etiology	Management
Inaccessible food or preparation difficulties	Social or health issues	Social service, homemaker, dietary supplements
Anorexia	Intercurrent illness HIV infection Depression	Treat Megestrol acetate, dronabinol Antidepressant therapy
Nausea, vomiting	Medications HIV gastroparesis	Discontinue Cisapride*
Mouth pain, dysphagia, odynophagia	Gingivitis, periodontitis Opportunistic diseases	Dental referral Specific therapy
Diarrhea, malabsorption	Opportunistic diseases HIV infection	Specific therapy Antiretroviral therapy

*Contraindicated for use with nonnucleoside reverse-transcriptase inhibitors and protease inhibitors.
Adapted from Libman H, Witzburg RA (eds). *HIV Infection: A Primary Care Manual*. Boston: Little Brown; 1996.

count of fewer than 200 cells/mm^3 and significant or persistent headaches, neuroimaging with a brain MRI or CT scan with contrast should be performed to rule out a mass lesion. If this is normal, lumbar puncture with CSF analysis (including cell count, chemistries, cryptococcal antigen, syphilis serology, cytology, and stains and cultures for pathogens) is indicated. Other useful tests include a serum cryptococcal antigen and toxo-

---

Table 7.9   Differential Diagnoses of Neurologic Syndromes

Headache

- Acute/chronic sinusitis
- Cryptococcal meningitis
- Lymphoma
- Toxoplasmosis
- TB meningitis
- Bacterial meningitis
- Syphilis
- Medication-related

Altered Mental Status

- Toxoplasmosis
- Cryptococcal meningitis
- HIV encephalopathy
- Progressive multifocal leukoencephalopathy
- CMV encephalitis
- Syphilis
- Medication-related

Painful Extremities

- Distal sensory polyneuropathy
- CMV polyradiculopathy
- HIV infection
- Syphilis
- Polymyositis

CMV = cytomegalovirus; TB = tuberculosis.

plasma IgG antibody, which will be positive in at least 90% of patients with cryptococcal meningitis and toxoplasma encephalitis, respectively.

The presence of a mass on radiologic imaging narrows the major differential diagnosis to toxoplasmosis or lymphoma. Toxoplasma lesions generally appear as multiple ring-enhancing lesions with minimal edema in the gray matter, whereas lymphomatous lesions are usually solitary, periventricular, nonenhancing, and have substantial surrounding edema. In patients who are positive for toxoplasma IgG, or in seronegative individuals with characteristic CNS lesions, empiric antitoxoplasma therapy usually is warranted. If a clinical and radiologic response is not seen within 10 to 14 days, a brain biopsy is indicated to establish definitive diagnosis.

Altered Mental Status

The evaluation of change in mental status in an HIV-infected patient should follow the approach to this condition in the general population, with the recognition of increased risk of infectious and neoplastic causes (Table 7.10). History should include the course, nature, and pattern of mental status change; presence of associated symptoms (e.g., fever, focal neurologic deficits); medications; drug use; recent trauma; and travel. All the CNS processes discussed previously can present with a change in mental status, and several other diagnoses also should be considered in the patient with advanced HIV disease. These include HIV encephalopathy (also known as AIDS dementia complex [ADC]), progressive multifocal leukoencephalopathy (PML), and CMV encephalitis (32) (Table 7.11).

A slowly progressive decline in cognitive function is the chief characteristic of ADC. Patients present with memory loss and altered thinking but also often have a slowing of motor skills and gait disturbances. PML manifests with seizure disorder, focal neurologic deficits, change in mental status, or a combination of the three. Characteristic neuroimaging findings should prompt either CSF PCR assay for the etiologic JC virus or brain biopsy, which remains the "gold standard" for diagnosis. CMV encephalitis is the least common of these disorders and classically presents with decreased cognitive function and markedly diminished sensorium. A positive CSF CMV DNA by PCR assay confirms the diagnosis.

Painful Extremities

Pain in the extremities is a common complaint in HIV-infected patients. The most common cause is distal sensory polyneuropathy presenting with numbness, tingling, burning, and pain in the feet or hands. Motor weakness is not a feature of this condition. The two most common causes are medication-related (e.g., didanosine [ddI], stavudine [d4T]) toxic neuropathy or HIV itself. In drug-induced neuropathy, early interruption of the

Table 7.10   Etiologies of Altered Mental Status ("MEND A MIND")

Etiology	Examples	Comments
Metabolic	Renal or hepatic dysfunction, electrolyte imbalances	Increased risk of chronic liver disease from HBV and HCV
Endocrine	Hyperglycemia, hypoadrenalism	Glucose intolerance and diabetes mellitus have been described on combination antiretroviral therapy
Neoplasia	Lymphomatous meningitis or primary CNS lymphoma	—
Drugs	Prescribed, complementary, or illicit	Medication levels can be affected by drug–drug interactions
Autoimmune	Systemic lupus erythematosus	—
Mechanical	Subdural hematoma, brain abscess	History or trauma, alcoholism, or injection drug use
Infections	Toxoplasmosis or CMV encephalitis, bacterial or fungal meningitis, sepsis	Requires prompt and aggressive evaluation
Neuropsychiatric	CVA, seizures, psychosis, schizophrenia	—
Dementia	HIV encephalopathy	Diagnosis of exclusion; may improve with combination antiretroviral therapy

CMV = cytomegalovirus; CNS = central nervous system; CVA = cerebrovascular accident; HBV = hepatitis B virus; HCV = hepatitis C virus.

medication usually leads to complete resolution of symptoms. CMV myelitis and polyradiculitis is a cause of pain in the lower extremities associated with weakness. These syndromes occur in individuals with CD4 counts of fewer than 100 cells/mm^3. Myopathy, related to HIV or medications (primarily ZDV), also presents with pain in the extremities and proximal weakness. It is associated with increased serum creatine phosphokinase (CPK) levels. Other causes of pain include non–HIV-related conditions such as disc disease and fibromyalgia syndrome.

History should include the nature, duration, and progression of symptoms, medications, and occupational exposures. Physical examination should include a neurologic and musculoskeletal assessment. If drug-related neuropathy is suspected, a trial period during which the medication is

Table 7.11   Characteristics of AIDS Dementia Complex, Progressive Multifocal Leukoencephalopathy, and Cytomegalovirus Encephalitis

Diagnosis	Radiologic Imaging	CSF Profile
ADC	Multifocal periventricular white-matter abnormalities	Mild lymphocytic pleocytosis; mildly increased protein
PML	Diffuse areas of nonenhancing white-matter abnormalities	Mild lymphocytic pleocytosis; mildly increased protein; positive JC virus DNA
CMV encephalitis	Diffuse periventricular white-matter enhancement	Moderate lymphocytic pleocytosis and increased protein

ADC = AIDS dementia complex; CMV = cytomegalovirus; CSF = cerebrospinal fluid; PML = progressive multifocal leukoencephalopathy.

withheld completely or reduced in dose is warranted. Evidence of weakness should be further evaluated with radiologic imaging of the spine by MRI or CT as appropriate. If CMV is suspected, lumbar puncture with examination of the CSF for CMV DNA by PCR—as well as for other causes (e.g., acid-fast bacillus, cytology)—is necessary. Other potentially useful tests for evaluation of painful extremities include vitamin B_{12} level, syphilis serology, thyroid stimulating hormone (TSH) level, CPK, and based on the clinical setting, electromyography, nerve conduction studies, and muscle biopsy.

Gynecologic Symptoms

Gynecologic complaints may be the initial manifestation of HIV infection in women (33). Many conditions, including vaginal candidiasis, cervical abnormalities, and cancer and pelvic inflammatory disease (PID), have an increased incidence or may be more difficult to treat.

Vaginal Discharge and Pelvic Pain

One of the most common complaints in HIV-infected women is vaginal discharge (3,34). This symptom can represent vaginitis or be the initial manifestation of a more significant problem, such as PID. Recurrent vaginal candidiasis, defined as at least four episodes in 1 year, is frequent in HIV disease. It is characterized by pruritus and a thick white discharge. Other causes of vaginal discharge, including bacterial vaginosis and trichomoniasis, are seen at the same rates in HIV-infected and seronegative women (34,35). Genital HSV infection, which is increased in frequency and severity in HIV disease, sometimes manifests with discharge but usually with localized discomfort.

Pelvic pain can be associated with PID, ectopic pregnancy, HSV infection, and other gynecologic abnormalities, including uterine fibroids, ovarian cysts, and endometriosis. Many studies have reported that HIV-infected women with PID may have fewer signs of acute infection and an increased risk of complications despite standard therapy (36). Women with HIV infection are also at increased risk for cervical dysplasia and neoplasia. Although usually asymptomatic, cervical lesions can present with vaginal symptoms in advanced cases (37).

Evaluation of women presenting with vaginal discharge or pelvic pain requires a careful history and abdominal and pelvic examinations. History should focus on the location and nature of symptoms, characteristics of any discharge, and the presence of fever and other associated symptoms. Testing for gonorrhea and chlamydia should be performed; any discharge should be examined with KOH for yeast and with normal saline for trichomoniasis or evidence of bacterial vaginosis (clue cells). A urine pregnancy test should be performed as clinically indicated. Other studies, including pelvic or abdominal ultrasound, and empiric treatment are determined by the clinical presentation and results of the initial investigation.

Menstrual Abnormalities

HIV-infected women may complain of menstrual abnormalities, but a recent study did not find an increased rate compared with seronegative controls (38). Evaluation of menstrual symptoms may include screening for pregnancy, uterine fibroids, and certain endocrinologic abnormalities. Referral to a gynecologist for consideration of endometrial biopsy is appropriate if initial studies are not revealing.

Dermatologic Symptoms

Dermatologic complaints affect over 90% of HIV-infected patients during the course of their illness (Table 7.12). These conditions range from the benign to life-threatening. Certain skin conditions are unique to HIV disease. These include dermatologic manifestations of the acute retroviral syndrome, OIs, and selected malignancies. Other conditions, which are seen in the general population as well, are more frequent (e.g., drug eruptions) and more severe or resistant to treatment (e.g., seborrheic dermatitis, xerotic eczema) (39,40). Some dermatologic conditions may have atypical

Table 7.12   Dermatologic Conditions in HIV Disease

Disease	Clinical Manifestations
Viral infections	
Acute HIV exanthem (primary HIV infection)	Fever, myalgias, urticaria; truncal, palmar, plantar maculopapules
Herpes simplex	May be relapsing with persistent erosions (*see* Fig. 8.11)
Varicella-zoster	May be recurrent; usually dermatomal (*see* Fig. 8.12)
Molluscum contagiosum	Clusters of white umbilicated papules
Oral hairy leukoplakia	Whitish, nonremovable verrucous plaques on sides of tongue
Warts (HPV)	Increased number and size of verrucous lesions
Fungal infections	
Candida albicans	Oral mucosal white plaques, sore throat, dysphagia, deep tongue erosions (*see* Fig. 8.5); intractable vaginal infection; nail infection
Tinea versicolor	Thick, scaly hypopigmented or light-brown plaques on trunk
Dermatophytes (tinea corporis, pedis, cruris)	Extensive involvement, especially groin and feet
Bacterial infections	
Staphylococcal	Superficial and subcutaneous infections; impetigo
Syphilis	Painless chancre; generalized plaques and papulosquamous lesions (*see* Fig. 8.3); incubation period for neurosyphilis may be very short (months)
Bacillary angiomatosis	Dome-shaped pedunculated solitary or multiple papules and nodules (4 mm–2 cm) (*see* Fig. 8.1); visceral involvement
Arthropod infestations	
Scabies	Generalized crusted papules and eczematous lesions
Miscellaneous disorders	
Seborrheic dermatitis	Red scaling plaques with yellow greasy scales and distinct margins on the face and scalp
Psoriasis	Activation of prior disease or no previous history
Xeroderma	Severe dry skin, possible erythroderma
Papular eruption	2–5-mm skin-colored papules on head, neck, upper trunk; pruritic, chronic
Eosinophilic and bacterial folliculitis	Groups of small vesicles and pustules that can become confluent
Thrombocytopenic purpura	Petechiae
Yellow nails	Yellow discoloration of nail plate; may be associated with *Pneumocystis carinii* pneumonia
Darkened nails	Dark blue appearance at bases of fingernails
Premature hair graying, long eyelashes	Usually with advanced HIV disease
Drug reactions	*See* Table 7.13
Kaposi's sarcoma	Pale to deep violaceous oval plaques and papules; oral lesions; visceral lesions (*see* Fig. 9.1)

Adapted from Libman H, Witzburg RA (eds). *HIV Infection: A Primary Care Manual*. Boston: Little Brown; 1996.

Table 7.12   *Continued*

Diagnosis	Treatment
HIV antibodies usually within 12 weeks of infection; low WBC count, thrombocytopenia, hypergammaglobulinemia	Symptomatic treatment
HSV culture, DFA, Tzanck smear for multinucleated giant cells	Acyclovir
VZV culture, DFA, Tzanck smear for multinucleated giant cells	Acyclovir
Biopsy or KOH preparations of soft central material show large viral inclusions	Cryosurgery
Clinical appearance	None generally necessary
Clinical appearance	Topical agents, cryosurgery, surgical excision
KOH slide preparation	Topical: nystatin suspension, clotrimazole troche Systemic: fluconazole
KOH slide shows numerous short hyphae and spores	Topical: selenium sulfide, miconazole, clotrimazole, sodium thiosulfate
KOH slide shows branched, septated hyphae	Topical: miconazole Oral: fluconazole
Culture	Dicloxacillin
Positive VDRL or RPR *and* FTA-Abs or MHA-TP	Penicillin
Biopsy	Erythromycin; chronic suppressive therapy may be necessary
KOH or oil preparation shows mites	Permethrin cream
Biopsy; KOH to rule out tinea	Ketoconazole cream; low-potency topical steroids
Biopsy	Treatment-resistant cases may respond to etretinate or zidovudine
Clinical presentation	Lactic acid emollients (Lac-Hydrin)
Biopsy shows lymphocytic perivascular infiltrate	Low-potency topical steroids; antipruritic lotions; antihistamines
Biopsy; negative culture for atypical organisms	Ultraviolet B phototherapy for EF; topical and/or systemic antibiotics for bacterial folliculitis
Complete blood count	Antiretroviral therapy
Clinical examination	None
Recent history of zidovudine treatment	None
Physical examination	None
Clinical examination	Alternative drugs
Biopsy	Localized disease: intralesional chemotherapy, radiation therapy Systemic disease: chemotherapy, interferon

DFA = direct fluorescent antibody; EF = eosinophilic folliculitis; FTA-Abs = fluorescent treponemal antibody, absorbed test; HSV = herpes simplex virus; HPV = human papillomavirus; MHA-TP = microhemagglutination–*Treponema pallidum*; RPR = rapid plasma reagin test; VDRL = Venereal Disease Research Laboratory test for syphilis; VZV = varicella-zoster virus; WBC = white blood cell.

presentations resulting in delay in diagnosis and treatment. Examples include ecthymatous varicella-zoster, which presents as heaped-up hyperkeratotic lesions; cryptococcosis presenting with skin lesions that mimic molluscum contagiosum; and others (10,39,41). The use of combination antiretroviral therapy has affected the presentation and course of a number of conditions, with the worsening of some (e.g., eosinophilic folliculitis) but improvement of many others (e.g., KS, molluscum contagiosum) (39).

The diagnosis of skin conditions relies on a complete history (including duration and distribution of lesions), associated local and systemic symptoms, and potential new exposures (e.g., medications, travel, jobs, pets, soaps, lotions). Physical examination should focus on skin, mucous membranes, abdomen for hepatosplenomegaly, and lymph glands for enlargement. Laboratory tests may include review of most recent CD4 cell count, CBC with differential, LFTs, and other serologies and blood cultures as determined by clinical presentation. If the diagnosis remains obscure or is associated with systemic symptoms, a skin biopsy may be indicated. Specimens should be examined using routine and special stains and should be cultured for bacteria, fungi, and mycobacteria.

Infectious Disorders

A wide range of infections, including OIs and other conditions that occur more frequently with HIV disease, can present with skin conditions. These include cryptococcosis (papular lesions resembling molluscum contagiosum), histoplasmosis (ulcers), *Candida* infection (thrush, angular chelitis, paronychia), syphilis, and bacterial infection (*S. aureus* pyomyositis). Other less common infectious causes include bacillary angiomatosis (cutaneous nodules associated with systemic symptoms) caused by *Rochilimaea* species and mycobacterial infections (14,42). A number of viral pathogens also can cause skin lesions including HSV, varicella-zoster virus (shingles), and poxviruses (molluscum contagiosum). Although parasitic infestations are unusual in the developed world, scabies can present as a severe crusting eruption known as Norwegian scabies, with biopsy specimen showing large numbers of mites (39).

Noninfectious Disorders

Drug Reactions

Drug reactions are common in HIV-infected patients and may limit the treatment of the virus and its complications (39,40) (Table 7.13). The most well-known reactions are to sulfa-containing medications, notably TMP-SMX in the treatment of PCP. Other commonly offending agents include ampicillin, NNRTIs, and amprenavir. Typically, drug reactions present as pruritic macular papular morbilliform or urticarial eruptions but also may

Table 7.13   Cutaneous Manifestations of Drug Toxicity

Drug	Manifestations	Comments
TMP-SMX	Exanthemous eruption, erythema multiforme, fixed drug eruption, toxic epidermal necrolysis, Stevens–Johnson syndrome	Increased frequency in HIV disease; eruption usually pruritic and associated with fever
Dapsone	Exanthemous eruption, Stevens–Johnson syndrome	May present as sulfone syndrome (fever, rash, hemolytic anemia, and fulminant hepatitis)
Zidovudine (ZDV)	Nail hyperpigmentation with mucous membranes and skin less commonly involved	—
Zalcitabine (ddC)	Oral ulcers	Less commonly associated with ddI
Abacavir	Rash accompanies hypersensitivity reaction in ~60% of cases	Usually associated with fever and worsening constitutional symptoms; drug rechallenge contraindicated
Nevirapine	Exanthemous eruption, Stevens–Johnson syndrome	Risk significantly decreased by dose escalation on initiation of therapy
Protease inhibitors	Acute exacerbation of chronic conditions (e.g., eosinophilic folliculitis); erythematous macular rash described with amprenavir	—
Foscarnet	Penile ulcers	Related to direct toxicity of drug on mucous membranes

ddI = didanosine; TMP-SMX = trimethoprim-sulfamethoxazole.

appear as erythema multiforme, erythema nodosum, and exfoliative dermatitis (toxic epidermal necrolysis and Stevens–Johnson syndrome). Manifestations of systemic involvement may include fever, abnormal LFTs, and interstitial nephritis. The management usually consists of drug discontinuation, symptomatic management, and careful observation.

Malignancies

The incidence of KS and anogenital squamous carcinomas related to human papillomavirus (HPV) are increased in HIV-infected patients. KS typically presents as reddish-purple macules, papules, nodules, or tumors on the skin or mucous membranes. Early lesions may resemble nevi or bruises, and diagnosis is established with biopsy. HPV-related squamous cancers are often suspected by physical examination of the cervix or rectum. They may be asymptomatic or present as a nonhealing lesion or mass. Diagnosis should be confirmed with biopsy. There is no evidence that other skin cancers are increased in frequency in HIV disease.

Other Conditions

A number of dermatologic conditions seen in immunocompetent hosts may be more severe or resistant to treatment in the context of HIV disease (39,41). Seborrheic dermatitis occurs in up to 80% of HIV-infected patients. It is characterized by scaly erythematous plaques primarily involving the eyebrows, scalp, and nasolabial folds. Other such conditions include xerotic eczema, psoriasis, and Reiter's syndrome (palmoplantar pustules associated with arthritis, urethritis and conjunctivitis) (39).

Eosinophilic folliculitis, which is seen generally in advanced HIV disease, presents as pruritic pustular lesions involving the chest above the nipples, the face, and the upper extremities (43). This condition often responds to ultraviolet light therapy. Another HIV-related condition known as "itchy red bump disease," is characterized by pruritic papular lesions that can involve any part of the body but classically begin on the trunk. It is difficult to treat and can result in the development of prurigo nodularis, lichen simplex chronicum, or secondary infection from persistent scratching (39).

■   ■   ■

Key Points

- With the introduction of combination antiretroviral therapy, the incidence of OIs has declined and other syndromes have begun to account for a greater proportion of the conditions seen in HIV-infected people.
- For the assessment of fever in patients with CD4 counts of fewer than 200 cells/mm^3, the differential diagnosis broadens to include HIV-related opportunistic diseases.
- *P. carinii* is the most common opportunistic pathogen responsible for pulmonary symptoms in HIV-infected people.
- Diarrhea is the most commonly reported HIV-related symptom. In patients with a CD4 count greater than 200 cells/mm^3, non–HIV-

related causes should be considered first. In patients with lower CD4 counts, medication toxicity or OIs may be responsible.

- Significant neurologic complications of HIV infection generally occur in patients with advanced disease.

- In women, gynecologic symptoms, such as recurrent *Candida* infection, may be the initial manifestation of HIV infection.

- Dermatologic conditions affect more than 90% of HIV-infected people and range from benign to life threatening. Some common dermatoses occur more often in patients with HIV disease and may be resistant to treatment.

■ ■ ■

REFERENCES

1. **Centers for Disease Control and Prevention.** Update: Trends in AIDS Incidence—United States, 1996. *Morbid Mortal Wkly Rep MMWR.* 1997;46:861–7.

2. **Moore RD, Chaisson RE.** Natural history of opportunistic disease in an HIV-infected urban cohort. *Ann Intern Med.* 1996;124:633–42.

3. **US Public Health Service, Infectious Disease Society of America.** 1999 USPHS/IDSA guidelines for the prevention of opportunistic infections in persons infected with human immunodeficiency virus. *Morbid Mortal Wkly Rep MMWR.* 1999;48(RR-10):1–66.

4. **Freedberg KA, Tosteson AN, Cotton DJ, Goldman L.** Optimal management strategies for HIV-infected patients who present with cough or dyspnea: a cost-effective analysis. *J Gen Intern Med.* 1992;7:261–72.

5. **Currier JS, Williams PL, Becker S, et al.** Incidence rates and risk factors for opportunistic infections in a randomized trial comparing AZT+3TC to the AZT+3TC+Indinavir (ACTG 320). In *Fifth Conference on Retroviruses and Opportunistic Infections.* Chicago: Infectious Diseases Society of America; 1998:abstract 257.

6. **Autran B, Carcelain G, Li TS, et al.** Positive effects of combined antiretroviral therapy on CD4+ T-cell homeostasis and function in advanced HIV disease. *Science.* 1997;277:112–6.

7. **Race EM, Adelson-Mitty J, Kriegel GR, et al.** Focal mycobacterial lymphadenitis following initiation of protease-inhibitor therapy in patients with advanced HIV-1 disease. *Lancet.* 1998;351:252–5.

8. **Gill VJ, Park CH, Stoch F, et al.** Use of lysis-centrifugation (Isolator) and radiometric (BUCTOUCHE) blood culture systems for the detection of mycobacteremia. *J Clin Microbiol.* 1985;22:543–6.

9. **Wolf DG, Spector SA.** Diagnosis of human cytomegalovirus central nervous system disease in AIDS patients by DNA amplification from cerebrospinal fluid. *J Infect Dis.* 1992;166:1412–5.

10. **Minamoto GY, Rosenberg AS.** Fungal infections in patients with acquired immunodeficiency syndrome. *Med Clin North Am.* 1997;81:381–409.

11. **Kovacs A, Leaf HL, Simberkoff MS.** Bacterial infections. *Med Clin North Am.* 1997;81:319–43.

12. **Bissuel F, Leport C, Perronne C, et al.** Fever of unknown origin in HIV-infected patients: a critical analysis of a retrospective series of 57 cases. *J Intern Med.* 1994; 236:529–35.

13. **Barat LM, Gunn JE, Steger KA, et al.** Causes of fever in patients infected with human immunodeficiency virus who were admitted to Boston City Hospital. *Clin Infect Dis.* 1996;3:320–8.

14. **Barnes PF, Bloch AB, Davidson PT, Snider DE.** Tuberculosis in patients with human immunodeficiency virus infection. *N Engl J Med.* 1991;324:1644–50.

15. **Pitchenik AE, Rubinson A.** The radiographic appearance of tuberculosis in patients with the acquired immune deficiency syndrome (AIDS) and pre-AIDS. *Am Rev Respir Dis.* 1985;31:393–6.

16. **de Kleijn EM, van Lier HJ, van der Meer JW.** Fever of unknown origin (FUO). Part II: Diagnostic procedures in a prospective multicenter study of 167 patients (the Netherlands FUO Study Group). *Medicine.* 1997;76:401–14.

17. **Duong TA.** Infection due to Penicillium marneffei, an emerging pathogen: review of 155 reported cases. *Clin Infect Dis.* 1996;23:125–30.

18. **Hetherington S, Steel HM, Lafon S, et al.** Safety and tolerance of abacavir (1592,ABC) alone and in combination therapy of HIV infection. In *Twelfth World AIDS Conference.* Geneva, Switzerland; 1998:abstract 12353.

18a. **Fineman DS, Palestro CJ, Kim CK.** Detection of abnormalities in febrile AIDS patients with in-III-labeled leukocyte and ga-67 scintography. *Radiology.* 1989; 170:677–80.

19. **Nichols L, Florentine B, Lewis W, et al.** Bone marrow examination for the diagnosis of mycobacterial and fungal infections in the acquired immunodeficiency syndrome. *Arch Pathol Lab Med.* 1991;115:1125–32.

20. **Cavicchi M, Pialoux G, Carnot F, et al.** Value of liver biopsy for the rapid diagnosis of infection in human immunodeficiency virus-infected patients who have unexplained fever and elevated serum levels of alkaline phosphatase or gamma-glutamyl transferase. *Clin Infect Dis.* 1995;20:606–10.

21. **Kielhofner M, Atmar RL, Hamill RJ, Musher DM.** Life-threatening Pseudomonas aeruginosa infections in patients with human immunodeficiency virus infection. *Clin Infect Dis.* 1992;14:403–11.

22. **Magnani G, Elia GF, McNeil MM, et al.** Rhodococcus equi cavitary pneumonia in HIV-infected patients: an unsuspected opportunistic pathogen. *J Acquir Immune Defic Syndr.* 1992;5:1059–64.

23. **Trachiotis GD, Hafner GH, Hix WR, Aaron BL.** Role of open lung biopsy in diagnosing pulmonary complications of AIDS. *Ann Thorac Surg.* 1992;54:898–901.

24. **Clayton F, Clayton CH.** Gastrointestinal pathology in HIV-infected patients. *Gastroenterol Clin North Am.* 1997;26:191–240.

25. **Wilcox CM, Rabeneck L, Friedman S.** AGA Technical Review: malnutrition and cachexia, chronic diarrhea, and hepatobiliary disease in patients with HIV infection. *Gastroenterology.* 1996;111:1724–52.

26. **Poles MA, Lew EA, Dieterich DT.** Diagnosis and treatment of hepatic disease in patients with HIV. *Gastroenterol Clin North Am.* 1997;26:291–321.

27. **Dubin G, Braffman MN.** Zidovudine-induced hepatotoxicity. *Ann Intern Med.* 1989;110:85–6.

28. **Ockenga J, Tillmann HL, Trautwein C, et al.** Hepatitis B and C in HIV-infected patients: prevalence and prognostic value. *J Hepatol.* 1997;27:18–24.

29. **Dieterich DT, Wilcox CM.** Diagnosis and treatment of esophageal disorders associated with HIV infection: Practice Parameters Committee of the American College of Gastroenterology. *Am J Gastroenterol.* 1996;91:2265–9.

30. **Silva M, Skolnik PR, Gorbach SL, et al.** The effect of protease inhibitors on weight and body composition in HIV-infected patients. *AIDS.* 1998;12:1645–51.

31. **Wheeler DA, Gilbert CL, Launer CA, et al.** Weight loss as a predictor of survival and disease progression in HIV infection. Terry Beirn Community Programs for Clinical Research on AIDS. *J Acquir Immune Defic Syndr.* 1998;18:80–5.

31a. **Holloway RG, Kieburtz KD.** Headache and the human immunodeficiency virus type 1 infection. Headache 1995;35:245–55.

32. **Price RW.** Neurologic complications of HIV infection. *Lancet.* 1996;348:445–52.

33. **Clark RA, Brandon W, Dumestre J, et al.** Clinical manifestations of infection with human immunodeficiency virus in women in Louisiana. *Clin Infect Dis.* 1993;17:165–72.

34. **Anastos K, Deneberg R, Solomon L.** Human immunodeficiency virus in women. *Med Clin North Am.* 1997;81:533–54.

35. **Greenblatt RM, Barkan S, Delapenha R, et al.** Lower genital tract infections among HIV-infected women and high-risk seronegatives: the women's interagency HIV study (WIHS). In *Eleventh International Conference on AIDS.* Vancouver, Canada; 1996:abstract We.C.3402.

36. **Wright TC, Ellerbock TV, Chaisson MA, et al.** Cervical intraepithelial neoplasia in women infected with human immunodeficiency virus: prevalence, risk factors, and validity of Papanicolaou smears: New York Cervical Disease Study. *Obstet Gynecol.* 1994;8:591.

37. **Barbosa C, Macasaet M, Brockmann S, et al.** Pelvic inflammatory disease and human immunodeficiency virus infection. *Obstet Gynecol.* 1997;89;65–70.

38. **Ellerbrock TV, Wright TC, Bush TJ, et al.** Characteristics of menstruation in women infected with human immunodeficiency virus. *Obstet Gynecol.* 1996;87:1030–4.

39. **Porras B, Costner M, Friedman-Klein AE, Cockerell CJ.** Update on cutaneous manifestations of HIV infection. *Med Clin North Am.* 1998;82:1033–80.

40. **Coopman SA, Johnson RA, Platt RE, et al.** Cutaneous disease and drug reactions in HIV infection. *N Engl J Med.* 1990;328:1670–4.

41. **Gilson IH, Barnett JH, Conans MA, et al.** Disseminated ecthymatous varicella-zoster infection in patients with acquired immunodeficiency syndrome. *J Am Acad Dermatol.* 1989;20:637–42.

42. **Koehler JE, Quinn FD, Berger TG, et al.** Isolation of Rochalimaea species from cutaneous and osseous lesions of bacillary angiomatosis. *N Engl J Med.* 1992;327:1625–31.

43. **Rosenthal D, Leboit PE, Lumpp L, et al.** Human immunodeficiency virus–associated eosinophilic folliculitis: a unique dermatitis associated with advanced human immunodeficiency virus infection. *Arch Dermatol.* 1992;127:206–9.

44. **Dover JS, Johnson RA.** Cutaneous manifestations of human immunodeficiency virus infection. *Arch Dermatol.* 1991;127:1381–91,1549–58.

8

■ ■ ■

Diagnosis and Management of Opportunistic Infections

Tamar Barlam, MD
Lori A. Panther, MD

The advent of effective combination antiretroviral therapy and improvement in primary prophylaxis has resulted in a significant reduction in the incidence of HIV-related opportunistic infections (OIs) over the past several years. However, they continue to occur with regularity in some populations, including in individuals who are unaware of their HIV-positive serostatus, have difficulty accessing care, are not adherent to medical regimens, and have not responded well to antiretroviral therapy. This chapter reviews the epidemiology, pathogenesis, clinical manifestations, diagnosis, and management of these conditions. Primary prophylaxis for these infections is discussed in Chapter 6.

Bacterial Infections

Bartonellosis

Epidemiology

The development of sophisticated molecular diagnostic techniques and the advent of the HIV epidemic resulted in better characterization and increased detection of *Bartonella* species infection. *Bartonella* infection in an AIDS patient was first suggested in 1983, manifesting as subcutaneous nodules with bacterial forms on Warthin–Starry stain and distinct from Kaposi's sarcoma in histopathology. In 1990, the organism was phylogenetically characterized as being related to *Rochalimaea quintana*, the agent of trench fever, and subsequently was named *R. henselae*. In 1993, *Rochalimaea* species was renamed *Bartonella* species. In 1991, the Armed Forces Institute of Pathology invoked their acronym to a newly described agent of cat scratch disease (CSD), *Afipia felis*, which was distinct from what was then the *Rochalimaea* species. Subsequent work in speciation has revealed that most of what we now know as CSD, or its systemic equivalent, bacillary angiomatosis (BA), is caused by *Bartonella henselae* or *B. quintana*.

Pathogenesis
Inoculation with *Bartonella* species via a lick or a bite from a cat or kitten evokes an inflammatory response and endothelial proliferation resulting in a nodule at the site of inoculation with associated regional lymphadenopathy (CSD). In HIV-infected patients, the organism can disseminate, resulting in inflamed, vascular nodules or cysts within the skin, lymph nodes, or viscera (BA).

Clinical Manifestations
In immunocompetent patients, CSD manifests as an ulcerated nodule at site of inoculation associated with regional lymphadenopathy. It usually resolves in 1 to 2 months without treatment and rarely is associated with systemic symptoms. In HIV-positive individuals, the cutaneous manifestation of BA occurs as rapidly proliferating papules or ulcerated nodules that easily bleed and that can be confused with Kaposi's sarcoma (Table 8.1 and Fig. 8.1). In addition, disseminated infection can occur. Fever is universal; abdominal pain and increased serum transaminase and alkaline phos-

Table 8.1   Features of Bacillary Angiomatosis and Kaposi's Sarcoma

Feature	Bacillary Angiomatosis	Kaposi's Sarcoma
Lesion appearance	Red papule/nodule, plaque rare; blanching; bleeds easily; painful	Purple papule/nodule/plaque; nonblanching; does not bleed easily; not painful
Progression in size and number of lesions	Often very rapid	Usually slow; occasionally rapid
Bone lesions	Sometimes	No
Systemic symptoms	Often	Rare
Histology	Round vascular space; plump endothelial cells; WBC infiltrate; stromal edema	Slit-like vascular space; spindled endothelial cells; no WBC infiltrate; no stromal edema

WBC = white blood cell.

phatase levels are common if there is liver involvement. Dissemination to other organs (e.g., meninges, brain, bones) also has been documented.

Diagnosis

Diagnosis of BA can be made histopathologically from tissue biopsy. Classic findings on hematoxylin and eosin stain are lobular proliferation of small blood vessels with plump endothelial cells, stromal edema, inflammation, and granular clumps of eosinophilic material representing clumps of organisms. Warthin–Starry stain is used to delineate the organisms. Electron microscopy shows trilaminar-walled bacillary organisms. *Bartonella* infection of the liver occurs histologically as *peliosis hepatis*. Peliosis occurs in infected tissues that do not have a continuous endothelium, such as liver, spleen, and lymph nodes. Histologic examination shows large lakes of blood-filled cavities with surrounding stromal edema and eosinophilic material, which represents collections of the organism.

Culture of blood and infected tissues is recommended. Although culture of tissues is particularly difficult, the yield of blood cultures is somewhat better when blood-enriched lysis-centrifuged media is used. The yield of blood cultures in BA is 50%. Serologic testing for *B. henselae*, available through the Centers for Disease Control and Prevention (CDC), is positive

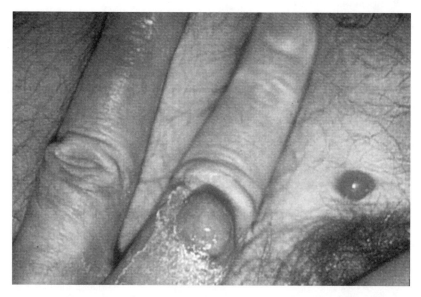

Figure 8.1   Characteristic skin lesions of bacillary angiomatosis. (Republished with permission from Koehler JE, LeBoit PE, Egbert BM, Berger TG. Cutaneous vascular lesions and disseminated cat-scratch disease in patients with the acquired immunodeficiency syndrome (AIDS) and AIDS-related complex. *Ann Intern Med.* 1988;109:449–55.)

in 88% of clinically suspected BA cases compared with 3% of healthy controls. Polymerase chain reaction (PCR) and speciation using either sequencing or molecular techniques are available in research settings.

Management
Because *Bartonella* infection is unusual in HIV disease, treatment recommendations are based on past experience and case reports. Standard doses of erythromycin, clarithromycin, azithromycin, and doxycycline all have been used with success. The length of therapy is based on the severity of illness, with 2 months recommended for isolated cutaneous disease, 3 months for bacteremia or suspected bacteremia, and 4 months for deep organ infection, osteomyelitis, or endocarditis. A clinical response usually is seen in 2 to 3 days. A Jarisch–Herxheimer reaction has been described on initiation of therapy.

A single episode of BA does not require maintenance therapy, but it is indicated for recurrent infection. Primary prevention is focused on proper advisement of HIV-positive patients regarding cat ownership. They should avoid licks, scratches, or bites from cats and contact with kittens and should pursue flea-control measures. In addition, when adopting a cat, patients should be advised to avoid those under one year of age.

Community-acquired Pneumonia

Epidemiology
Community-acquired pneumonia (CAP) is common in HIV-infected patients, with the highest risk in injection-drug users. Most frequent causative agents include *Streptococcus pneumoniae*, *Staphylococcus aureus*, *Haemophilus influenzae*, *Klebsiella pneumoniae*, and *Pseudomonas aeruginosa*. A few reports also have noted *Legionella* species at an increased frequency compared with the general population. Two thirds of all HIV-infected patients presenting with CAP have a CD4 count of fewer than 200 cells/mm^3. The risk of pneumococcal pneumonia is approximately five to 15 times that of seronegative individuals. Pneumococcal bacteremia is 100 times as frequent, but mortality rates are similar.

Pathogenesis
The increased risk of bacterial pneumonia in HIV disease probably is related to diminished immune function rather than increased exposure or colonization. Decreased B-cell activation, opsonizing ability, and antibody-dependent cytotoxicity all seem to contribute.

Clinical Manifestations
Symptoms of CAP in HIV-infected patients are similar to those of the general population, with acute onset of fever, productive cough, pleuritic chest pain,

and dyspnea. Atypical pneumonia with *Legionella* species, *Mycoplasma pneumoniae*, and respiratory viruses should be considered in patients with a nonproductive cough. There is the added risk of a coincident infection with opportunistic pathogens, such as *Pneumocystis carinii* or *Mycobaterium tuberculosis*, and this possibility should be considered if the patient fails to improve.

Diagnosis

Sputum examination establishes a presumptive microbiologic diagnosis in 50% of patients with pneumococcal pneumonia. The sputum Gram stain is most helpful when there are fewer than 10 epithelial cells and greater than 25 leukocytes per high-power field, with a predominant bacterial population present. Sputum cultures are less helpful because of overgrowth of oropharyngeal flora. Blood cultures are positive in 60% of HIV-infected patients compared with 15% to 30% of seronegative individuals.

Ninety percent of patients have a unilateral infiltrate on chest radiograph; pleural effusions and cavitary lesions are less common. In patients with diffuse infiltrates, atypical pathogens or *P. carinii* pneumonia (PCP) should be considered. Laboratory abnormalities are similar to the HIV-negative population, with leukocytosis and hypoxemia being common.

Management

The response to antibiotic therapy is similar to that of seronegative individuals. A 10- to 14-day course of antibiotics is recommended. Penicillin-resistant *S. pneumoniae* does not seem to occur at greater frequency. Initial therapy with ceftriaxone, with or without erythromycin *or* levofloxacin, is recommended. Concomitant pulmonary infections should be considered if the patient does not show improvement over 3 to 5 days.

The recurrence rate of pneumococcal disease is 13% in HIV-infected patients compared with 7% of controls, with the risk increasing as the CD4 cell count declines. Immunization against pneumococcus is recommended in all HIV-infected patients, with 85% of clinical isolates included in the 23-valent pneumococcal polysaccharide vaccine. In addition, chronic oral antibiotic prophylaxis with trimethoprim-sulfamethoxazole (TMP-SMX) or another antibiotic active against pneumococcus also is effective. It is debatable whether *H. influenzae* vaccine should be administered routinely to HIV-infected patients, because type b strains comprise a minority of invasive infections.

Mycobacterium avium Complex Infection

Epidemiology

Mycobacterium avium and *M. intracellulare*, referred to as *M. avium* complex (MAC), are atypical mycobacteria that cause disseminated disease in HIV-infected patients with CD4 counts of fewer than 50 to 75 cells/mm^3.

Before the widespread use of primary prophylaxis, MAC was the initial OI in 24% of patients and was found at autopsy in over 75% of cases.

Ubiquitous in the environment, MAC is found particularly in water sources, including fresh and sea water, tap water, and steam heat. Both respiratory and gastrointestinal colonization precede MAC infection, and positive local cultures are predictive of systemic infection. However, routine surveillance cultures are not recommended because 62% of individuals with MAC infection have negative results.

Clinical Manifestations

MAC infection manifests with fever, night sweats, and diarrhea with weight loss. On physical examination, patients may have lymphadenopathy, hepatosplenomegaly, and evidence of wasting. Unlike tuberculosis (TB), MAC does not cause pulmonary disease often; cavitary and nodular pulmonary infiltrates occur in approximately 2.5% of patients.

MAC lymphadenitis has been reported after the institution of combination antiretroviral therapy. Patients develop fever, adenitis, leukocytosis, and necrotizing granulomata 1 to 3 weeks into therapy. The syndrome is thought to represent an exuberant inflammatory response of subclinical infection to immune system reconstitution.

Diagnosis

Laboratory examination may reveal anemia, leukopenia, and/or thrombocytopenia; an increased serum alkaline phosphatase level also may be revealed. Lysis centrifugation isolator blood cultures are used to diagnose MAC infection but may take several weeks to become positive. These cultures, which are sensitive for intracellular organisms, are performed by lysing mononuclear cells and plating them to solid media on which colony counts can be quantified. Less commonly, bone marrow or liver biopsy is necessary for diagnosis.

Pathology of infected sites shows distended histiocytes filled with acid-fast bacilli, minimal inflammatory response, and poorly formed granulomata (Fig. 8.2). M. genavense is a poorly growing, fastidious mycobacterium. It has similar manifestations as MAC infection and responds to the same therapeutic agents. It, as well as extrapulmonary TB, should be considered in patients with positive acid-fast smears consistent with MAC but who have negative culture results.

Management

Therapy for MAC infection was marginally effective before the availability of the macrolides clarithromycin and azithromycin. Medical regimens today generally consist of three drugs: clarithromycin or azithromycin in combination with ethambutol and rifabutin (Table 8.2). Ciprofloxacin and amikacin sometimes are used as alternative agents as part of a multidrug regimen. Previous prophylaxtic therapy with macrolides should be taken into account when choosing a treatment.

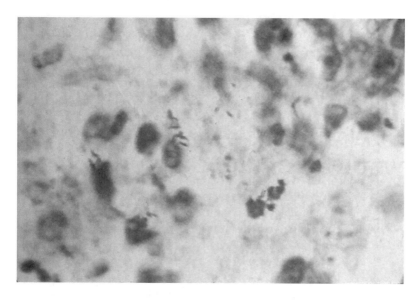

Figure 8.2   *Mycobacterium avium* complex infection diagnosed by liver biopsy. (From *Hospital Physician.* Turner White communications; Apr 1988.)

Azithromycin prophylaxis selects for macrolide resistance to a lesser degree than clarithromycin. Ethambutol has minimal toxicity at current dosing recommendations and is additive or synergistic with other agents. Rifabutin drug interactions must be considered carefully. For example, therapy with clarithromycin and rifabutin increases rifabutin levels by 100% and decreases clarithromycin levels by 50%. Concomitant treatment with fluconazole independently increases rifabutin levels. Uveitis (e.g., ocular pain, redness, photophobia, hypopyon) is uncommon when patients are given rifabutin 300 mg/d. A dose reduction is necessary if rifabutin is given with ritonavir, indinavir, nelfinavir, or amprenavir and a dose increase is necessary if given with efavirenz. Rifabutin is contraindicated with the other protease inhibitors. Fluoroquinolones, such as ciprofloxacin, have activity against 20% to 30% of MAC isolates. Amikacin can be used in severe cases and in patients who are not responding to treatment. Clofazimine, previously a component of MAC treatment regimens, has been associated with increased mortality and is no longer recommended. The use of adjunctive steroids in end-stage patients with MAC infection may result in improved constitutional symptoms and weight gain without significant risks.

Response to treatment for MAC infection may be gradual and take several weeks. Secondary antimicrobial prophylaxis should be maintained indefinitely. There are insufficient data at this time to know whether therapy for MAC can be discontinued safely in patients on combination antiretroviral therapy who have a sustained rise in their CD4 count over 100 cells/mm^3. Studies are ongoing to address this question. MAC lymphadenitis related to initiation of combination antiretroviral therapy should be

Table 8.2   Drugs Used in the Treatment of Mycobacterial Infections

Drug	Usual dose	Major toxicities
Amikacin	7.5 mg/kg every 12–24 hours IM or IV	Nephrotoxicity Ototoxicity
Azithromycin	500 mg/d orally	Gastrointestinal intolerance Hepatotoxicity Rash Headache Dizziness Reversible hearing loss
Ciprofloxacin	500–750 mg twice daily orally	Gastrointestinal intolerance Neurotoxicity Rash
Clarithromycin	500 mg twice daily orally	Gastrointestinal intolerance Hepatotoxicity Rash Headache Dizziness Reversible hearing loss
Ethambutol	15–25 mg/kg/d orally	Optic neuritis Rash Gastrointestinal intolerance Hepatotoxicity
Isoniazid	300 mg/d orally	Hepatotoxicity Fever Rash Peripheral neuropathy
Pyrazinamide	25 mg/kg/d orally	Hepatotoxicity Hyperuricemia Rash
Rifabutin	300–450 mg/d orally	Gastrointestinal intolerance Hepatotoxicity Rash Orange discoloration of secretions Uveitis
Rifampin	600 mg/d orally	Gastrointestinal intolerance Hepatotoxicity Rash Orange discoloration of secretions
Streptomycin	15 mg/kg/d IM	Ototoxicity Vestibular toxicity

IM = intramuscularly; IV = intravenously.

treated specifically. Antiviral agents can be continued, and consideration should be given to the addition of anti-inflammatory therapy.

Salmonellosis

Epidemiology

Although *Salmonella* bacteremia accounts for less than 1% of all OIs, recurrent bacteremia in HIV-infected patients occurs at 20-fold the incidence of seronegative individuals. All patients with recurrent *Salmonella* infection should be screened for HIV infection. Nontyphoidal species predominate. Transmission is generally from food or animal sources, but unusual sources such as marijuana have been reported. Unlike *Campylobacter* and *Shigella*, *Salmonella* is not an organism primarily acquired via sexual transmission; low socioeconomic status is the most common risk factor. Bacteremia occurs in almost one half of all HIV-infected patients with *Salmonella* enteritis.

Pathogenesis

HIV-induced defects in local mucosal and systemic humoral and cell-mediated immunity lead to bloodstream invasion once the organism establishes an infection in the gastrointestinal mucosa. These same defects may lead to its persistence in macrophages and a resultant increased risk of recurrent bacteremia.

Clinical Manifestations

Recurrent salmonellosis is a CDC-defined criterion for AIDS. Most patients present with fever, chills, sweats, anorexia, and weight loss. Gastrointestinal complaints are also common. Co-existence of other gastrointestinal diseases, such as cytomegalovirus (CMV) or parasitic infections and Kaposi's sarcoma, predispose to bacteremia. Local suppurative complications (e.g., abscesses in spleen, brain, meninges, lung, urinary tract) have been described. Relapse is common and increased in patients who have bacteremia and in those who did not receive quinolone therapy for their previous infection.

Diagnosis

Blood cultures provide the highest yield for diagnosis of invasive salmonellosis and should be performed in HIV-infected patients who have either systemic or gastrointestinal symptoms of infection. Commonly isolated strains include *Salmonella enteritidis*, *S. typhimurium*, *S. heidelberg*, *S. arizonae*, and *S. dublin*. Approximately one third of patients with gastroenteritis will have bacteremia. Laboratory studies may show leukocytosis and increased liver function tests.

Management

A 2-week course of therapy for *Salmonella* bacteremia is recommended. Ciprofloxacin is the drug of choice, but ceftriaxone or TMP-SMX can be used if quinolones are contraindicated. Quinolones have superior penetration into macrophages in which the organism persists and, by this mechanism, may decrease the risk of recurrent disease.

Long-term suppressive oral antibiotic therapy is recommended if *Salmonella* infection recurs. Patient education should performed regarding food handling, travel, health risks of keeping reptiles as pets, and proper needle cleaning.

Syphilis

Epidemiology
Since the late 1980s, the overall incidence of syphilis has decreased appreciably, although recently there has been an increase in syphilis in young urban adolescents. The incidence of syphilis is almost 20-fold higher in African emigrants. There is a definite link between genital ulcer diseases, such as syphilis, and the risk of acquiring HIV infection. One study reported that all HIV-positive individuals presenting to a sexually transmitted diseases clinic had evidence of active syphilis at five times the rate of HIV-negative controls.

Pathogenesis
The causative agent of syphilis, *Treponema pallidum*, is a spirochete appearing as slender helical cells with three cilia at each end. Syphilis usually is spread via sexual contact but can be transmitted by kissing, direct inoculation (needle stick), and transplacentally. The organism at first proliferates locally in the inoculated area and regional lymph nodes, after which a bacteremia occurs in which organs and tissues of the reticuloendothelial system are seeded.

Clinical Manifestations
The natural history of syphilis is divided into primary, secondary, early latent, late latent, and tertiary stages. Primary syphilis begins with a skin chancre after an incubation period of a few weeks to months from inoculation. The chancre is classically nontender, clean-based, and associated with regional lymphadenopathy. In the HIV-infected patient, chancres may be multiple.

The secondary stage occurs at approximately 6 weeks after contact and is associated with disseminated skin and mucosal lesions and generalized lymphadenopathy (Fig. 8.3). If primary syphilis is untreated, 60% to 90% of patients will go on to the secondary stage. In a minority of cases, the secondary stage may develop while the chancre is still present. Dissemination to the central nervous system (CNS) is common, although symptomatic acute syphilitic meningitis occurs in only 1% to 3% of patients. Patients with both primary and secondary syphilis are potentially infectious to their sexual partners.

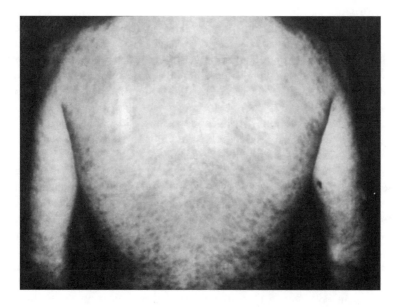

Figure 8.3   Generalized cutaneous eruption of secondary syphilis. (From *Ann Intern Med.* 1987;107:492–5.)

Latent syphilis is an asymptomatic stage, divided up into early latency (designated as within the first year after the secondary stage when relapses of secondary syphilis are common) and late latency (designated as beyond the first year). In the latent stage of syphilis, perinatal transmission is still possible.

Tertiary syphilis is rare, occurring 10 to 45 years after initial acquisition and is characterized by an obliterative endarteritis affecting multiple organs, such as the heart and great vessels, brain, skin, bone, and viscera.

Neurosyphilis is seen in 10% of untreated patients and can occur at any stage. HIV-infected patients are no more likely to present with neurosyphilis than seronegative individuals, although symptomatic meningeal and meningovascular syphilis may be more common. Syphilitic meningitis presents within 5 years of infection. Meningovascular syphilis can occur in the first 10 years after infection, presenting with multiple small infarcts of the brain and spinal cord and similar cerebrospinal fluid (CSF) abnormalities. *Tabes dorsalis* and parenchymatous neurosyphilis are associated with tertiary syphilis.

Our knowledge of syphilis in the context of HIV disease is based on numerous case reports and series but few prospective data. These cases have suggested that HIV-infected patients with syphilis may have atypical clinical presentations, altered serologic response to infection, an increased frequency of neurosyphilis, and an inadequate clinical response to standard therapy. However, clinical experience suggests that most HIV-infected patients with syphilis have typical disease manifestations.

Diagnosis

Diagnosis of syphilis usually is based on serologic evidence, because culture of the organism is not possible in the clinical laboratory. Serologic tests in HIV-positive individuals should be interpreted as for the general population, although there are a few case reports of seronegativity or delayed serologic response due to defects in B-cell function. In these instances, consider either repeating the serology or performing a biopsy of skin or mucous membrane lesions if clinical suspicion for syphilis remains high. Diagnosis of syphilis can be made by darkfield examination of serous fluid or immunofluorescent staining of skin lesions.

Nonspecific treponemal tests (rapid plasma reagin [RPR] and Venereal Disease Research Laboratory test for syphilis [VDRL]) are quantitative, less specific, and indicate the degree of disease activity. Specific treponemal tests (fluorescent treponemal antibody [FTA], *Treponema pallidum* hemagglutination [TPHA], and microhemagglutination–*Treponema pallidum* [MHA-TP]) are qualitative, specific, and indicate whether the patient has ever been exposed to syphilis. The nonspecific treponemal test becomes positive 4 to 7 days after the primary lesion appears. Although the nonspecific test can be negative in both primary and tertiary syphilis, it is almost always positive in secondary syphilis.

The role of lumbar puncture (LP) in the evaluation of HIV-positive patients with syphilis is controversial; the CDC does not recommend it for all patients. Because CSF abnormalities occur in 40% of the HIV-positive population overall, the clinical utility of performing a LP in this setting remains to be defined. LP is recommended for any patient with inexplicable neurological symptoms, a serum VDRL greater than 1:32, treatment failure (*see* below), late latent syphilis, or syphilis of unknown duration.

In neurosyphilis, CSF examination usually shows a positive VDRL, modest pleocytosis, increased protein level, and a moderately low glucose. Although a positive CSF VDRL confirms active neurosyphilis, a negative CSF VDRL does not exclude it. If the CSF VDRL is negative and CSF indices are suggestive of neurosyphilis, a CSF MHA-TP can be performed. If the CSF MHA-TP is negative, CNS syphilis is ruled out but a positive CSF MHA-TP is not diagnostically helpful.

Management

The treatment regimens for syphilis by stage are presented in Table 8.3. They are the same in HIV-infected and seronegative patients. Penicillin remains the drug of choice. For penicillin-allergic patients, doxycycline 100 mg orally twice daily for 14 days can be considered in early-stage syphilis. Penicillin should be used to treat neurosyphilis, with desensitization performed if there is a history of drug allergy.

A dilemma in the treatment of syphilis is the persistently positive serum VDRL. The serum VDRL ideally should become negative within 1 year for primary, 2 years for secondary, and 5 years for tertiary syphilis. If this does

Table 8.3   Treatment of Syphilis

Primary, secondary, and early latent (<1 year duration) syphilis

Recommended regimen: 2.4 mIU benzathine penicillin G IM once
Doxycycline, 100 mg twice weekly orally for 2 weeks, if penicillin allergic

Late latent (>1 year duration) and cardiovascular syphilis

Recommended regimen: 2.4 mIU/wk benzathine penicillin G IM for 3 weeks
  (total 7.2 mIU)
Doxycycline, 100 mg twice weekly orally for 4 weeks, if penicillin allergic

Neurosyphilis*

Recommended regimen: 18–24 mIU/d aqueous penicillin G IV for 10–14 days
Alternative: 2.4 mIU/d procaine penicillin IM plus 50 mg probenecid four times
  daily for 10–14 days
If patient is penicillin allergic, skin test and desensitize as necessary

IM = intramuscularly; IV = intravenously.
*Note: Following completion of a neurosyphilis regimen, many authorities recommend the administration of 2.4 mIU/wk benzathine penicillin for 3 weeks.
Adapted from Centers for Disease Control. 1998 Sexually transmitted disease treatment guidelines. *MMWR Morbid Mortal Wkly Rep.* 1998;47(RR-1):28–40.

not occur, three possibilities should be considered: persistent infection, re-infection, and a false-positive test. Serum VDRL should be followed at 3, 6, 9, 12, and 24 months for early and 6, 12, 18, and 24 months for late latent or neurosyphilis. Failure is defined as 1) an inability of VDRL to be reduced fourfold or greater, or 2) a fourfold increase in VDRL at any time during follow-up. In these cases, an LP should be performed, and the patient should be treated for neurosyphilis if indicated or retreated with three weekly doses of benzathine penicillin if the CSF examination is negative.

Because one third of all sexual contacts of patients with early syphilis contract the infection, contact tracing should be performed on confirmed cases. All sexual contacts of a primary-stage syphilis patient within 3 months of the index case diagnosis should be given penicillin. All contacts of patients with secondary and tertiary syphilis should be evaluated and treated as appropriate.

Tuberculosis

Epidemiology and Microbiology

Tuberculosis (TB) is one of the most significant infectious diseases in the world. The alarming increase in cases of active TB noted in the United States in the mid-1980s was multifactorial, but HIV infection was an important association. At least half the patients with positive cultures for TB in New York City from 1992 to 1995 were co-infected with HIV and had a median CD4 count of 71 cells/mm^3. By mid-1995, 6 million people worldwide were co-infected with HIV and TB. By the year 2000, 14% of all new TB infections (1.4 million cases) will be in the setting of HIV disease. It is unknown whether HIV-infected patients are more susceptible to acquisition of TB, but once infected they are at much higher risk for progression to active disease. In one study, 15% of HIV-infected injection-drug users with a reactive skin test (PPD) developed active TB within 2 years compared with none in the control group.

Multidrug-resistant TB also markedly increased in the 1980s, and most documented outbreaks occurred in HIV-infected patients. Infection usually is contracted during clinic visits or hospitalizations on units specializing in HIV care. Rapid progression from infection to active disease has been observed, with a median survival of only 66 days. Immediate treatment with at least two active drugs improves prognosis; however, patients with low CD4 counts had poor treatment response. Restoration of strict infection control practices and use of directly observed therapy have curtailed this epidemic.

Clinical Manifestations

In HIV-infected patients with higher CD4 cell counts, TB is most often the result of reactivation of previous infection, and the usual presentation consists of fever and pulmonary symptoms. Chest radiograph shows localized pulmonary infiltrates or cavities. At lower CD4 counts, the presentation of TB is more likely to be atypical. Chest radiograph can show diffuse alveolar and interstitial infiltrates (60%), focal consolidation (30%), or pleural effusion (10%). Twenty-five percent have mediastinal and intrathoracic adenopathy, which may caseate and form abscesses that erode into adjacent structures. There is less cavitary and upper lobe disease. Up to 70% of TB patients with advanced HIV disease have extrapulmonary infection, which can involve the skin, lymph nodes, CNS, liver, bone marrow, and/or genitourinary tract (Fig. 8.4).

Diagnosis

It is more difficult to diagnose TB in HIV-infected patients than in the general population because of atypical clinical presentations, lower yield of sputum cultures, and cutaneous anergy. As HIV infection progresses and cellular immunity declines, the PPD often becomes nonreactive, and chest radiograph findings are more nonspecific. All patients with possible TB should have a PPD placed; control tests are no longer necessary. A positive PPD in the context of HIV disease is defined as 5 mm of induration or greater. Examination of the sputum for acid-fast organisms should be performed if there is evidence of pulmonary disease. However, HIV-infected patients are more

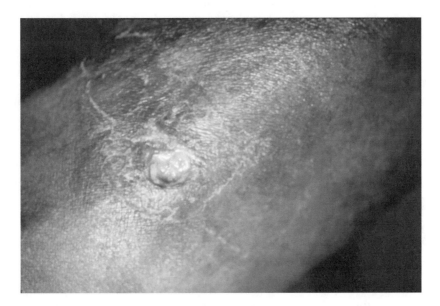

Figure 8.4   Cutaneous tuberculosis in patient with advanced HIV disease. (For color reproduction, *see* Plate 1 at back of book.)

likely to have negative smears than are seronegative individuals. If the smear demonstrates acid-fast bacilli, PCR techniques are available to distinguish *Mycobacterium tuberculosis* from atypical mycobacteria.

It is important to culture the organism for identification and susceptibility testing. Systems using liquid rather than solid media and radiometric methodology to identify positive cultures (e.g., BACTEC) provide reliable culture results in 1 to 2 weeks and sensitivity data 1 week later. Patients with disseminated TB often have positive blood cultures using either the BACTEC system or lysis centrifugation isolator cultures.

Management
Bacteriologic response to TB treatment is similar in HIV-infected patients and seronegative individuals. Historically, however, survival is shortened in HIV disease once active TB develops. Viral loads do not return to baseline despite successful therapy, which is possibly secondary to cytokine activation.

Table 8.2 lists the commonly used antimycobacterial agents. Most patients should receive four-drug therapy with isoniazid (INH), rifampin (RIF), pyrazinamide (PZA), and a fourth drug (e.g., ethambutol, streptomycin) for 2 months until culture sensitivity is known. If the strain is susceptible, therapy should continue with INH and RIF daily or biweekly for at least 6 months after cultures are negative. Some studies suggest that relapse is lower if treatment continues for 12 months total. Extrapulmonary disease is often treated for longer periods. If multidrug-resistant TB is suspected, initial therapy should be with six or more drugs, depending on the susceptibility data for strains prevalent in the particular region. Infectious disease consultation is recommended.

There is growing evidence that rifabutin can be substituted for rifampin. This has particular relevance because rifabutin has different drug interactions and can be used with some protease inhibitors. Rifabutin also is occasionally of use in rifampin-resistant strains. Rifapentine, a long-acting rifamycin with activity against *M. tuberculosis* and MAC, recently has been approved for use. Although results are encouraging, patients treated with once-weekly INH and rifapentine who relapsed had a higher rate of rifampin resistance.

The use of the tumor necrosis factor inhibitors, such as pentoxifylline, and thalidomide has been studied as an adjunct in the treatment of TB in HIV-infected patients. Pentoxifylline did not show a significant clinical effect, but anemia improved while on therapy. Patients treated with thalidomide showed significant weight gain and improvement in viral load assays. However, this effect reversed as soon as therapy was discontinued. A significant number of severe rashes were associated with thalidomide therapy.

Fungal Infections

Candidiasis

Epidemiology
Mucosal infections with *Candida* species are extremely common in HIV disease. Virtually all HIV-infected patients experience oral candidiasis at some time in their disease process, and both oral and esophageal candidiasis can be a manifestation of primary HIV infection. Vulvovaginal candidiasis usually presents earlier than oral candidiasis in women. The incidence of esophageal candidiasis, which is an AIDS-defining diagnosis, is approximately 15%.

Pathogenesis
Candida species live as commensals in the oral cavity and the female genital tract. Decreased lymphocyte proliferative response to *Candida* antigen and decreased specific mucosal antibodies may predispose to mucosal infection in the setting of HIV disease.

Clinical Manifestations
Vulvovaginal candidiasis initially presents in women with a CD4 count of approximately 500 cells/mm^3, which is higher than for other mucosal *Candida* infections. Patients present with vulvar itching and a thick, white vaginal discharge.

Oral candidiasis initially occurs in patients with a CD4 count between 200 and 500 cells/mm³ and may involve part or all of the mucosa of the mouth and pharynx. Presenting symptoms may include oral discomfort and altered taste sensation. Generally, a white exudate is seen on physical examination, but an atrophic form, manifested by glistening mucosa, also has been described (Fig. 8.5). Another type of oral candidiasis is angular cheilitis, which is composed of painful fissures at the corners of the mouth.

Esophageal candidiasis presents in patients with a CD4 count of fewer than 200 cells/mm³. Symptoms include dysphagia, odynophagia, and retrosternal pain with swallowing. Although 30% of patients do not have associated oral candidiasis, esophageal symptoms occurring in its presence usually indicate contiguous spread of infection.

Despite the frequent occurrence of mucosal candidiasis, candidemia (or deep tissue involvement) is unusual. It is hypothesized that the presence of antibody directed against *Candida* species is more prevalent in HIV-infected individuals as a result of polyclonal B-cell activation, which may prevent dissemination. Disseminated *Candida* infection, when it occurs, is associated with classic risk factors, such as neutropenia, intravascular line infection, or chronic corticosteroid therapy.

Diagnosis

It is important to confirm diagnosis of vulvovaginal candidiasis by potassium hydroxide (KOH) preparation of vaginal fluid obtained during pelvic examination. Invasive forms, which exhibit pseudohyphae, can be distinguished from commensal organisms, which exist in oval yeast forms.

The diagnosis of oral candidiasis is suspected clinically and confirmed by KOH preparation of pharyngeal lesions. Differential diagnosis includes hairy leukoplakia, which manifests as white plaques on the tongue or buccal mucosa and cannot be removed by a tongue blade.

In esophageal candidiasis, esophagogastroduodenoscopy (EGD) demonstrates a white exudate overlying friable mucosa, and definitive diagnosis requires biopsy. In cases in which the clinical suspicion for esophageal symptoms is high, empiric antifungal therapy is initiated; EGD is reserved for those cases in which there is no clinical response to treatment. Barium swallow is not useful for diagnosis. Differential diagnosis of esophageal symptoms includes esophageal CMV, HSV, lymphoma, and Kaposi's sarcoma.

Management

Treatment for candidiasis is presented in Table 8.4. For vulvovaginal candidiasis, topical therapy with clotrimazole 2%, miconazole 1%, butaconazole 1%, or terconazole 0.5% cream is usually successful. A useful alternative medication is oral fluconazole. In rare situations, intravenous amphotericin B has been necessary.

For oral candidiasis, recommended topical therapy consists of 10-mg troches of clotrimazole or 100,000-U vaginal tablets of nystatin taken orally

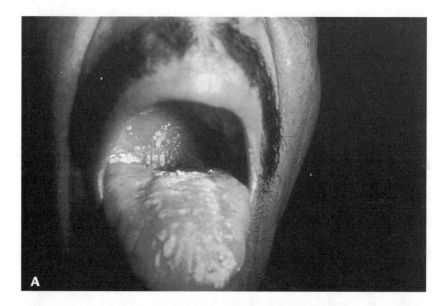

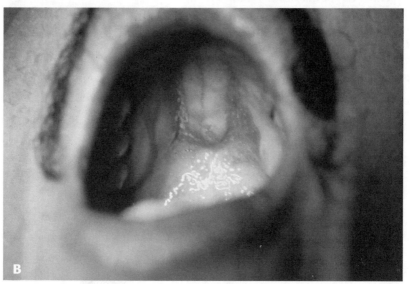

Figure 8.5   Pseudomembranous (A) and atrophic (B) variants of oral candidiasis. (For color reproduction, *see* Plates 2 and 3 at back of book.)

four to five times daily for 7 to 10 days; systemic therapy with fluconazole 100 mg/d is reserved for refractory cases. Therapy for esophageal candidiasis consists of fluconazole 100–200 mg/d. If there is no response within 7 to 10 days of initiating treatment, a diagnostic EGD is recommended. In re-

Table 8.4   Treatment of Candidiasis

Type of infection	Treatment
Thrush	Nystatin suspension swish and swallow, 5 mL five times daily *or* Clotrimazole troche 10 mg five times daily
Cutaneous infection	Clotrimazole or other antifungal cream
Vaginitis	Clotrimazole or other antifungal cream or troches
Oral, cutaneous, or vulvovaginal infection; refractory to topical therapy or frequently recurrent	Fluconazole 100 mg/d orally
Esophagitis	Fluconazole 100–200 mg/d orally
Fungemia or disseminated infection	Amphotericin B 0.6 mg/kg/d IV

IV = intravenously.

fractory cases, itraconazole suspension or intravenous amphotericin B therapy may be necessary.

Generally, maintenance therapy is not recommended for mucosal candidiasis in HIV-infected patients because of the potential for side effects, drug interactions, and the risk of emergence of resistance. However, it may be necessary in advanced HIV disease; fluconazole 50–200 mg/d is usually effective.

Cryptococcosis

Epidemiology
Cryptococcal disease is the most common life-threatening fungal infection in HIV-positive patients, with a mortality rate of approximately 20%. Between 5% and 10% of HIV-infected patients worldwide develop cryptococcal disease. Most of them have advanced immunodeficiency, with a CD4 count fewer than 100 cells/mm^3. Meningoencephalitis is the most common presentation, although pulmonary and cutaneous infections also have been described. The incidence of cryptococcosis is highest in injection-drug users, Africans, African-Americans, and Haitians.

Pathogenesis
Cryptococcus neoformans exists in a yeast form and is ubiquitous in soil. Its primary mode of acquisition is probably via the respiratory route, with sec-

ondary spread hematogenically to the brain, lungs, bone marrow, liver, and spleen. HIV-related abnormalities in opsonization, cell-mediated immunity, and humoral immunity permit its growth and dissemination. The polysaccharide capsule of *Cryptococcus* is poorly immunogenic, and minimal inflammation generally is observed in pathologic specimens.

Clinical Manifestations

Symptoms and signs of cryptococcal meningoencephalitis are often indolent and nonspecific. In HIV-positive patients, the mean time from onset of symptoms to diagnosis is 31 days. Fever is present in 60% to 80% of cases, headache in over 70%, altered mental status in 25%, meningismus in 20%, seizure in 5%, and focal neurological deficits in 6% to 11%. Extraneural cryptococcal disease occurs in 50% of patients. Features on presentation that portend a poor prognosis include extraneural disease, altered mental status, hyponatremia, CSF cryptococcal antigen (CRAG) greater than 1:1024, CSF white blood cell count (WBC) of fewer than 20 cells/mm^3, and CSF opening pressure greater than 30 cm H$_2$O.

Diagnosis

The serum CRAG is positive in 99% of patients who have cryptococcal meningoencephalitis. Rare false-positive tests occur from cross-reactivity with rheumatoid factor or concomitant systemic infection with *Trichosporon beigelii*. Rare false-negative CRAG tests occur in patients with poorly encapsulated strains.

A positive CSF CRAG is essential for diagnosis. Other indices are nonspecific and in rare cases may be entirely normal. CSF WBC usually shows a lymphocytosis of fewer than 100 cells/mm^3, and CSF glucose and protein levels vary widely. India ink examination of CSF is positive in 75% to 80% of cases showing 4 to 6 µM narrow-based, budding, round yeast cells with a distinct capsule (Fig. 8.6). Culture of the yeast from the CSF remains the "gold standard" for diagnosis, although rarely it may be negative if the organism load is low.

Brain imaging with computed tomography (CT) or magnetic resonance imaging (MRI) should be performed in all cases of suspected cryptococcal disease to rule out a space-occupying lesion. Differential diagnosis includes other subacute meningitides from mycobacterial or other fungal pathogens, partially treated bacterial meningitis (if the patient is on chronic antibiotics), viral meningoencephalitis, CNS syphilis, toxoplasmosis, and lymphoma.

Management

If the patient presents with severe cryptococcal disease manifested by altered mental status, cranial nerve palsy, high opening CSF pressure, or CSF CRAG titer greater than 1:64, then intravenous amphotericin B at 0.5–1.0 mg/kg/d is recommended (Table 8.5). It is administered until a total dose of 15 mg/kg is reached or symptoms resolve. The clinical response rate is

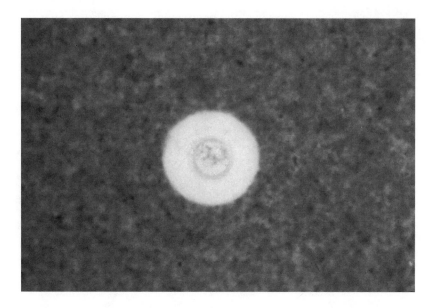

Figure 8.6   *Cryptococcus neoformans* on India ink stain of cerebrospinal fluid.

approximately 70%. Side effects of amphotericin B include phlebitis, fever, rigors, nausea, vomiting, anemia, hypokalemia, hypomagnesemia, and renal tubular acidosis. The addition of flucytosine to amphotericin B often is not well tolerated in HIV-infected patients because of hematologic and renal toxicity. Liposomal amphotericin B has less renal toxicity and can be used as an alternative agent in patients with underlying renal dysfunction. The effectiveness of liposomal amphotericin B in the treatment of cryptococcal disease in HIV-positive patients is still under investigation.

Compared with amphotericin B, fluconazole as initial therapy is associated with more early deaths, slower CSF organism clearance, and a lower response rate to treatment. Based on these observations, fluconazole generally is reserved for continuation of initial therapy once symptoms improve and for lifelong maintenance therapy to prevent relapse. An initial regimen of fluconazole only should be considered in patients with mild cryptococcal disease (normal mental status, nonfocal examination, normal opening pressure, CSF CRAG < 1:64). It is given in the dosage of 800 mg/d for 3 days, followed by 400 mg/d for 10 to 12 weeks. The role of itraconazole in the management of cryptococcal infection is not yet well defined.

Initial treatment regimens are changed to maintenance therapy after 10 to 12 weeks once clearance of *Cryptococcus* from CSF is documented by culture. Generally, oral fluconazole 200 mg/d is recommended. Relapse of cryptococcal meningoencephalitis while on maintenance therapy is a sig-

Table 8.5   Treatment of Cryptococcosis

Drug	Usual Dosage	Major Toxicities
Amphotericin B	Primary treatment: 0.5–1.0 mg/kg/d IV	Lower doses, especially when used alone, have not been very effective
	Maintenance treatment: generally fluconazole (see entry below)	Combination with flucytosine is not recommended Patients should be kept well hydrated Nonsteroidal anti-inflammatory drugs (e.g., ibuprofen) may decrease fever, chills, and rigors caused by amphotericin B
Fluconazole	Primary treatment: 400–800 mg/d orally Maintenance treatment: 200 mg/d orally	Measurement of serum fluconazole concentrations may be indicated in selected cases

IV = intravenously.

nificant predictor of mortality and may indicate persistent infection in sequestered sites such as the prostate gland.

Data are insufficient at this time to know whether secondary prophylaxis for cryptococcal infection can be discontinued safely in patients on combination antiretroviral therapy who have a sustained rise in their CD4 count to over 100 cells/mm^3. Studies are ongoing to address this question.

Histoplasmosis

Epidemiology and Pathogenesis
Histoplasmosis is a relatively common diagnosis in HIV-infected patients from endemic areas, such as the Ohio and Mississippi River valleys, Haiti, Puerto Rico, and South and Central America. Cases in patients who have not visited endemic areas for many years likely represent reactivation of latent infection.

The yeast *Histoplasma capsulatum* is found in soil. Primary histoplasmosis occurs when dust is stirred up and spores are aerosolized. HIV-infected patients, especially those with advanced disease, are at increased risk of disseminated infection. Histoplasmosis is not transmitted from person to person.

Clinical Manifestations
Disseminated histoplasmosis usually manifests as subacute constitutional symptoms, including fever, weight loss, and respiratory complaints (e.g.,

dyspnea, cough). Physical examination may reveal lymphadenopathy or splenomegaly. Chest radiography often reveals bilateral diffuse nodular infiltrates with or without adenopathy. However, dissemination to the spleen, liver, lymph nodes, bone marrow, or brain may occur in the absence of pulmonary involvement.

Diagnosis
The diagnostic yield of bronchoscopy is approximately 80% in the presence of pulmonary infiltrates. Bone marrow biopsy or blood culture has a sensitivity of approximately 90% in disseminated disease. Serologic testing of blood for *Histoplasma* antigen is also clinically useful.

Mangement
Amphotericin B (0.5–1.0 mg/kg/d IV for 7–14 days) is given as initial therapy for severe cases of histoplasmosis; itraconazole (300 mg po bid for 3 days then 200 mg po bid for 12 weeks) is used for mid to moderate infections. Itraconazole 200 mg/d should be given indefinitely for maintenance therapy. Primary prophylaxis with itraconazole should be considered in patients who live in an endemic area and have a CD4 cell count of fewer than 100 cells/mm^3.

Pneumocystis carinii Pneumonia

Epidemiology
The widespread use of primary and secondary prophylaxis for PCP has had a significant impact on the course of HIV disease. Mortality related to PCP has improved greatly since the onset of the epidemic, with survival rates increasing from approximately 50% to 90%. The incidence of PCP as an AIDS-indicator disease is decreasing in the United States and Europe, and PCP has always been relatively uncommon in developing countries. Patients presenting with PCP generally have a CD4 count of fewer than 200 cells/mm^3.

Pathogenesis
Historically, *Pneumocystis carinii* has been classified as a protozoan, although recent ribosomal RNA sequencing has shown it to be more closely related to fungi, specifically *Saccharomyces* species. However, antifungal agents are not effective against *P. carinii* because its cyst wall sterols are unlike those of most fungi. The organism is acquired via the respiratory route, but it is not thought to be transmitted from person to person. Ninety-five percent of people are colonized with *P. carinii* by age 5, and it is felt that most cases in adults are a result of reactivation of latent cyst forms attached to alveolar epithelium. On reactivation, sporozoites form within the cyst and emerge as mature trophozoites, which lead to inflammation and increased alveolar permeability.

Clinical Manifestations

Patients with PCP usually have a nonproductive cough, dyspnea on exertion, and fever for several days to weeks before presentation. Those who smoke may have a productive cough from an underlying bronchitis or a secondary infection with an encapsulated bacterial organism. Physical examination may show dry rales on chest auscultation, although it is often normal.

Patients on PCP prophylaxis may have an altered clinical presentation. The use of aerosol pentamidine (AP) has increased the risk of extrapulmonary pneumocystosis, which can involve the lymph nodes, bone marrow, spleen, liver, gastrointestinal tract, sinuses, and retina. Disseminated calcifications of lymph nodes and visceral organs should raise suspicion of extrapulmonary pneumocystosis.

Diagnosis

Chest radiograph shows bilateral interstitial infiltrates in 90% of patients on presentation, although it may be normal early in the course of infection (Fig. 8.7). Pneumothorax or focal infiltrates are unusual but have been reported; pleural effusions are rare and should raise the suspicion of another process, such as pulmonary Kaposi's sarcoma. Patients receiving AP prophylaxis may present with upper lobe infiltrates, pneumothorax, or intraparenchymal cysts. All patients should have a room-air arterial blood gas (ABG) or oximetry for the purpose of establishing the severity of disease. The serum lactate dehydrogenase (LDH) level is increased in over 90% of cases but is a nonspecific finding. A diffusion capacity for carbon monoxide (DLCO) of less than 80% suggests the diagnosis of PCP but is also not specific.

Given the broad differential diagnosis of interstitial pneumonias in HIV infection, every attempt should be made to diagnose PCP. Induced sputum

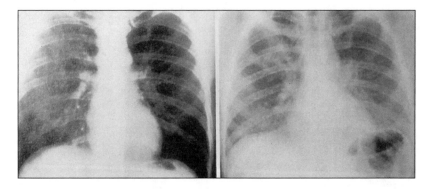

Figure 8.7   Serial chest radiographs showing the development of *Pneumocystis carinii* pneumonia. (From *Western J Med.* 1982;137:400–7.)

using monoclonal antibody testing is the diagnostic test of choice; if unavailable, bronchoalveolar lavage (BAL) can be performed. The mean yield of an induced sputum test is approximately 60% and depends on technical expertise in preparation of sample and the organism burden. BAL, with its 90% sensitivity, generally is reserved for cases when the sputum induction is negative. It is acceptable to start empiric PCP therapy before obtaining a diagnosis because the yield of the sputum examination does not decrease for at least several days. Transbronchial biopsy (TbBx) usually is not necessary to diagnose PCP. However, if no diagnosis is forthcoming from BAL, TbBx is indicated to rule out other possibilities. The use of AP decreases the sensitivity of sputum induction and BAL and results in lower organism load when the sputum induction is positive. However, the organism yield of TbBx does not decrease.

Management
Oral or intravenous TMP-SMX is the mainstay of treatment, but alternative regimens are available (Table 8.6). Side effects of TMP-SMX may include fever, rash, neutropenia, and increased liver function tests. If the drug rash is mild, it may be possible to "treat through" it with antihistamines, but other

---

Table 8.6   Treatment of *Pneumocystis carinii* Pneumonia

Oral Regimens

TMP-SMX 2 DS tablets orally every 8 hours for 21 days

TMP 15 mg/kg/d divided into 3–4 doses *and* dapsone 100 mg/d orally for 21 days

Clindamycin 450 mg orally four times daily *and* primaquine base 15 mg/d orally for
    21 days

Atovaquone suspension 750 mg orally twice daily for 21 days

Intravenous Regimens

TMP-SMX 15–20 mg (TMP component per kilogram per day divided into 3–4 IV
    doses) for 21 days

Pentamidine 3–4 mg/kg/d IV for 21 days

Clindamycin 600 mg IV four times daily *and* primaquine base 15 mg/d orally for
    21 days

Trimetrexate 45 mg/m^2/d IV for 21 days *and* folinic acid 20 mg/m^2 (IV or orally)
    four times daily for 24 days

*Adjunctive Use of Corticosteroids**

Prednisone 40 mg orally twice daily for 5 days, followed by 40 mg/d orally for
    5 days, followed by 20 mg/d orally for 11 days

DS = double-strength; IV = intravenously; TMP-SMX = trimethoprim-sulfamethoxazole.
* Only if partial pressure of arterial blood (PaO$_2$) is less than 70 or alveolar-arterial gradient is greater than 35.

toxicities may necessitate a change in therapy. Pentamidine should be given to patients who require intravenous therapy and who cannot tolerate TMP-SMX. Toxicities of intravenous pentamidine may include hypotension, hypoglycemia, rash, neutropenia, and azotemia. Adjunctive corticosteroid therapy is recommended in patients presenting with a room-air partial pressure of oxygen (PO_2) of less than 70 or an alveolar-arterial gradient greater than 35. The benefit of steroid therapy in patients who do not meet these criteria, or in patients who worsen during therapy, is unknown. Steroids act by decreasing inflammatory cytokines in the lung, stabilizing capillary permeability, and thus improving oxygenation. Patients may experience a recurrence of herpes simplex virus infection or oral candidiasis during steroid therapy.

On initiation of antimicrobial therapy, respiratory function sometimes worsens transiently in relation to cytokine release, but clinical improvement should occur within 5 days. Survival drops to approximately 50% in those who have to switch therapies because of drug failure. Intubation should be considered in patients with PCP who present with or progress rapidly to respiratory failure.

Secondary prophylaxis is essential because 70% to 80% of patients with PCP who do not take prophylaxis eventually have recurrence. The most effective prophylactic therapy remains TMP-SMX; dapsone, AP, and atovaquone are alternative agents (see Table 6.1). AP is a useful alternative in those who are unable to take TMP-SMX or dapsone. PCP prophylaxis regimens that are also effective for prevention of toxoplasmosis include TMP-SMX, dapsone with pyrimethamine, and atovaquone. In patients with a history of nonanaphylactoid reaction to TMP-SMX, desensitization to the drug should be considered (see Table 6.2). Desensitization protocols have been successful in approximately 75% of patients.

There are insufficient data at this time to know whether secondary prophylaxis for PCP can be discontinued safely in patients on combination antiretroviral therapy who have a sustained rise in their CD4 count to over 200 cells/mm^3. Studies are ongoing to address this question.

Parasitic Infections

Gastrointestinal Parasite Infection

Epidemiology and Microbiology
Diarrheal illness secondary to intestinal parasites is more common in HIV-infected patients living in or traveling to developing countries. The major pathogens include *Cryptosporidium*, Microsporidia, and *Isospora* species. Contaminated water is frequently the source of infection. Routine methods for water purification are not effective against *Cryptosporidium* because these organisms are too small to be filtered by common water systems and are resistant to chlorine and ozone. Cryptosporidial infection is associated

with animal contact and fecally contaminated environmental surfaces as well. Person-to-person transmission is possible. *Cryptosporidium* can undergo a complete developmental cycle in a single host and increase the organism load via autoinfection. Microsporidia is responsible for one third to one half of the chronic diarrhea in AIDS, and it is the sole pathogen in cholangitis in 38% of cases. The two major types of Microsporidia are *Enterocytozoon bieneusi* and *Encephalitozoon intestinalis* (formerly *Septata intestinalis*). *Encephalitozoon bellum* has been associated with many of the cases of keratoconjunctivitis. The life cycle of *Isospora* is also in a single host, but the oocyst must enter the environment for sporulation.

Clinical Manifestations

After a 2- to 14-day incubation period, *Cryptosporidium parvum* causes profuse watery diarrhea with low-grade fever, abdominal cramps, nausea, vomiting, and malabsorption. Patients have been reported to have up to 17 liters of liquid stool per day. The organism less often invades the common bile duct and causes acalculous cholecystitis. Patients with a CD4 count of fewer than 50 cells/mm^3 are at increased risk for biliary symptoms and death. Cryptosporidial infection involving the respiratory tract also is well described.

Microsporidiosis is mainly caused by *Enterocytozoon bieneusi*. The organism concentrates in the proximal jejunum and duodenum, producing a chronic nonbloody diarrhea associated with anorexia, bloating, and weight loss. Biliary tract involvement also has been described. Keratoconjunctivitis, often caused by *Encephalitozoon bellum*, is associated with foreign body sensation, ocular pain, excessive tearing, blurred vision, and photophobia.

Isospora infects enterocytes of the proximal small intestine, causing mucosal changes and inflammatory cells in the lamina propria. Symptoms develop within 1 week of oocyst ingestion. There is low-grade fever, anorexia, profuse watery diarrhea, and abdominal cramping. Colitis, acalculous cholecystitis, and extra-intestinal manifestations all have been described.

Cyclospora species is associated with a brief prodrome of fever and malaise, then explosive watery diarrhea, abdominal cramps, bloating, and flatulence that may abate and recur over time. *Blastocystis bominis* frequently is found in stool samples, but its pathogenicity is unclear. Low-grade fever and gastrointestinal symptoms have been attributed to it in some cases. Other causes of intestinal infection in HIV disease include giardiasis and amebiasis, with symptomatology and response to treatment similar to those described in seronegative patients. Case reports of HIV disease and strongyloidiasis have been published, but the infection is no more prevalent in this context.

Diagnosis

Examination of stool samples should be the initial strategy for diagnosing gastrointestinal parasites. Stool examination with a modified acid-fast stain will identify *Cryptosporidium*, Microsporidia, *Isospora*, and *Cyclospora* species.

Chemofluorescent stains can be used to look for microsporidial spores but are less specific than a modified trichrome stain (in which spores appear as pinkish red, ovoid structures with a belt-like stripe) or a Giemsa stain. Similar techniques can be used to identify spores in other body fluids. PCR techniques are being developed for *Enterocytozoon bieneusi* and *Encephalitozoon intestinalis*. Routine ova and parasite examination of the stool will identify *Giardia lamblia, Entamoeba histolytica, B. hominis*, and *Strongyloides stercoralis*. If stool samples are nondiagnostic, endoscopic procedures with biopsy should be considered (Fig. 8.8).

Management

Management of gastrointestinal parasites is summarized in Table 8.7. Therapy for *Cryptosporidia* has been disappointing and is primarily supportive, consisting of hydration and antimotility agents. Azithromycin and paromomycin have been used therapeutically, but studies show marginal benefit. Octreotide, a somatostatin-like agent, given 50 µg three times a day subcutaneously, increasing in 100 µg increments to a maximum dosage of 500 µg/d, can be used for symptomatic control. Nitazoxanide and hyperimmune bovine colostrum (cryptosporidial IgA) have been studied and demonstrate variable responses.

Microsporidial infection is also difficult to treat. *Encephalitozoon intestinalis* responds well to albendazole with eradication of the organism, but is a less common pathogen than *Enterocytozoon bieneusi*. *E. bieneusi* can be treated partially with albendazole, but relapse occurs if the drug is stopped. Atovaquone also can give symptomatic relief. Fumagillin can be used topically for corneal infection but is toxic if given systemically. A new analogue of fuma-

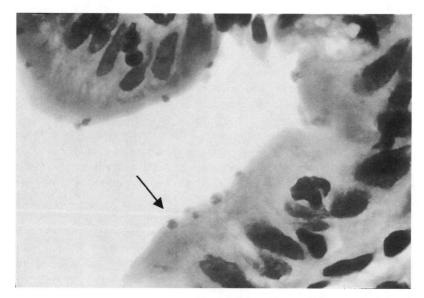

Figure 8.8 *Cryptosporidium* cysts on small bowel biopsy. (From CDC, Atlanta, GA.)

Table 8.7   Diagnosis and Treatment of Gastrointestinal Parasites

Organism	Diagnostic Studies	Therapy	Alternatives	Comments
Cryptosporidiosis	Acid-fast stain of stool; oocysts 4–5 µm; monoclonal antibody study of stool	Azithromycin 1200 mg/d orally for 14 days, then 600 mg/d orally	Paromomycin 500–750 mg orally three times daily *or* clarithromycin 500 mg orally twice daily	Minocycline and pyrimethamine synergistic *in vitro* with the macrolides
Microsporidiosis				
Enterocytozoon bieneusi	Chemofluorescent, Giemsa, or trichrome stain of stool	Albendazole 400 mg orally twice daily for 30 days, then 200–400 mg/d orally for maintenance	Atovaquone 750 mg orally three times daily	Albendazole gives only symptomatic relief
Encephalitozoon intestinalis	As with *E. bieneusi* above	As with *E. bieneusi* above	Fumagillin and new analogues	Albendazole eradicates infection
Cyclospora infection	Acid-fast stain of the stool; oocysts 8–10 µm	TMP-SMX DS orally twice daily for 10 days, followed by one orally three times weekly for maintenance	—	Fluoroquinolones under study
Isosporiasis	Acid-fast stain of the stool; oocysts 30 × 12 µm	TMP-SMX DS orally four times daily for 10 days, then twice daily for 3 weeks for maintenance	Pyrimethamine 75 mg/d orally for 14 days with folinic acid	Fluoroquinolones under study
Giardiasis	Stool for ova and parasites, monoclonal antibody test or *Giardia* antigen test	Metronidazole 250 mg orally three times daily for 5–10 days	Tinidazole 2 g orally (one-time dose)	—
Blastocystis hominis	Stool ova and parasites	Metronidazole 750 mg orally three times daily for 10–20 days	Iodoquinol 650 mg orally three times daily for 10–20 days	Pathogenicity is uncertain
Entamoeba histolytica	Stool ova and parasites	Metronidazole 750 mg orally three times daily for 10 days *or* tinidazole 2 g/d orally for 3 days	—	Acute treatment is followed by iodoquinol 650 mg orally three times daily for 20 days *or* paromomycin 500 mg orally three times daily for 7 days
Strongyloides stercoralis	Stool ova and parasites	Albendazole 400 mg/d orally for 3 days *or* ivermectin 200 µg/kg/d orally for 2 days	Thiabendazole 25 mg/kg orally twice daily for 2 days	

DS = double strength; TMP-SMX = trimethoprim-sulfamethoxazole.

gillin being used in breast cancer clinical trials seems promising for treatment.

Papillary stenosis and sclerosing cholangitis, which sometimes occurs with cryptosporidiosis or microsporidiosis, are not easily treatable. Endoscopic retrograde cholangiopancreatography (ERCP) with sphincterotomy offers pain relief, but symptoms may recur.

Isosporiasis can be managed effectively with TMP-SMX. If patients are TMP-SMX intolerant, pyrimethamine should be used. *Cyclospora* infection responds to TMP-SMX, and the efficacy of ciprofloxacin is being studied. Drugs with activity against *B. hominis* include metronidazole and TMP-SMX.

The risk of contracting cryptosporidial infection can be minimized by microstraining filters (0.1–1 µm) that are kept clean to avoid bacterial overgrowth, boiling water for 1 minute, and using high-quality bottled water. Well and spring water are safer than river and lake water. Infection with other parasites can be reduced by using similar measures.

MAC prophylaxis with clarithromycin or rifabutin decreases the incidence of cryptosporidial infection by greater than 75%. Combination antiretroviral therapy has been associated with symptomatic improvement of cryptosporidial and microsporidial infections.

Toxoplasmosis

Epidemiology
Toxoplasmosis is the most common CNS OI in HIV-infected patients and is the diagnosis in 60% of those presenting with mass lesions on brain imaging. Patients tend to have advanced immunodeficiency, the vast majority with a CD4 count of fewer than 100 cells/mm^3. Approximately one third of all HIV-positive individuals in the United States exhibit serologic evidence of previous exposure to toxoplasmosis by positive toxoplasma IgG antibody test; Europe and the developing world have higher rates. Of seropositive patients, there is a 24% risk of developing active toxoplasmosis within 2 years of AIDS diagnosis.

Pathogenesis
Toxoplasma gondii is an obligate intracellular parasite acquired via ingestion of viable oocysts excreted in cat feces or present in undercooked meat. The oocysts transform into replicating trophozoites that disseminate through the body and encyst in tissues. Lack of containment because of HIV-related defects in T-cell and macrophage immunity permits emergence of tachyzoites, the proliferative form of the organism, which is found with cyst forms in tissue specimens during active infection. The organism's predilection for infection in the brain may reflect "sequestering" from immune surveillance in the CNS. Because the vast majority of toxoplasmosis cases are associated with a positive serum IgG antibody test, most are thought to represent reactivated latent infection.

Clinical Manifestations

Patients with toxoplasmosis usually present with fever and neurological complaints. Headache is present in approximately 55% of cases, confusion in 52%, fever in 47%, seizures in 29%, and focal neurological deficits in 69%. Ocular and pulmonary disease has been described but is rare. Patients who have had PCP as their AIDS-defining diagnosis and who have lymphopenia on presentation have a relatively poor prognosis.

Diagnosis

Demonstration of serum antibodies to *T. gondii* is important for diagnosis. Over 95% of patients with toxoplasmosis will have detectable antibodies, with a median IgG titer of 1:256; serum IgM antibody is almost invariably negative. In asymptomatic patients, an IgG titer of greater than 1:128 is predictive of eventual development of CNS infection. In patients followed longitudinally, there is no appreciable change in serum IgG titer when CNS infection reactivates. The incidence of toxoplasmosis in IgG-negative patients is 1% to 3%.

Brain imaging with CT with contrast or MRI is recommended in all patients who are suspected of having CNS toxoplasmosis. Most lesions are located in the cerebral hemispheres, mainly in the frontoparietal area at the gray-white junction, although lesions also can be seen in the deep white matter or basal ganglia (Fig. 8.9). Head CT shows a median of two enhancing hypodense lesions in 91% of patients; 75% of these have associated cerebral

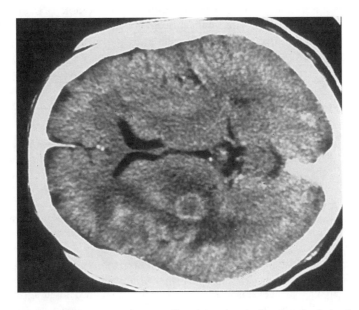

Figure 8.9 Computed tomography scan of head showing single enhancing lesion in patient with toxoplasmosis.

edema. Approximately 25% of patients have solitary lesions on CT. MRI is more sensitive than CT for the detection of toxoplasmic lesions and should be performed if the CT is negative or if it shows only one lesion. Solitary lesions on MRI are far less common than with CT and should raise suspicion for an alternative diagnosis. Differential diagnosis of a patient presenting with CNS complaints who has an abnormal brain imaging study includes bacterial abscess, cryptococcoma or other fungal infection, mycobacterial infection, septic emboli, and lymphoma.

Examination of the CSF should be performed only in the absence of a significant mass lesion and is helpful in excluding other infectious and malignant processes. The CSF indices associated with toxoplasmosis are variable, although there is usually a mononuclear pleocytosis, mildly increased protein, and normal or low glucose level. CSF IgG is positive in 88% of patients with a median titer of 1:4.

Management

The standard of care in a patient with suspected toxoplasmosis is institution of empiric antimicrobial therapy. Brain biopsy should be considered if there is no clinical or radiographic improvement within 10 to 14 days. If the patient does not have detectable IgG antibody or has an MRI showing a single mass lesion or nonenhancing lesion(s), brain biopsy should be performed immediately.

Effective drug combinations for toxoplasmosis include sulfadiazine with pyrimethamine *or* clindamycin with pyrimethamine (Table 8.8). Both regimens are commonly associated with side effects. Alternative regimens include TMP-SMX, clarithromycin or azithromycin with pyrimethamine, doxycycline

---

Table 8.8   Treatment of Toxoplasmosis

Initial Regimen

Sulfadiazine 1–2 g orally four times daily *and* pyrimethamine 50–100 mg/d orally after loading with 100–200 mg pyrimethamine for 1 day; folinic acid 10–50 mg/d orally should be administered to prevent leukopenia

or

Clindamycin 300–450 mg orally four times daily *and* pyrimethamine 50–100 mg/d orally; folinic acid 10–50 mg/d orally should be administered concurrently

Maintenance Regimen

Sulfadiazine 0.5–1 g orally four times daily *or* clindamycin 300–450 mg orally 3–4 times daily with pyrimethamine 25–75 mg/d orally; folinic acid 10 mg/d orally should be administered concurrently; both regimens are commonly associated with side effects, including rash and diarrhea with pyrimethamine, clindamycin with flucytosine, and atovaquone. Adjunctive corticosteroid therapy should be used only if indicated for cerebral edema.

Maintenance therapy for toxoplasmosis is important to prevent relapse. There are insufficient data at this time to know whether secondary prophylaxis for toxoplasmosis can be discontinued safely in patients on combination antiretroviral therapy who have a sustained rise in their CD4 count to over 100 cells/mm^3. Studies are ongoing to address this question.

Viral Infections

Cytomegalovirus Infection

Epidemiology
Cytomegalovirus (CMV) infection has been a cause of significant morbidity and mortality in patients with advanced HIV disease. Before the advent of combination antiretroviral therapy, CMV disease occurred in 20% to 40% of HIV-infected individuals, generally in those with a CD4 count of fewer than 50 cells/mm^3. In recent years, there has been a dramatic decrease in the number of new cases. CMV disease is usually the result of a chronic latent infection becoming clinically manifest rather than of acute infection.

Clinical Manifestations
Retinitis comprises 75% to 85% of the end-organ disease caused by CMV infection and is characterized by yellow to white areas of necrosis and edema along a vascular distribution (Fig. 8.10). Hemorrhagic areas also are seen. With healing, CMV lesions leave atrophic scars. Retinal detachment is a well-described complication and is more common with prolonged infection.

CMV causes significant gastrointestinal tract disease as well. The most common manifestations are esophagitis and colitis, but ulcers and mass lesions also have been described. Patients with esophagitis present with dysphagia and odynophagia, and those with colitis have abdominal pain and diarrhea. Papillary sclerosis and sclerosing cholangitis also have been associated with CMV infection.

Many neurological syndromes attributable to CMV infection have been described. Polyradiculopathy manifests as urinary retention, progressive bilateral leg weakness, and ascending paraparesis with areflexia similar to Guillain–Barré syndrome. This can progress rapidly over several weeks, leading to flaccid paraplegia and a loss of bowel and bladder function. Encephalitis presents with lethargy, apathy, confusion, nystagmus, ataxia, and unilateral or bilateral cranial nerve palsies. Ventriculoencephalitis is a severe form of encephalitis characterized by 1) necrosis of cranial nerves and periventricular parenchyma, 2) a fulminant course, and 3) death at a median of 5 weeks.

Other less common CMV disease manifestations include interstitial pneumonitis, adrenal disease, and viremia associated with constitutional symptoms.

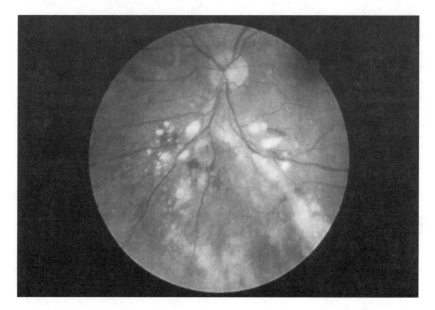

Figure 8.10   Retinal photograph of patient with cytomegalovirus retinitis. (From *Ann Intern Med.* 1988;109:963–9.) (For color reproduction, *see* Plate 4 at back of book.)

Diagnosis

Generally, the diagnosis of CMV retinitis is made on clinical grounds. Gastrointestinal and pulmonary disease is diagnosed by tissue biopsy revealing CMV intracellular inclusions. A respiratory CMV culture may be positive without clinical disease. Diagnosis of CMV polyradiculopathy can be confirmed by LP. CSF examination typically reveals increased protein, decreased glucose, and pleocytosis with a predominance of leukocytes. A positive CSF PCR for CMV is diagnostic. Diagnosis of encephalitis is supported by MRI findings of multifocal parenchymal disease and/or periventricular involvement with contrast enhancement. CSF PCR is occasionally positive, and the CSF profile is often normal.

CMV antigen assays are now generally available. Monoclonal antibody-based stains detect a CMV-specific 65-kD matrix protein in infected polymorphonuclear leukocytes. The assay measures the number of infected cells per 200,000 cells, and is therefore a quantitative technique. It is more sensitive and rapid than CMV culture of the blood. It can be positive in patients without evidence of CMV infection, but studies suggest that a high number of infected cells predicts clinical disease within 3 months. This assay is useful for predicting relapse in patients on CMV therapy. PCR techniques are more sensitive, but they have poorer predictive value, are more expensive, and are more difficult to perform.

Management

Before the advent of combination antiretroviral therapy, patients with CMV retinitis on systemic therapy had a median survival of 8.5 to 12.6 months. Therapy for newly diagnosed retinitis is presented in Table 8.9. Initial treatment is 14 to 21 days with ganciclovir or foscarnet, which is followed by maintenance therapy at a lower dose. Alternatively, a ganciclovir implant can be placed surgically by an ophthalmologist, with oral ganciclovir prescribed to prevent systemic disease and retinitis in the other eye.

Table 8.9   Treatment of Cytomegalovirus Infection

Drug	Route	Dose	Toxicity
Ganciclovir			
Induction	Intravenous	5 mg/kg every 12 hours	Neutropenia Anemia
Maintenance	Intravenous	5 mg/kg/d 5–7 d/wk	Thrombocytopenia Nausea/diarrhea
	Oral	1 g thrice daily	Less neutropenia than intravenous
Intravitreal implant*		Every 6 months	No systemic toxicity
Foscarnet			
Induction	Intravenous	60 mg/kg every 8 hours *or* 90 mg/kg every 12 hours	Nephrotoxicity Hypocalcemia Hypophosphatemia Hypomagnesia
Maintenance	Intravenous	90–120 mg/kg/d	Anemia Nausea Seizure
Cidofovir			
Induction	Intravenous	5 mg/kg/wk for 2 weeks with probenecid 2 g orally 3 hours before each dose and 1 g orally 2 and 8 hours after dose	Nephrotoxicity Neutropenia
Maintenance	Intravenous	5 mg/kg every other week with probenecid as above	

* Consider co-administration of oral ganciclovir to prevent systemic infection.

Ganciclovir is associated primarily with hematologic toxicity, including neutropenia and thrombocytopenia. Granulocyte colony-stimulating factor (GCSF) is sometimes required to treat these complications. Foscarnet is an effective alternative treatment for CMV retinitis but has significant toxicities. These include nausea, malaise, neurological symptoms, electrolyte imbalances (e.g., decreased calcium, magnesium, and phosphate), and renal dysfunction. The infusion takes 2 hours and requires a pump. A ganciclovir implant provides intravitreal drug levels four times those obtained with systemic therapy. Surgical risks associated with the implant procedure include blurred vision lasting several weeks, and retinal detachment, hemorrhage, and endophthalmitis occur infrequently. The implant is generally effective for 6 months, when active drug is depleted and a new implant is required. Time to relapse with the implant in one study was 221 days compared with only 71 days in patients on intravenous ganciclovir.

Cidofovir is also effective against the herpesviruses including CMV. It is synergistic with ganciclovir and foscarnet *in vitro*. Unlike ganciclovir, it does not require viral enzymes for activation and is active in uninfected cells, thereby preventing the spread of CMV. However, it causes proximal tubular necrosis, proteinuria, and renal dysfunction; probenecid and intravenous hydration are necessary to reduce this risk.

Patients with relapsing disease should receive another course of initial treatment followed by maintenance therapy. It is not clear whether there is a benefit to using foscarnet if ganciclovir was initially given and vice versa, but this approach is typical. Combination therapy with both ganciclovir and foscarnet is another option. Implants also should be considered in patients who have relapsing disease, particularly if the infection is sight-threatening. Cidofovir is effective salvage therapy, with a median of 115 days until the next relapse. However, CMV strains resistant to both ganciclovir and foscarnet are resistant to cidofovir over 80% of the time.

There are data suggesting that maintenance therapy for CMV retinitis can be discontinued safely in patients on combination antiretroviral therapy whose CD4 count has risen to greater than 100–150 cells/mm^3 for 3 to 6 months and whose viral load is well suppressed. Such patients should be monitored regularly by an ophthalmologist.

Patients with gastrointestinal disease respond to induction therapy but may require a longer course of treatment. Maintenance therapy is sometimes deferred. With no maintenance therapy, patients with colitis relapse in a median of 9 weeks. However, a subset of patients continues to do well for up to 1 year after induction therapy without maintenance. Pulmonary disease should be treated with 3 weeks of induction therapy, but only 60% to 70% of patients will respond.

Herpes Simplex Virus Infection

Epidemiology and Microbiology

Herpes simplex virus types 1 (HSV-1) and 2 (HSV-2) are closely related herpesviruses. In the United States, their incidence is over 80% and approximately 20%, respectively. HSV latently infects trigeminal or sacral sensory ganglia; it reactivates periodically, causing symptoms. Patients with advanced HIV disease may have frequent and severe recurrences. HSV, as a genital ulcer disease, increases the risk of HIV transmission. In addition, symptomatic HSV infection increases HIV transcription and replication, and this also may promote transmission.

Clinical Manifestations

Lesions caused by HSV begin as vesicles on an erythematous base that are often preceded by pain and tingling at the site, usually the genitals or mouth (Fig. 8.11). Over several days, they begin to form a crust. HSV can be more aggressive in HIV-infected patients, causing prolonged ulcerative lesions and significant morbidity. HSV is also a cause of esophagitis in HIV disease, with approximately one half of the patients having predisposing factors, such as a nasogastric procedure, corticosteroid therapy, or chemotherapy. HSV encephalitis and meningitis are not increased in frequency in HIV-infected patients. HSV can cause retinal necrosis but less often than can varicella-zoster virus (see below).

Diagnosis

Diagnosis of HSV infection is best made by direct immunofluorescence assay (DFA) of vesicular fluid with a fluorescein isothiocyanate-labeled monoclonal antibody. This study has a 90% diagnostic yield compared with 65% with culture. A fresh vesicle without crusting should be sampled. The

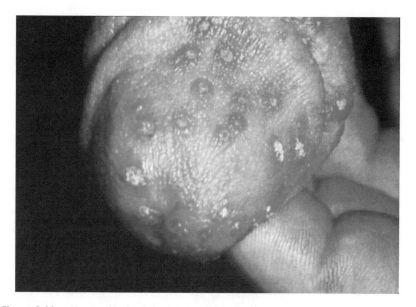

Figure 8.11   Herpes simplex infection involving penile glans.

Tzanck smear, which is a Giemsa or Wright stain of vesicular fluid to demonstrate multinucleated giant cells, is a useful alternative but less sensitive and dependent on the skill of the observer.

Management

Oral acyclovir is the drug of choice; 400 mg given three times daily for 7 to 10 days usually is adequate (Table 8.10). Famciclovir and valacyclovir, which are newer agents, are more expensive and offer no advantages. Severe cases of HSV infection can be treated intravenously with acyclovir 5 mg/kg every 8 hours. Acyclovir-resistant HSV may require a course of intravenous foscarnet. Chronic suppression with acyclovir 400 mg twice daily should be considered in patients with frequent or severe recurrences.

Varicella-Zoster Virus Infection

Epidemiology and Microbiology

Varicella-zoster virus (VZV) is a herpesvirus that causes chicken pox (primary infection) and zoster or "shingles" (reactivation infection). HIV-in-

---

Table 8.10   Treatment of Herpes Simplex Virus and Varicella Zoster Virus Infections

HSV Infection	
Primary or recurrent mucocutaneous disease	Acyclovir 400 mg thrice daily orally
Extensive mucocutaneous disease	Acyclovir 5 mg/kg every 8 hours for 7–14 days IV
Visceral	Acyclovir 10 mg/kg IV every 8 hours for 14–21 days IV
Prevention of relapse	Acyclovir 400 mg twice daily orally
Infection with acyclovir-resistant HSV strain	Topical trifluridine 5% or foscarnet 40 mg/kg every 8 hours IV
VZV infection	
Localized infection (shingles)	Acyclovir 800 mg orally every 4 hours while awake (5 times daily) *or* Famciclovir 500 mg thrice daily orally *or* Valacyclovir 1 g thrice daily orally
Disseminated infection (cutaneous or visceral)	Acyclovir 10 mg/kg every 8 hours for 7–14 days IV
Prevention of relapse	No therapy indicated
Infection with acyclovir-resistant VZV strain	Foscarnet 40 mg/kg every 8 hours IV

HSV = herpes simplex virus; IV = intravenous; VZV = varicella-zoster virus.

fected individuals are at risk for zoster as their immune function diminishes, but it does not have independent prognostic significance. The risk of zoster increases as the CD4 cell count declines.

Clinical Manifestations
Zoster typically involves a single dermatome, although it also may cause disseminated disease. The lesions present as grouped vesicles on an erythematous base, and they are often uncomfortable (Fig. 8.12). Postherpetic neuralgia is uncommon in HIV-infected patients. VZV infection infrequently has neurological manifestations including motor neuropathy, meningitis, encephalitis, ventriculitis, transverse myelitis, radiculomyelitis, cerebral vasculitis, and cranial nerve palsies.

Varicella-zoster virus is a major cause of acute retinal necrosis (ARN) and rapidly progressive herpetic retinal necrosis (RPHRN). ARN is defined

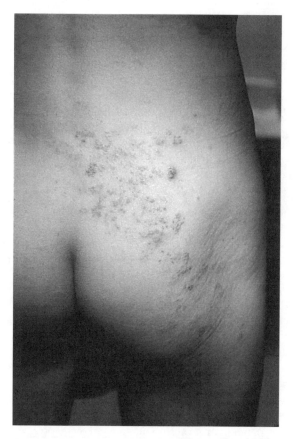

Figure 8.12   Shingles (varicella-zoster infection) involving lumbar dermatomes.

by focal, well-demarcated areas of necrotizing retinitis involving the retinal periphery anterior to vascular arcades. There is circumferential progression with associated occlusion of the retinal vessels, vitritis, and anterior uveitis. RPHRN occurs more frequently in advanced HIV disease than ARN and is characterized by early macular involvement, bilateral multifocal disease, outer retinal opacification, minimal inflammatory changes, and retinal detachment (with multiple ragged retinal tears that lead to blindness). In most patients, an episode of zoster will precede the eye disease.

Diagnosis

Zoster can be diagnosed by DFA of vesicular fluid, which is more sensitive and rapid than culture. Early lesions are more often positive than lesions that have begun to crust. ARN and RPHRN are diagnosed clinically by ophthalmologic examination. Neurological disease can be diagnosed by PCR of the CSF. There are occasional false-positive results, perhaps related to subclinical reactivation of VZV associated with other neurological diseases.

Management

Acyclovir 800 mg five times daily is given for 7 days (see Table 8.10). Patients with shingles usually do well with resolution of the rash and no complications. Maintenance therapy is not necessary. Famciclovir 500 mg three times daily also is effective in treating zoster, as is valacyclovir 1 g three times daily. If the patient is extremely ill or has neurological disease, intravenous acyclovir 10 mg/kg every 8 hours should be given instead. Acyclovir-resistant VZV is treated with intravenous foscarnet. Although patients with ARN usually respond well to intravenous acyclovir, those with RPHRN typically do not.

Viral Hepatitis

Epidemiology

Hepatitis A, B, and C infections are common in HIV disease. Because hepatitis A virus (HAV) is transmitted via the fecal-oral route, it is seen mainly in gay men. Hepatitis B virus (HBV), which can be spread sexually or through exposure to infected blood, occurs in gay men, heterosexuals, and injection drug users. Hepatitis C virus (HCV), which is transmitted primarily through exposure to infected blood, is seen in injection drug users, hemophiliacs, and other individuals who acquired HIV infection through blood products.

Hepatitis A causes acute infection only. Hepatitis B is self-limited in 96% of HIV-seronegative patients, with the remainder chronically infected and having a variable clinical course. Hepatitis C is a chronic infection in the majority of patients and often is associated with progressive liver disease. Twenty to fifty percent of patients with chronic HCV infection develop cirrhosis within 10 years. Eighty to ninety percent of patients with HIV disease have serologic evidence of previous HBV infection. Seroprevalence studies in injection-drug users and hemophiliacs report a 50% to 90% rate of HCV infection.

Clinical Manifestations

Acute viral hepatitis is characterized by anorexia, nausea, vomiting, upper abdominal pain, and jaundice; fever is common with HAV infection. Rarely, fulminant hepatitis occurs with rapidly progressive hepatic dysfunction. Physical examination may show a jaundiced patient with tender hepatomegaly. Liver function tests, particularly serum transaminases and bilirubin levels, are increased. Symptoms and signs of acute hepatitis often persist for several weeks before resolving. Patients with hepatitis B or C who develop chronic infection may be asymptomatic or have exacerbations of these same symptoms with variable frequency. Over years, they become at risk for cirrhosis and hepatoma.

The clinical course of HAV infection does not seem to be altered in the context of HIV disease. HBV infection is several times more likely to become chronic in HIV-infected patients, but its course tends to be less aggressive. This observation may be related to the role of the immune system in mediating liver damage associated with HBV infection. Chronic HBV infection has been noted to flare when combination antiretroviral therapy is initiated, perhaps representing an immune reconstitution syndrome. It also may do so if lamivudine (3TC), which has action against this virus as well as HIV, is discontinued. In contrast to HBV infection, HCV is often more aggressive in HIV-infected patients, especially in those with advanced disease.

Diagnosis

Acute viral hepatitis is suggested by the clinical presentation in association with abnormal liver function tests. Differential diagnosis includes hepatotoxicity related to alcohol and medications and biliary tract disease. Diagnosis of viral hepatitis is established by serologic tests, including IgM anti-HAV for hepatitis A, hepatitis B surface antigen (HBsAg) for hepatitis B, and anti-HCV for hepatitis C. If anti-HCV is positive, the diagnosis of active hepatitis C infection should be verified with recombinant immunoblot assay or PCR for HCV RNA test. Chronic hepatitis is defined as lasting 6 months or longer. Liver biopsy may be recommended to establish the extent of disease in patients with chronic hepatitis and to identify those who are candidates for pharmacologic treatment. In general, liver function test abnormalities do not correlate well with histologic findings.

Management

The management of acute hepatitis is supportive. Patients should be asked to maintain adequate oral intake to prevent dehydration and to rest as needed. Interferon-α and 3TC have been effective in patients with chronic HBV infection, and interferon-α in combination with ribavirin has been useful for the treatment of chronic HCV infection. However, the experience with these agents in HIV-infected patients has been variable. Toxicity from interferon (e.g., constitutional complaints, neuropsychiatric symptoms, gastrointestinal intolerance) is common. Viral load assays are helpful in monitoring response to therapy. Patients with chronic hepatitis should be cautioned about the use of alcohol, acetaminophen, and other potentially hepatotoxic agents.

All HIV-infected patients should be tested serologically for HAV, HBV, and HCV infections. Immunization against hepatitis A and B is recommended in those without previous exposure to these pathogens, although the response to these vaccines may be diminished, particularly in advanced HIV disease.

■   ■   ■

Key Points

- Bacillary angiomatosis, caused by *Bartonella* species, is manifested by skin lesions resembling those of Kaposi's sarcoma and occasionally visceral involvement.

- Recurrent pneumococcal pneumonia and salmonellosis are two conventional bacterial infections that have been described in HIV-infected patients.

- MAC infection presents with constitutional symptoms in the context of advanced HIV disease. Diagnosis is by isolator blood culture or tissue biopsy. Treatment consists of a multidrug antimicrobial regimen.

- Syphilis is common in HIV-infected patients and sometimes has unusual features and an atypical response to therapy.

- The risk of HIV-infected patients with a positive PPD developing active TB is much higher than that of the general population. Diagnosis may be difficult because of atypical clinical presentations and cutaneous anergy.

- Recurrent mucosal candidiasis is common in patients with HIV disease. Treatment is with topical antifungal agents or oral fluconazole.

- Cryptococcal infection, which involves the meninges and/or lungs, is the most frequent serious fungal infection in HIV-infected patients. Treatment consists of intravenous amphotericin B followed by oral fluconazole.

- Disseminated histoplasmosis is reported in HIV-infected patients from endemic regions such as the midwestern United States. It is managed with amphotericin B.

- Common clinical features of PCP include fever, weight loss, non-productive cough, and dyspnea on exertion. Treatment is with TMP-SMX or intravenous pentamidine. Corticosteroids are added if there is significant pulmonary compromise.

- Gastrointestinal parasitic infections, such as cryptosporidiosis and microsporidiosis, cause chronic diarrhea and weight loss, especially in patients with advanced HIV disease.

- Toxoplasmosis, which is the most common CNS OI in HIV-infected patients, presents with focal lesions on brain-imaging studies. Treatment is sulfadiazine in combination with pyrimethamine.

- CMV infection manifests as retinitis, gastrointestinal disease, or neurological syndromes in advanced HIV disease. Treatment of retinitis consists of ganciclovir (implant or intravenous) or intravenous foscarnet.

- HSV and VZV are responsible for recurrent mucocutaneous disease in HIV-infected patients. Treatment is with acyclovir, with a higher dose necessary for VZV infection.

- Chronic hepatitis from HCV is frequent in injection-drug users and may be difficult to manage in the context of HIV disease.

■   ■   ■

SUGGESTED READINGS

General

U.S. Public Health Service, Infectious Disease Society of America. 1999 guidelines for the prevention of opportunistic infections in persons infected with human immunodeficiency virus. *Morbid Mortal Wkly Rep MMWR.* 1999;48(RR-10):1–66.

Bacillary Angiomatosis

Adal KA, Cockerell CJ, Petri WA. Cat scratch disease, bacillary angiomatosis, and other infections due to *Rochalimaea. N Engl J Med.* 1994;330:1509–15.

Perkocha LA, Geaghan SM, Yen TSB. Clinical and pathological features of bacillary peliosis hepatis in association with HIV infection. *N Engl J Med.* 1990;3232:1581–6.

Community-Acquired Pneumonia

Bush CE, Donovan RM, Markowitz NP, et al. A study of HIV RNA viral load in AIDS patients with bacterial pneumonia. *J Acquir Immune Defic Syndr Hum Retrovirol.* 1996;13:23–6.

Garcia-Leoni ME, Moreno S, Rodeno P, et al. Pneumococcal pneumonia in adult hospitalized patients infected with HIV. *Arch Intern Med.* 1992;152:1808–12.

Gebo KA, Moore RD, Keruly JC, Chaisson RE. Risk factors for pneumococcal disease in HIV-infected patients. *J Infect Dis.* 1996;173:857–62.

Hirschtick RE, Glassroth J, Jordan MC, et al. Pneumococcal disease during HIV infection: epidemiologic, clinical, and immunologic perspectives. *Ann Intern Med.* 1992; 117:314–24.

Markowitz N, Rosen MJ, Mangura BT, et al. Bacterial pneumonia in persons infected with HIV. *N Engl J Med.* 1995;333:845–51.

Steinhart R, Steingold AL, Taylor F, et al. Invasive *Haemophilus influenzae* infections in men with HIV infection. *JAMA.* 1992;268:3350–2.

Mycobacterium avium Complex Infection

Hoover DR, Graham NMH, Bacellar H, et al. An epidemiologic analysis of *Mycobacterium avium* complex disease in homosexual men infected with HIV type 1. *Clin Infect Dis.* 1995;20:125–8.

Race EM, Adelson-Mitty J, Kriegel GR, et al. Focal mycobacterial lymphadenitis following initiation of protease-inhibitor therapy in patients with advanced HIV-1 disease. *Lancet.* 1998;351:252–5.

Rubin DS, Rahal JJ. *Mycobacterium avium* complex. *Infect Dis Clin North Am.* 1994; 8:413–26.

Shafran SD, Singer J, Zarowny DP, et al. A comparison of two regimens for the treatment of *Mycobacterium avium* complex bacteremia in AIDS: rifabutin, ethambutol, and clarithromycin versus rifampin, ethambutol, clofazimine, and ciprofloxacin. *N Engl J Med.* 1996;335:377–83.

Salmonellosis

Asperilla MO, Smego RA, Scott LK. Quinolone antibiotics in the treatment of *Salmonella* infections. *Rev Infect Dis.* 1990;12:873–89.

Levine WC, Buehler JW, Bean NH, Tauxe RV. Epidemiology of nontyphoidal *Salmonella* bacteremia during the HIV epidemic. *J Infect Dis.* 1991;164:81–7.

Nelson MR, Shanson DC, Hawkins DA, Gazzard BG. *Salmonella, Campylobacter,* and *Shigella* in HIV-seropositive patients. *AIDS.* 1992;6:1495–8.

Syphilis

Gordon SM, Eaton ME, George R, et al. The response of symptomatic neurosyphilis to high-dose intravenous penicillin G in patients with HIV infection. *N Engl J Med.* 1994;331:1469–73.

Hook EW III, Marra CM. Acquired syphilis in adults. *N Engl J Med.* 1992; 326:1060–9.

Hutchinson CM, Hook EW III, Shepard M, et al. Altered clinical presentation of early syphilis in patients infected with HIV infection. *Ann Intern Med.* 1994;121:94–9.

Lukehart SA, Hook EW III, et al. Invasion of the central nervous system by *Treponema pallidum*: implications for diagnosis and therapy. *Ann Intern Med.* 1988;109:855–62.

Marra CM, Critchlow CW, Hook EW III, et al. The role of CSF treponemal antibodies in the diagnosis of asymptomatic neurosyphilis. *Arch Neurol.* 1995;52:68–72.

Musher DM. Syphilis, neurosyphilis, penicillin, and AIDS. *J Infect Dis.* 1991;152:1201–6.

Musher DM, Hamill RJ, Baughn RE. Effect of HIV infection on the course of syphilis and on the response to treatment. *Ann Intern Med.* 1990;113:872–81.

Tuberculosis

Alpert PL, Munsiff SS, Gourevitch MN, et al. A prospective study of tuberculosis and HIV infection: clinical manifestations and factors associated with survival. *Clin Infect Dis.* 1997;24:661–8.

Shafer RW, Edlin BR. Tuberculosis in patients infected with HIV: perspective on the past decade. *Clin Infect Dis.* 1996;22:683–704.

Candidiasis

Imam N, Carpenter C, Mayer KH, et al. Heirarchical pattern of mucosal candida infections in HIV-seropositive women. *Am J Med.* 1990;89:142–6.

Maenza JR, Keruly JC, Moore RD, et al. Risk factors for fluconazole-resistant candidiasis in HIV-infected patients. *J Infect Dis.* 1996;173:219–25.

Powderly WG, Finkelstein D, Feinberg J, et al. A randomized trial comparing fluconazole with clotrimazole troches for the prevention of fungal infections in patients with advanced HIV infection: NIAID AIDS Clinical Trials Group. *N Engl J Med.* 1995; 332:700–5.

Reef SE, Mayer KH. Opportunistic candidal infections in patients infected with HIV: prevention issues and priorities. *Clin Infect Dis.* 1995;21(S1):S99–102.

Cryptococcosis

Chuck SL, Sande MA. Infections with *Cryptococcus neoformans* in AIDS. *N Engl J Med.* 1989; 321:794–9.

Nelson MR, Fisher M, Cartledge J, et al. The role of azoles in the treatment and prophylaxis of cryptococcal disease in HIV infection. *AIDS.* 1994;8:651–4.

Powderly WG. Therapy for cryptococcal meningitis in patients with AIDS. *Clin Infect Dis.* 1992;4(S1):S54–9.

Powderly WG, Finkelstein D, Feinberg J, et al. A randomized trial comparing fluconazole with clotrimazole troches for the prevention of fungal infections in patients with advanced HIV infection. *N Engl J Med.* 1995;332:700–5.

Powderly WG, Saag MS, Cloud G, et al. A controlled trial of fluconazole or amphotericin B to prevent relapse of cryptococcal meningitis in patients with AIDS. *N Engl J Med.* 1992;326:793–8.

Saag MS, Powderly WG, Cloud GA, et al. Comparison of amphotericin B with fluconazole in the treatment of acute AIDS-associated cryptococcal meningitis. *N Engl J Med.* 1992;326:83–9.

Histoplasmosis

Wheat LJ, Connolly-Stringfield PA, Baker RL, et al. Disseminated histoplasmosis in the acquired immune deficiency syndrome: clinical findings, diagnosis and treatment, and review of the literature. *Medicine.* 1990;69:361–74.

Wheat LJ, Hafner R, Wulfsohn M, et al. Prevention of relapse of histoplasmosis with itraconazole in patients with the acquired immunodeficiency syndrome. *Ann Intern Med.* 1993;118:610–6.

Pneumocystis carinii Pneumonia

Bozette SA, Finkelstein DM, Spector SA, et al. A randomized trial of three antipneumocystis agents in patients with advanced HIV infection. *N Engl J Med.* 1995;332:693–9.

Gluckstein D, Ruskin J. Rapid oral desensitization to trimethoprim-sulfamethoxizole (TMP-SMZ): use in prophylaxis for *Pneumocystis carinii* pneumonia in patients with AIDS who were previously intolerant to TMP-SMZ. *Clin Infect Dis.* 1995;20:849–53.

Jules-Elysee KM, Stover DE, Zaman MB, et al. Aerosolized pentamidine: effect on diagnosis and presentation of *Pneumocystis carinii* pneumonia. *Ann Int Med.* 1990; 112:750–7.

Masur H. Prevention and treatment of *Pneumocystis* pneumonia. *N Engl J Med.* 1992; 327:1853–60.

National Institutes of Health, University of California Expert Panel for Corticosteroids as Adjunctive Therapy for *Pneumocystis* Pneumonia. Special report: consensus statement on the use of corticosteroids as adjunctive therapy for *Pneumocystis* pneumonia in AIDS. *N Engl J Med.* 1990;323:1500–4.

Simonds RJ, Hughes WT, Feinberg J, Navin T. Preventing *Pneumocystis carinii* pneumonia in persons with HIV. *Clin Infect Dis.* 1995;21(S1):S44–8.

Gastrointestinal Parasite Infection

Carr A, Marriott D, Field A, et al. Treatment of HIV-1-associated microsporidiosis and cryptosporidiosis with combination antiretroviral therapy. *Lancet.* 1998;351:256–61.

Didier ES. Microsporidiosis. *Clin Infect Dis.* 1998;27:1–8.

McGowan I, Hawkins AS, Weller IVD. The natural history of cryptosporidial diarrhoea in HIV-infected patients. *AIDS.* 1993;7:349–54.

Toxoplasmosis

Dannemann B, McCutchan A, Israelski D, et al. Treatment of toxoplasmic encephalitis in patients with AIDS: a randomized trial comparing pyrimethamine plus clindamycin to pyrimethamine plus sulfadiazine. *Ann Intern Med.* 1992;116: 33–43.

Girard P-M, Landman R, Gaudebout C, et al. Dapsone-pyrimethamine compared with aerosolized pentamidine as primary prophylaxis against *Pneumocystis carinii* pneumonia and toxoplasmosis in HIV infection. *N Engl J Med.* 1993;328:1514–20.

Jacobson MA, Besch CL, Child C, et al. Efficacy of atovaquone in treatment of toxoplasmosis in patients with AIDS. *Lancet.* 1992; 340:637–8.

Luft BJ, Hafner R, Korzun AH, et al. Toxoplasmic encephalitis in patients with AIDS. *N Engl J Med.* 1993;329:995–1000.

Luft BJ, Remington JS. Toxoplasmic encephalitis in AIDS. *Clin Infect Dis.* 1992;15: 211–22.

Porter SB, Sande MA. Toxoplasmosis of the central nervous system in AIDS. *N Engl J Med.* 1992;327:1643–8.

Wallace MR, Rossetti RJ, Olson PE. Cats and toxoplasmosis risk in HIV-infected adults. *JAMA.* 1993;269:76–7.

Cytomegalovirus Infection

Jacobson MA. Treatment of cytomegalovirus retinitis in patients with AIDS. *N Engl J Med.* 1997;337:105–14.

Jacobson MA, Zegans M, Pavan PR, et al. Cytomegalovirus retinitis after initiation of highly active antiretroviral therapy. *Lancet.* 1997;349:1443–5.

Whitley RJ, Jacobson MA, Friedberg DN, et al. Guidelines for the treatment of cytomegalovirus diseases in patients with AIDS in the era of potent antiretroviral therapy. *Arch Intern Med.* 1998;158:957–69.

Herpes Simplex Virus Infection

Stewart JA, Reef SE, Pellett PE, et al. Herpesvirus infections in persons infected with HIV. *Clin Infect Dis.* 1995;21(Suppl 1):S114–20.

Varicella-Zoster Virus Infection

Glesby MJ, Moore RD, Chaisson RE. Clinical spectrum of herpes zoster in adults infected with HIV. *Clin Infect Dis.* 1995;21:370–5.

Ormerod LD, Larkin JA, Margo CA, et al. Rapidly progressive herpetic retinal necrosis: a blinding disease characteristic of advanced AIDS. *Clin Infect Dis.* 1998;26:34–45.

Veenstra J, van Praag RME, Krol A, et al. Complications of varicella zoster virus reactivation in HIV-infected homosexual men. *AIDS.* 1996;10:393–9.

Viral Hepatitis

Gross JB Jr. Clinician's guide to hepatitis C. *Mayo Clin Proc.* 1998;73:355–60.

Main J, McCarron B, Thomas HC. Treatment of chronic viral hepatitis. *Antiviral Chem Chemother.* 1998;9:449–60.

9

■ ■ ■

Diagnosis and Management of Opportunistic Cancers

Kaposi's Sarcoma
Bruce J. Dezube, MD
Jerome E. Groopman, MD

AIDS-Related Lymphomas
John P. Doweiko, MD

Anogenital Squamous Cell Cancer
John P. Doweiko, MD

KAPOSI'S SARCOMA
Bruce Dezube
Jerome Groopman

Epidemiology

Kaposi's sarcoma (KS), an AIDS-defining condition, is the most common neoplasm arising in HIV-infected patients. In the United States, it is over 20,000 times more frequent in individuals with AIDS than in the general population and over 300 times more common than in other immunosuppressed patients.

Although KS has been associated with all risk behaviors for HIV infection, it usually occurs in men who have sex with men. As reported by the Centers for Disease Control and Prevention (CDC), KS is an AIDS-defining diagnosis in 20% to 30% of homosexual men, which contrasts sharply with

9% of Haitians, 3% of heterosexual injection-drug uses, 3% of transfusion recipients, 3% of women and children, and 1% of hemophiliacs. The risk of KS is greatest in geographic areas in the United States where the AIDS epidemic originated. For example, the proportion of gay or bisexual men with AIDS who have KS ranges from 30% in New York or California to approximately 5% in Kansas or Iowa. KS is four times more common in an HIV-infected woman with a sexual partner who is a bisexual man than one who is an injection-drug user. The percentage of AIDS cases presenting as KS has decreased over time. For example, among gay or bisexual AIDS patients in the United States, the proportion with KS decreased from 40% in 1983 to 13% in 1988.

These epidemiologic observations suggested that the etiology of KS is infectious and transmitted mainly by sexual contact. Since then, a landmark study has demonstrated the presence of herpesvirus-like DNA sequences, not only in AIDS-associated KS but also in classic KS and in KS that occurs in seronegative homosexual men. The discovery of KS herpes virus (KSHV), also known as human herpes virus-8 (HHV8), has altered our understanding of this neoplasm. The prevalence of KSHV/HHV8 infection strongly correlates with the number of homosexual partners. Among HIV-infected patients who are seropositive for KSHV/HHV8 antigen, the 10-year probability of developing KS is approximately 50%.

Pathogenesis

The pathogenesis of AIDS-related KS has been an area of active investigation. The cell of origin is believed to be lymphatic endothelium based on surface characteristics of neoplastic KS spindle cells. Histology of KS lesions shows whorls of such spindle cells with neovascularization, white cell infiltration, and microhemorrhage with hemosiderin deposition. The findings in AIDS-KS are similar to those of the classical form of indolent KS seen predominantly in elderly individuals of Southern European descent and the aggressive form described in Africa and in patients undergoing immunosuppressive therapy for organ transplantation.

The intimate relationship that exists between the integrity of the cellular immune system and development of KS is highlighted by the observation that effective combination antiretroviral therapy has been associated with a decreased proportion of new AIDS cases presenting with KS. Previous anecdotal reports described spontaneous regression of KS on discontinuation of immunosuppressive therapy for patients with organ transplantation.

Recent studies have examined the question of whether KS is a monoclonal or polyclonal proliferative disorder. There is evidence to support both hypotheses. What transforms the normal lymphatic endothelial cell into a malignant spindle cell is still not fully understood. There has been an effort to relate past information on the roles of cytokines and HIV *tat* protein in KS pathogenesis to recent data on KSHV/HHV8.

HIV *tat* is a multifunctional protein that not only acts as a transcriptional activator within the cell but also is secreted and can act as a cytokine-like molecule. There are two major domains of the HIV *tat* protein that have been defined: 1) a basic domain that has some homology to growth factors (e.g., vascular endothelial growth factor [VEGF]), and 2) a domain containing an arginine-glycine-aspartic acid (RGD) sequence that mirrors the active domain of extracellular matrix protein (e.g., fibronectin).

A number of recent studies have documented that HIV *tat* can activate the surface receptor for VEGF as well as surface adhesion receptors of the J-integrin family. Thus, one could imagine the lymphatic endothelial cell being exposed to HIV *tat* in proximity to infected T lymphocytes and macrophages. The growth signals mediated by HIV *tat* via activation of the VEGF surface receptor and certain J-integrin receptors might promote excessive and dysregulated cellular proliferation. Indeed, a transgenic mouse model that expresses human *tat* has developed pathologic lesions that have some resemblance to KS.

Other investigations have revealed a variety of biologically active proteins of the cytokine family that are able to stimulate KS spindle growth *in vitro*. These include interleukin-6 (IL-6), Oncostatin M, tumor necrosis factor (TNF), and platelet-derived growth factor (PDGF). More recently, it has been demonstrated that a number of chemokines—low-molecular-weight, biologically active molecules that primarily mediate cell migration—also affect KS spindle cells. Most prominent among these are members of the macrophage inhibitory protein (MIP) family.

Against this background of KS spindle cell proliferation—either by native cytokines or cytokine-like properties of HIV *tat*—is the discovery of KSHV/HHV8. Serologic evidence of infection with this virus is high among both AIDS-related and classic KS cases, with a lower prevalence in the general population. KSHV/HHV8 infects not only endothelial cells but also hematopoietic cells, particularly B lymphocytes. Biologically active molecules released by these cells may drive KS spindle cell transformation and proliferation.

The concept of "molecular piracy" comes into play when one examines the genetic elements carried by KSHV/HHV8. That is, KSHV/HHV8 encodes proteins that have homology to 1) the MIP-1 family of chemokines, 2) active cell cycle regulators of the cyclin family, and 3) activated receptors of the chemokine family. Thus, KSHV/HHV8 infection could result in both the release in a disordered fashion of biologically active proteins with cytokine properties *and* expression of a switched-on chemokine receptor that would drive cell proliferation. Recent work on this constitutively activated chemokine receptor *in vitro* reveals that it has the properties of an oncogene and therefore could be an important contributor to the neoplastic transformation of lymphatic endothelium to malignant KS spindle cells.

The disproportionate frequency with which KS is diagnosed in men suggests that sex hormones could have a role in enhancing neoplasm development. There are some data that androgenic hormones stimulate KS spindle cell development and that female hormones inhibit it; however, this area is still controversial.

Corticosteroid therapy has been associated with the induction of KS and with the exacerbation of pre-existing KS. This association needs to be kept in mind because of the not uncommon use of steroids in HIV-infected patients for immune thrombocytopenic purpura and *Pneumocystis carinii* pneumonia. KS lesions may regress on reduction or withdrawal of steroids. Opportunistic infections also have been associated with the induction of KS and with the exacerbation of pre-existing KS similar to that described with corticosteroid therapy. High levels of pro-inflammatory cytokines that result from opportunistic infections may account for these effects.

Clinical Manifestations

AIDS-related KS has a variable clinical course, ranging from minimal disease that presents as an incidental finding to explosive growth that results in significant morbidity and mortality. Skin lesions are usually papular, ranging in size from several millimeters to centimeters in diameter. They appear in a symmetrical distribution, most often on the lower extremities, face (especially the nose), oral mucosa, and genitalia. These may be arranged in a linear fashion along skin "tension lines." Early lesions may be mistaken for purpura, hematomas, angiomas, dermatofibromas, or nevi. Colors include many hues of pink, red, purple, and brown (Fig. 9.1B), and yellow perilesional halos are sometimes seen (Fig. 9.1C). KS lesions, especially on the thighs and soles of the feet, are infrequently plaque-like or exophytic with breakdown of overlying skin (Fig. 9.1A). Lymphedema, particularly of the face, genitalia, and lower extremities, may be out of proportion to the extent of disease. The psychosocial effects of KS may be profound and includes emotional distress, guilt, anger, ostracism, and loss of employment.

Extracutaneous spread of KS is common. Oral cavity KS occurs in approximately one third of patients and is the initial site of the disease in approximately 15%. The palate is most often affected followed by the gingiva. Intra-oral lesions may become traumatized during normal chewing, causing pain, bleeding, ulceration, and secondary infection. They may interfere with nutrition and speech.

Gastrointestinal involvement is found in 40% of cases at the time of initial diagnosis and in up to 80% at autopsy. Gastrointestinal lesions cause weight loss, abdominal pain, nausea, vomiting, bleeding, or diarrhea in some patients but are asymptomatic in others. Testing the stool for occult blood is the usual way to screen for gastrointestinal involvement. Typically, lesions on endoscopic examination are hemorrhagic nodules that can be isolated or confluent (Fig. 9.1D). Because they tend to be submucosal, biopsies may not demonstrate KS.

Pulmonary involvement may present with fever, dyspnea, cough, hemoptysis, or chest pain, or it can be an asymptomatic finding on chest radiograph. Radiographic findings vary greatly and can include nodular, interstitial and/or alveolar infiltrates; pleural effusion, hilar, and/or mediastinal adenopathy; or an isolated pulmonary nodule. A presumptive diagnosis of pulmonary KS usually can be made by the characteristic appearance of slightly raised cherry-red lesions on bronchoscopy. Gallium-thallium scanning may be helpful in evaluating an abnormal radiograph; KS is usually positive by thallium and negative by gallium, whereas infection is generally the reverse.

Other organs less frequently involved with KS include the lymphatic system, liver, pancreas, heart, and bone marrow.

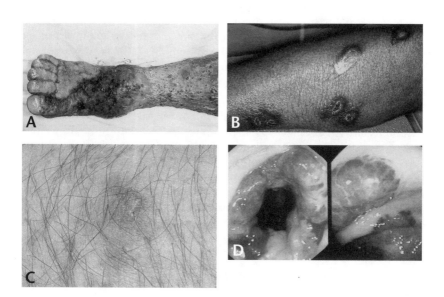

Figure 9.1   Manifestations of Kaposi's sarcoma, including plaque-like lesion with breakdown of overlying skin (A), multiple colored lesions on leg (B), lesion with yellow halo (C), and annular masses with circumferential infiltration and luminal obstruction in the colon and rectum (D). (Reprinted with permission from van den Brink MR, Dezube BJ. AIDS-related Kaposi's sarcoma. *J Clin Oncol.* 1997;15:1283-4.) (For color reproduction, *see* Plates 5–8 at back of book.)

Diagnosis

Although the presumptive diagnosis of KS often can be made readily by an experienced clinician, a skin biopsy is confirmatory. It is especially important to biopsy any lesions that are less typical of KS and associated with constitutional symptoms to rule out bacillary angiomatosis (BA) (*see* Fig. 8.1). Skin lesions of BA usually appear as numerous red round papules or nodules. KS and BA can occur simultaneously in the same patient. Less commonly, KS can be mimicked by extrapulmonary pneumocystosis, even in the absence of evident lung infection.

Staging and Prognosis

The initial evaluation of a patient with KS consists of a physical examination with special attention to those areas typically affected, such as the lower extremities, face, oral mucosa, genitalia, gastrointestinal tract, and lungs. Checking the stool for occult blood is performed to screen for gastrointestinal lesions, with endoscopy reserved for those patients who test positive or have gastrointestinal symptoms. Chest radiography is performed to screen for pulmonary lesions. Bronchoscopy can be reserved in those with persistent respiratory symptoms or an abnormal radiograph not explained by other causes. Computed tomography (CT) scanning of the chest, abdomen, and pelvis is typically not necessary but may be helpful in some cases. The CD4 cell count and HIV viral load are important for staging and treatment decisions.

The most commonly used staging system for AIDS-related KS was developed by the AIDS Clinical Trial Group (ACTG) of the National Institutes of Health (Table 9.1). Patients are categorized as belonging to a good or poor risk group according to three parameters: extent of tumor (T), immune status (I), and severity of systemic illness (S). This classification system has been shown to predict survival prospectively. However, it predated HIV viral load testing, which might be expected to refine further the staging of this tumor.

Treatment

Combination antiretroviral therapy, which is associated with a regression in the size of KS lesions in many patients, should be prescribed with the goal of maximally suppressing HIV viral load. The major objectives of treatment of KS are palliation of symptoms; shrinkage of tumor to alleviate edema, organ compromise, or psychological stress; and prevention of disease progression. Treatment options are individualized based on the extent of and rate of growth of the tumor and the patient's HIV disease status.

Table 9.1   Staging Classification for AIDS-Related Kaposi's Sarcoma

	Good Risk (all of the following)	Poor Risk (any of the following)
Tumor (T)	Confined to skin and/or lymph nodes and/or minimal oral disease (non-nodular KS confined to palate)	Tumor-associated edema or ulceration; extensive oral KS; gastrointestinal KS; KS in other non-nodal viscera
Immune system (I)	CD4 count ≥200 cells/mm³	CD4 count <200 cells/mm³
Systemic illness (S)	No history of OI or thrush; no "B" symptoms*; Karnofsky performance status ≥70	History of OI and/or thrush; "B" symptoms* present; Karnofsky performance status <70; other HIV-related illness (e.g., neurological disease, lymphoma)

OI = opportunistic infection; KS = Kaposi's sarcoma.
* "B" symptoms are unexplained fever, night sweats, weight loss, and diarrhea persisting more than 2 weeks.
Adapted from Dezube BJ. Clinical presentations and natural history of AIDS-related KS. *Hematol Oncol Clin North Am.* 1996;10:1023–9.

Local Therapy

Local treatments (e.g., intralesional chemotherapy, radiation therapy, laser therapy, cryotherapy, topical applications of various drugs) can all be effective at controlling local tumor growth. Vinblastine is the most widely used intralesional agent and has an excellent response rate. It can be injected directly into a KS lesion as a 0.2–0.3 mg/mL solution with a volume of 0.1 mL per 0.5 cm² of lesion. Multiple injections may be necessary for larger lesions. A second series of injections often is administered 3 to 4 weeks later. Treated lesions will fade and regress but typically will not resolve completely. Radiation therapy can effectively palliate symptomatic disease that is too extensive to be treated with intralesional chemotherapy but that is not extensive enough to warrant systemic therapy. A large lesion on the sole of the foot would be one such example.

Alitretinoin gel 0.1% (PanRetin) is the only topical, patient-administered therapy approved for KS. Alitretinoin is a naturally occurring retinoid that binds both to retinoic acid receptors and to retinoid X receptors. In two phase III studies, alitretinoin gel compared with placebo was associated with a greater duration of response and more prolonged time to disease progression. Most patients require 4 to 8 weeks of treatment. Skin irritation is the most common side effect.

Chemotherapy

Although many older chemotherapeutic agents have been found to be active against KS both alone or in combination therapy, current systemic treatment generally involves the newer liposomal anthracyclines and paclitaxel. The liposomal formulation of the anthracyclines provides the theoretical advantage of longer plasma half-life, higher tumor concentrations of drug, and less toxicity in nontargeted organs; in other words, a much better benefit-to-risk ratio when compared with conventional chemotherapy.

The two currently approved liposomal anthracyclines, liposomal doxorubicin (Doxil) and liposomal daunorubicin (DaunoXome), have become the first-line treatment for KS. In randomized multicenter trials, each of these liposomal agents has been found to be superior to conventional chemotherapy (bleomycin and vincristine with or without nonliposomal doxorubicin) in terms of response rates and toxicity profiles. The dosage of Doxil is 20 mg/m^2 every 3 weeks; the dosage of DaunoXome is 40 mg/m^2 every 2 weeks.

Each of these products can reliably shrink tumors, lessen edema, and cause the color of lesions to fade. Moreover, Doxil is effective even in patients whose tumors have progressed while receiving conventional doxorubicin. Generally, side effects from these liposomal products are mild. Alopecia and neuropathies in particular are unusual with liposomal products compared with conventional chemotherapies. Even at higher cumulative doses, these agents have not typically been associated with the cardiomyopathy that has limited the use of nonliposomal anthracyclines.

Paclitaxel (Taxol) is the newest systemic chemotherapeutic agent approved for KS. Although potentially more toxic than the liposomal anthracyclines, paclitaxel has demonstrated striking efficacy as a second-line treatment for KS. Recommended dosing schedules are 100 mg/m^2 over 3 hours every 2 weeks or 135 mg/m^2 over 3 hours every 3 weeks. Because of concern about the use of steroids in HIV-infected patients, the dexamethasone premedication is typically 10 mg (instead of the usual 20 mg) administered orally at both 12 and 6 hours before chemotherapy. Diphenhydramine and ranitidine also are given.

Interferon-α

Interferon-α (Intron A, Roferon-A) is a biological-response modifier that produces clinically significant responses in approximately 20% to 40% of AIDS-KS patients, especially in those with higher CD4 cell counts and a disease limited to the skin. Although low dosages of interferon-α (<10 million U/m^2/d) can be used in combination with HIV nucleoside reverse-transcriptase inhibitors, this therapy often is associated with significant toxicity, including fever, chills, cognitive impairment, neutropenia, and hepatic dysfunction.

Future Directions

Recent advances in understanding the pathogenesis of KS are uncovering many potential targets for KS therapies. These include angiogenesis, sex hormones, and cellular differentiation. Angiogenesis inhibitors (fumagillin and thalidomide), preparations of human chorionic gonadotropin, and the differentiating agent 9-*cis*-retinoic acid all have caused tumor regression in early trials. Identifying the etiologic agent of KS may lead to the development of targeted therapies 1) to inhibit the specific protein products of KSHV/HHV8 that contribute to KS spindle cell growth, and 2) to block the switched-on chemokine receptor.

SUGGESTED READINGS

Reviews

Biggar RJ, Rabkin CS. The epidemiology of AIDS-related neoplasms [Review]. *Hematol Oncol Clin North Am.* 1996;10:997-1010

Miles SA. Pathogenesis of AIDS-related KS: evidence of a viral etiology [Review]. *Hematol Oncol Clin North Am.* 1996;10:1011-21

Dezube BJ. Clinical presentations and natural history of AIDS-related KS [Review]. *Hematol Oncol Clin North Am.* 1996;10:1023-9

Karp JE, Pluda JM, Yarchoan R. AIDS-related KS: a template for the translation of molecular pathogenesis into targeted therapeutic approaches [Review]. *Hematol Oncol Clin North Am.* 1996;10:1031-49

Lee F-C, Mitsuyasu RT. Chemotherapy of AIDS-related KS [Review]. *Hematol Oncol Clin North Am.* 1996;10:1051-68.

Other References

Albini A, Soldi R, Giunciuglio D, et al. The angiogenesis induced by HIV-1 *tat* protein is mediated by the Flk-1/KDR receptor on vascular endothelial cells. *Nat Med.* 1996;2:1371–5.

Beral V, Peterman TA, Berkelman RL, Jaffe HW. KS among persons with AIDS: a sexually transmitted infection? *Lancet.* 1990;335:123–8.

Barillari G, Gendelman R, Gallo RC, Ensoli B. The *tat* protein of HIV type 1, a growth factor for AIDS Kaposi's sarcoma and cytokine-activated vascular cells, induces adhesion of the same cell types by using integrin receptors recognizing the RGD amino acid sequence. *Proc Natl Acad Sci U S A.* 1993;90:7941–5.

Dezube BJ, Von Roenn JH, Holden-Wiltse J, et al. Fumagillin analog in the treatment of KS: a phase I AIDS clinical trial group study. *J Clin Oncol.* 1998;16:1444–9.

Fiorelli V, Gendelman R, Samaniego F, et al. Cytokines from activated T cells induce normal endothelial cells to acquire the phenotypic and functional features of AIDS–Kaposi's sarcoma spindle cells. *J Clin Invest.* 1995;95:1723–34.

Friedman SL, Wright TL, Altman DF. Gastrointestinal KS in patients with the acquired immune deficiency syndrome: endoscopic and autopsy findings. *Gastroenterology.* 1985;89:102–8.

Gill PS, Lunardi-Iskandar Y, Louie S, et al. The effects of preparations of human chorionic gonadotropin on AIDS-related KS. *N Engl J Med.* 1996;335:1261–9.

Gill PS, Wernz J, Scadden DT, et al. Randomized phase III study of liposomal daunorubicin versus doxorubicin, bleomycin, and vincristine in AIDS-related KS. *J Clin Oncol.* 1996;14:2353–64.

Gruden JF, Huang L, Webb WR, et al. AIDS-related KS of the lung: radiographic findings and staging system with bronchoscopic correlation. *Radiology.* 1995;195:545–52.

Holland JC, Tross S. Psychosocial considerations in the therapy of epidemic KS. *Semin Oncol.* 1987;14(Suppl 3):48–53.

Ioachim HL, Adsay V, Giancotti FR, et al. KS of internal organs: a multiparameter study of 86 cases. *Cancer.* 1995;75:1376–85.

Koehler JE, Sanchez MA, Garrido CS, et al. Molecular epidemiology of Bartonella infections in patients with bacillary angiomatosis-peliosis. *N Engl J Med.* 1997;337:1876–83.

Krown SE, Test MA, Huang J. AIDS-related KS: prospective validation of the AIDS Clinical Trials Group Staging Classification. *J Clin Oncol.* 1997;15:3085–92.

Martin JN, Genom DE, Osmond DH, et al. Sexual transmission and the natural history of HHV-8 infection. *N Engl J Med.* 1998;338:948–54.

Moore PS, Chang Y. Detection of herpesvirus-like DNA sequences in KS in patients with and without HIV infection. *N Engl J Med.* 1995;332:1181–5.

Murphy PM. Pirated genes in Kaposi's sarcoma. *Nature.* 1997;385:296–9.

Stewart S, Jablonowski H, Goebel FD, et al. Randomized comparative trial of pegylated liposomal doxorubicin versus bleomycin and vincristine in the treatment of AIDS-related KS. *J Clin Oncol.* 1998;16:683–91.

AIDS-RELATED LYMPHOMAS

John Doweiko, MD

Conditions that alter cellular immunity predispose to the development of neoplasms (1,2,3). These include congenital disorders (e.g., ataxia-telangiectasia, Wiskott–Aldrich syndrome), drug-induced immunosuppression for organ transplantation, and some chronic autoimmune diseases. It has been estimated that 30% to 40% of HIV-infected patients will develop a malignancy over time (1,4). However, this percentage is likely to become greater as survival lengthens (5).

Some malignancies encountered in the HIV-infected population are AIDS-defining (Table 9.2). These include Kaposi's sarcoma (KS), B-cell lymphomas, and epithelial squamous cell cancers, particularly of the anogenital epithelium and uterine cervix (6). Other malignancies occur

Table 9.2   Malignancies in HIV Disease

AIDS-defining

• Kaposi's sarcoma

• B-cell lymphoma

• Anogenital squamous cell carcinoma

Other

• Hodgkin's disease

• Plasma cell dyscrasia

• B-cell acute lymphocytic leukemia

• T-cell lymphoma

• Testicular cancer

• Lung cancer

with greater frequency in the context of HIV disease, but are not considered AIDS-defining. Most important of these is Hodgkin's disease (7). The incidence of B-cell acute lymphocytic leukemia and plasma cell dyscrasias also is increased, with relative risks approximately sixfold and 12-fold higher, respectively, than those of the general population (6). T-cell lymphoma may occur more frequently in the HIV-infected population (6). The incidence of testicular cancer (7) and lung cancer (8,9) also is higher.

Hodgkin's Disease

Previous controversy as to whether HIV infection is associated with a higher incidence of Hodgkin's disease has been resolved by recent studies that have shown a frequency that is greater than 18 times that of the HIV-seronegative population (6,7). Hodgkin's disease occurs most often in patients whose HIV risk behaviors include injection-drug use (10). Its onset is relatively late in the course of the HIV infection, when the median CD4 count has declined to 300 cells/mm^3 or fewer (10).

Hodgkin's disease in HIV-infected patients differs from that in the general population. Constitutional symptoms occur in over 80% of cases on presentation (6,10), a much higher proportion than that encountered in seronegative patients. The disease is typically more advanced at the time of presentation, with over 75% of patients in stage III or IV (10,11), and is more aggressive in its course (10). Extranodal disease occurs in over 65% of HIV-infected patients (12), and over 50% have bone marrow involvement (6).

The histologic spectrum of HIV-related Hodgkin's disease differs from that of the general population (6,12,13). Pathologic types associated with poorer prognosis, such as mixed cellularity and lymphocyte depleted, are encountered in a higher proportion of HIV-infected patients (Table 9.3). In Hodgkin's disease occurring in the general population, involved tissues are infiltrated with T lymphocytes. The cellular infiltrate in HIV-associated Hodgkin's disease is relatively poor in T cells. This finding may account for its more aggressive nature (6,10,11). Epstein–Barr virus (EBV) may play a greater role in the pathogenesis of HIV-related Hodgkin's disease; 83% to 100% of these Hodgkin's disease cases have EBV genome within the Reed–Sternberg cells (a much higher proportion than that encountered in the general population) (12,13). Despite these differences in the nature of Hodgkin's disease in the context of HIV infection, the rate of complete remission may be as high as 80% with standard treatment regimens (10).

Non-Hodgkin's Lymphoma

HIV infection increases the risk of lymphoma 60- to 100-fold over that of the general population (14–17). Approximately 10% of HIV-infected patients will develop a non-Hodgkin's lymphoma (15). As with the other malignancies, the occurrence of lymphomas is expected to increase as survival lengthens related to better control of HIV infection and the prevention of opportunistic infections (15,17–19). There does not seem to be any correlation between the risk behavior for HIV infection and the likelihood of developing non-Hodgkin's lymphoma.

Table 9.3   Distribution of Histologic Types of Hodgkin's Disease

Histology	HIV-Infected Population	Seronegative Population
Lymphocyte predominant	1%	5%
Nodular sclerosing	27%	70%
Mixed cellularity	55%	22%
Lymphocyte depleted	12%	1%
Unclassifiable	5%	2%

Primary Central Nervous System Lymphoma

Primary central nervous system (CNS) lymphomas comprise 20% of all AIDS-related lymphomas but only account for 2% of lymphomas in the general population (20). Primary CNS lymphomas tend to occur relatively late in the course of HIV disease, with a mean CD4 count of 30 cells/mm^3 compared with 190 cells/mm^3 for systemic lymphomas (20,21). Most of these tumors are immunoblastic-plasmacytoid or large cell histology (20), and they are always monoclonal (21). Primary CNS lymphomas rarely spread outside of the nervous system and are typically multifocal.

Unlike systemic lymphomas that have secondarily spread to the CNS wherein cerebrospinal fluid (CSF) cytology is positive in at least 80% with the first lumbar puncture, leptomeningeal involvement with primary CNS lymphomas is uncommon (22,23). Here the CSF cytology is positive for malignant lymphocytes in only 15% of cases (21,22). However, these tumors all contain genomic material from EBV (21,22,24,28) that, when detected via polymerase chain reaction on CSF analysis, may be a surrogate marker for primary CNS lymphoma (25). Compared with biopsy, the sensitivity of this test is approximately 84%, with a positive predictive value of nearly 100%, and a negative predictive value of 93% (25).

Primary CNS lymphomas are the second most common brain mass lesions in patients with AIDS after toxoplasmosis (26) (Table 9.4). At the time

Table 9.4   Comparison of Characteristics of Toxoplasmosis and Central Nervous System Lymphoma

Toxoplasmosis	CNS Lymphoma
In 15% of AIDS patients	In 5% of AIDS patients
Subacute illness	More chronic illness
Predominance of focal symptoms and signs	50% have nonfocal symptoms and signs
Variable location in the CNS	75% are supratentorial
Basal ganglia commonly are involved	80% are located deep in the brain (white matter and periventricular regions)
Multiple lesions on MRI scan in 85% of cases	50% are multifocal on MRI scan
Over 90% enhance, typically in an even pattern	Variable enhancement pattern but generally less intense
Lesions of 1–3 cm is more consistent with toxoplasmosis	Lesion >3.0 cm is more consistent with lymphoma

CNS = central nervous system; MRI = magnetic resonance imaging.

of presentation, they are often at least 3 cm in size, growing in a perivascular distribution (27). On magnetic resonance imaging (MRI) scan, over one half of patients have multiple lesions that are hypo- or isodense on T1- and T0-weighted imaging (28). The most common locations are the cerebral hemispheres, followed by the basal ganglia, cerebellum, and brain stem. Unlike primary CNS lymphomas in the general population, these tumors may ring-enhance because more rapid growth results in central necrosis (27,28).

Pathogenesis

AIDS-related lymphomas have a different pathogenesis and behavior than lymphomas of similar histology that occur in the general population (25,29–32). They result from a combination of factors (Table 9.5). During the course of HIV infection, there is chronic stimulation of B cells (24,33,34), the early effects of which include hypergammaglobulinemia and persistent generalized lymphadenopathy (24). Lymphocytes are the only cells that rearrange their DNA during the normal course of adult life—a process necessary to provide for the range of antibody specificity required (24,33,34). The chronic B-cell stimulation and proliferation that occurs with HIV disease increases the chances that a genetic error will occur during this process. The immunosuppression from HIV infection results in a loss of immune surveillance, allowing aberrant B cell clones to proliferate instead of being eliminated by the cellular immune system (24,34,35).

The dysregulation of cytokines that occurs during HIV infection is a major driving force for B-cell proliferation (33,36,37). Two cytokines in particular have special importance (33). Interleukin-6 (IL-6) levels increase early during the course of HIV infection (38); their duration and amplitude predict the likelihood of lymphoma developing over time. In addition, there is an inverse relationship between IL-6 levels and the response of a

---

Table 9.5   Pathogenic Factors in AIDS-Related Lymphomas

- Chronic stimulation of B cells

- Immunosuppression and loss of immune surveillance

- Proto-oncogenes and tumor-suppressor genes

- Destruction of lymph nodes

- Cytokines

- Other viral infections

lymphoma to therapy (38). Interleukin-10 (IL-10) levels also are increased markedly in HIV disease (39). This cytokine acts as an autocrine growth factor for lymphomas while simultaneously inhibiting cellular immune response (39). High levels of IL-10 are associated with a poor prognosis for AIDS-related lymphomas (39).

Coinciding with chronic stimulation of B cells is the destruction of the dendritic reticulum network of the germinal centers of lymph nodes (23,24,33). These dendritic cells exert a control over B-cell apoptosis and participate in antigen presentation. The loss of these cells from HIV infection compromises the control of B-cell proliferation and interferes with the ability to mount a specific humeral response because of defective antigen presentation.

The DNA rearrangements that occur during B-cell development may activate proto-oncogenes, inactive tumor-suppressor genes, or both (29,40,41). Proto-oncogenes are normal growth-promoting genes that, when translocated to other areas of the genome, may result in unregulated proliferation of cells (31,42). Over 75% of AIDS-related lymphomas have alterations of at least one proto-oncogene (41–44). Tumor-suppressor genes normally prevent unregulated cellular growth via control of apoptosis (31,40,41,45,46). Over 90% of AIDS-related lymphomas have alterations in at least one tumor-suppressor gene (43,46).

Two other viruses may affect the risk of lymphomas in HIV-infected patients. EBV replication induces a polyclonal B-cell proliferation and simultaneously dysregulates tumor-suppressor genes and proto-oncogenes (47–52). KS herpesvirus (KSHV/HHV8) possesses genes homologous to human genes that control cell cycling (53–57).

Histology

Three histologic types comprise almost all AIDS-related lymphomas (33,40,58) but account for only approximately 10% of all non-Hodgkin's lymphomas in the general population. Over 95% are B-cell neoplasms, with the remaining being of T-cell or indeterminate origin (27). Overall, approximately 90% are monoclonal tumors (27) (Table 9.6).

Small, noncleaved cell lymphomas (Burkitt's or non-Burkitt's types) constitute approximately 40% of all AIDS-related lymphomas (40). These tumors tend to present at CD4 counts greater than 200 cells/mm^3 (33). Small, noncleaved cell lymphomas are almost always monoclonal.

Large cell lymphomas account for approximately 30% of AIDS-related lymphomas. These are the most heterogenous of the lymphomas encountered, forming a spectrum that contains various proportions of B-cell, T-cell, and macrophage antigens; approximately 10% contain a malignant lymphocytic proliferation that is polyclonal (40).

Table 9.6   Clonality of AIDS-Related Lymphomas

Histology	Proportion of Cases	Monoclonal
Small, noncleaved cell	40%	>95%
Large cell	30%	~90%
Immunoblastic-plasmacytoid	30%	~80%

The remaining 30% of AIDS-related lymphomas are immunoblastic-plasmacytoid lymphomas. These may be polyclonal in up to 20% of cases. Rare types of lymphoma sometimes encountered in HIV-infected individuals include Ki-1 anaplastic lymphoma, angiotrophic large cell lymphoma, mucosa-associated lymphoid tissue, and Sézary syndrome (33).

Clinical Manifestations

Non-Hodgkin's lymphoma may present with a mass lesion, organ failure from tumor infiltration, obstruction, or bleeding. Fever, particularly if it persists for over 2 weeks, also may be a sign of this tumor (59,60). Overall, approximately 65% of patients present with extranodal tumor, and over 95% eventually will develop extranodal spread. The sites of involvement are noted in Table 9.7. The bone marrow is involved in approximately one third of patients at the time of presentation (61).

The gastrointestinal tract is the most frequent site of extranodal disease (62,63) and the presenting site in up to 45% of cases. Of these, the colon is involved in 46%, the ileum in 39%, the stomach in 23%, and the other areas in the remainder (62,63). The features of gastrointestinal tract disease include abdominal pain and/or weight loss; life-threatening complications (e.g., bleeding, perforation, obstruction) may occur in approximately 40% of cases (63). Studies have shown that those with gastrointestinal tract lymphoma tend to survive longer and are more likely to respond to therapy than those with extra–gastrointestinal tract disease (62).

Secondary spread to the CNS—almost always as lymphomatous meningitis (64)—is present in 20% to 40% of patients at the time of presentation. Headache, cranial nerve palsies, and meningeal signs sometimes occur even though almost one quarter of patients with leptomeningeal disease have no symptoms (64). Leptomeningeal spread, per se, is not associated with a poorer prognosis. Therapy with intrathecal cytarabine given concur-

Table 9.7   Sites of Involvement of AIDS-Related Lymphomas*

Site	Involvement
Lymph nodes	38%
Lung	33%
Liver	33%
Bone marrow	30%
Central nervous system	27%
Spleen	23%
Small bowel	22%
Large bowel/rectum	21%

* Total is greater than 100% because some patients have multiple sites of involvement.

rently with systemic chemotherapy is often successful in eradicating meningeal disease (64).

Primary effusion lymphomas, also known as body cavity lymphomas, are a distinct clinical and pathologic subtype of AIDS-related non-Hodgkin's lymphoma (58,65–69). These tumors originate in the pleura, pericardium, peritoneum, serosal surfaces, and, rarely, the meninges (66). They present with a serous (lymphomatous) effusion but no detectable mass lesion (65). Although primary effusion lymphomas have little propensity to disseminate, they cause local destruction and have a uniformly poor outcome to therapy (65). Primary effusion lymphomas are high-grade neoplasms that may lack surface expression of T- or B-cell lymphocyte antigens, but they do express CD-45 and the activation antigens CD-30, CD-38, CD-71, and HLA-DR (65,66). They consistently have material from EBV, and almost all contain genomic material from KSHV/HHV8 (65,69).

Diagnosis

Diagnosis of lymphoma is made by excisional lymph node biopsy or by biopsy of an involved extranodal site. Routine staging also should include computed tomography (CT) or MRI of the head, chest, abdomen, and pelvis; gallium scan; lumbar puncture with cytologic analysis of cerebrospinal fluid (CSF); and bone marrow examination. Gastrointestinal symptoms should be investigated endoscopically.

Therapeutic Strategies

Optimal management for AIDS-related lymphomas has yet to be defined, but the standard therapy consists of "CHOP," i.e., cyclophosphamide, doxorubicin, vincristine, and prednisone. Complete responses occur less often and are less durable in HIV-infected patients than in the general population (70). Comparison between standard-dose and low-dose chemotherapeutic regimens reveals complete responses, time to progression, and median survival to be similar in both treatment arms, but there is less toxicity in the low-dose regimen (71,72). There seems to be a trade-off between the response rate achieved with a standard-dose regimen and the greater immunosuppression that is induced by it (72–83). Furthermore, several anticancer agents contained in current treatment regimens for lymphomas may induce or enhance the expression of HIV (78,83). Conversely, HIV infection may render lymphocytes resistant to the cytotoxic activity of some antineoplastic agents (78,83–86).

Zidovudine (ZDV), originally developed in 1964 as an antineoplastic agent, has antiproliferative activity when combined with drugs that disrupt thymidylate synthesis, such as 5-fluorouracil and methotrexate. In small studies, response rates as high as 80% have been achieved. Other nucleoside reverse-transcriptase inhibitors have not been shown to have this effect (86,87).

Methyl-glyoxal, bis-guanlhydrazone (mitoguazone, or MGBG) is a non–cell-cycle–specific cytotoxic agent. This compound inhibits the biosynthesis of polyamines—short peptides that are important to DNA, RNA, and membrane integrity (5,88,89). The drug has produced response rates of 29% to 49% in relapsed or refractory systemic AIDS-related lymphomas, with a median survival of 21.5 months for complete responders (5). MGBG has the advantage of good CNS penetration and a relative lack of bone marrow toxicity (5,89) but may cause mucositis, gastrointestinal symptoms, paresthesias, somnolence, and vasodilation (88,89). Studies using this drug for initial therapy and in combination with other agents are ongoing.

Daily, low-dose subcutaneous interleukin-2 infusions have been shown to promote expansion of immune effectors, such as natural killer cells. Small studies have demonstrated that this effect may result in down-regulation of lymphoproliferative disorders in HIV-infected patients (90). Combination antiretroviral therapy must be given concurrently to prevent augmentation of HIV replication (90).

Another line of investigation for therapy of AIDS-related lymphomas involves monoclonal antibodies. The prototype is anti-B4–blocked ricin (85). The "A" chain of ricin is an enzyme that inactivates ribosomes, and B4 (CD-19) is a B-lineage–restricted surface antigen expressed in over 95% of AIDS-related B-cell lymphomas. This antibody is given with multi-agent chemotherapy. Toxicities include fever, allergic reactions, hepatic dysfunction, and capillary leak syndrome (85).

Therapy for primary CNS lymphomas, which consists of radiation therapy with corticosteroids and/or alkylating agents, may increase the length of survival but rarely results in an extended remission. Survival without therapy is 2 to 3 months from the time of presentation compared with 6 to 8 months with therapy (34,36,39,40). However, palliation of these tumors for up to 18 months has been reported with aggressive radiation therapy and control of HIV infection (34,36,39,63).

Prognosis

Given appropriate therapy, patients with AIDS-related lymphomas with good prognostic features may attain complete remission rates exceeding 50%, with median survival of at least 18 months (60,91,92). Prognosis is not affected by leptomeningeal disease at the time of diagnosis, the size of the mass lesion, or the presence of constitutional symptoms (60,91,92). However, several adverse prognostic features have been identified, including age greater than 40 years, a CD4 count below 100 cells/mm^3, and a high serum lactate dehydrogenase (LDH) level at the time of diagnosis (Table 9.8). These characteristics independently increase the hazard ratio by 1.6, 1.7, and 1.8, respectively (72,93,86). Other adverse prognostic features in-

Table 9.8   Adverse Prognostic Features of AIDS-Related Lymphomas

- Age >40 years
- History of injection drug use
- Previous therapy with adriamycin or vincristine
- Multiple sites of disease
- CD4 count <100 cells/mm^3
- High (>1000 U/dL) serum LDH level

No. of Adverse Prognostic Features	Complete Response Rate	Median Survival
Zero	80%	18 months
One	67%	14 months
Two	57%	11 months
Four	13%	4 months

clude a history of injection-drug use; previous therapy with adriamycin, vincristine, or both; and more than one disease site. Combinations of these characteristics are associated with a lessening of the complete response rate and median survival (93).

REFERENCES

1. **Levine AM.** AIDS-related malignancies. *Curr Opin Oncol.* 1994;6:489–91.

2. **Conant MA.** Management of human immunodeficiency virus-associated malignancies. *Recent Results Cancer Res.* 1995;139:423–32.

3. **Rabkin CS.** Epidemiology of AIDS-related malignancies. *Curr Opin Oncol.* 1994;6:492–6.

4. **White DA.** Pulmonary complications of HIV-associated malignancies. *Clin Chest Med.* 1996;17:755–61.

5. **Levine'AM, Tulpule A, Tessman D, et al.** Mitoguazone therapy in patients with refractory or relapsed AIDS-related lymphoma: results from a multicenter phase II trial. *J Clin Oncol.* 1997;15:1094–103.

6. **Levine AM, Pieters AS.** Non–AIDS-defining cancer. In *Summaries of the First National AIDS Malignancy Conference.* Bethesda, MD: National Cancer Institute; 1997:18–20.

7. **Koblin BA, Hessol NA, Zauber AG, et al.** Increased incidence of cancer among homosexual men, New York City and San Francisco, 1978–1990. *Am J Epidemiol.* 1996;144:916–23.

8. **Gabutti G, Vercelli M, De Rosa MG, et al.** AIDS-related neoplasms in Genoa, Italy. *Eur J Epidemiol.* 1995;11:609–14.

9. **Biggar RJ, Rabkins CS.** The epidemiology of AIDS-related neoplasms. *Hematol Oncol Clin North Am.* 1996;5:997–1010.

10. **Andrieu JM, Roithmann S, Tourani JM, et al.** Hodgkin's disease during HIV-1 infection: the French registry experience. *Ann Oncol.* 1993;4:635–41.

11. **Gerald M, Adler R.** Hodgkin's disease as an indicator of AIDS. *Med Hypotheses.* 1995;45:76–82.

12. **Tearily U, Errant D, Dulcet R, et al.** Hodgkin's disease and HIV infection: clinicopathologic and virologic features of 114 patients from the Italian Cooperative Group on AIDS and Tumors. *J Clin Oncol.* 1995;13:1758–67.

13. **De Re V, Boiocchi M, De Vita S, et al.** Subtypes of Epstein-Barr virus in HIV-1-associated and HIV-1-unrelated Hodgkin's disease cases. *Int J Cancer.* 1993;54:895–8.

14. **Biggar RJ, Rosenberg PS, Cote T.** Kaposi's sarcoma and non-Hodgkin's lymphoma following the diagnosis of AIDS: Multistate AIDS/Cancer Match Study Group. *Int J Cancer.* 1996;68:754–8.

15. **Tearily U, Franceschi S, Carbone A.** Malignant tumours in patients with HIV infection. *Br Med J.* 1994;308:1148–53.

16. **Irwin D, Kaplan L.** Clinical aspects of HIV-related lymphoma. *Curr Opin Oncol.* 1993;5:852–60.

17. **Goplen AK, Dunlop O, Liestrol K, et al.** The impact of primary central nervous system lymphoma in AIDS patients: a population-based autopsy study from Oslo. *J Acquir Immune Defic Syndr Hum Retrovirol.* 1997;14:351–4.

18. **Rabkin CS, Hilgartner MW, Hedberg KW, et al.** Incidence of lymphomas and other cancers in HIV-infected and HIV-uninfected patients with hemophilia. *JAMA.* 1992;267:1090–4.

19. **Monoz A, Schrager LK, Bacellar H, et al.** Trends in the incidence of outcomes defining AIDS in the Multicenter AIDS Cohort Study: 1985–1991. *Am J Epidemiol.* 1993;137:423–38.

20. **McCarty M.** HIV and cancer. *Lancet.* 1994;343:1032.

21. **Roberts TC, Storch GA.** Multiplex PCR for diagnosis of AIDS-related central nervous system lymphoma and toxoplasmosis. *J Clin Microbiol.* 1997;35:268–9.

22. **Przybylski GK, Goldman J, Ng VL, et al.** Evidence for early B-cell activation preceding the development of Epstein–Barr virus–negative AIDS-related lymphoma. *Blood.* 1996;88:4620–9.

23. **MacMahon EM, Glass JD, Hayward SD, et al.** Association of Epstein–Barr virus with primary central nervous system lymphoma in AIDS. *AIDS Res Hum Retroviruses.* 1992;8:740–2.

24. **Koopman G, Pals ST.** Cellular interactions in the germinal center: role of adhesion receptors and significance for the pathogenesis of AIDS and malignant lymphoma. *Immunol Rev.* 1992;126:21–45.

25. **Levine AM, Pieters AS.** Clinical aspects of AIDS-related lymphoma. In *Summaries of the First National AIDS Malignancy Conference.* Bethesda, MD: National Cancer Institute; 1997:40–44.

26. **Ruiz A, Post MJ, Bundschu C, et al.** Primary central nervous system lymphoma in patients with AIDS. *Neuroimaging Clin North Am.* 1997;7:281–96.

27. **Chapell ET.** Guthrie B, Orenstein J. The role of stereotactic biopsy in the management of HIV-related focal brain lesions. *Neurosurgery.* 1992;30:825–9.

28. **Johnson BA, Fram EK, Johnson PC, Jacobowitz R.** The variable MR appearance of primary lymphoma of the central nervous system: comparison with histopathologic features. *Am J Neuroradiol.* 1997;18:563–72.

29. **Ometto L, Menin C, Masiero S, et al.** Molecular profile of Epstein–Barr virus in HIV type 1–related lymphadenopathies and lymphomas. *Blood.* 1997;90:313–22.

30. **Herndier B, McGrath M, Abbey N, et al.** A nonlymphoma idiotype is indicative and predictive for B-cell malignancies in AIDS. *Hybridoma.* 1993;12:529–37.

31. **Schlaifer D, Krajewski S, Galoin S, et al.** Immunodetection of apoptosis-regulating proteins in lymphomas from patients with and without HIV infection. *Am J Pathol.* 1996;149:177–85.

32. **Komanduri KV, Luce JA, McGrath MS, et al.** The natural history and molecular heterogeneity of HIV-associated primary malignant lymphomatous effusions. *J Acquir Immune Defic Syndr Hum Retrovirol.* 1996;13:215–26.

33. **Sandler AS, Kaplan L.** AIDS lymphoma. *Curr Opin Oncol.* 1996;8:377–85.

34. **Wang CY, Snow JL, Su WP.** Lymphoma associated with HIV infection. *Mayo Clin Proc.* 1995;70:665–72.

35. **Gerdes J, Flad HD.** Follicular dendritic cells and their role in HIV infection. *Immunol Today.* 1992;13:81–3.

36. **Marsh JW, Herndier B, Tsuzuki A, et al.** Cytokine expression in large cell lymphoma associated with AIDS. *J Interferon Cytokine Res.* 1995;15:261–8.

37. **Lai CF, Ripperger J, Morella KK, et al.** Receptors for interleukin (IL)-10 and IL-6-

type cytokines use similar signaling mechanisms for inducing transcription through IL-6 response elements. *J Biol Chem.* 1996;271:13968–75.

38. **Sandler AS, Kaplan L.** AIDS lymphoma. *Curr Opin Oncol.* 1996;8:377–85.

39. **Masood R, Zhang Y, Bond MW, et al.** Interleukin-10 is an autocrine growth factor for AIDS-related B-cell lymphoma. *Blood.* 1995;85:3423–30.

40. **Foreman KE, Bacon PE, Hsi ED, Nickoloff BJ.** *In situ* polymerase chain reaction–based localization studies support role of human hervesvirus-8 as the cause of two AIDS-related neoplasms: Kaposi's sarcoma and body cavity lymphoma. *J Clin Invest.* 1997;99:2971–8.

41. **Xerri L, Parc P, Brousset P, et al.** Predominant expression of the long isoform of Bcl-x (Bcl-xL) in human lymphomas. *Br J Haematol.* 1996;92:900–6.

42. **Ambinder R, Harrington M.** EBV: how the kissing virus becomes deadly. In *Summaries of the First National AIDS Malignancy Conference.* Bethesda, MD: National Cancer Institute; 1997:45–50.

43. **Gaidano G, Carbone A, Pastore C, et al.** Frequent mutation of the 5′ noncoding region of the BCL-6 gene in AIDS-related non-Hodgkin's lymphomas. *Blood.* 1997;89:3755–62.

44. **Gaidano G, Pastore C, Capello D, et al.** Involvement of the *bcl-6* gene in AIDS-related lymphomas. *Ann Oncol.* 1997;8(Suppl 2):105–8.

45. **Martin A, Magne G, Stefanuto S, Feuteun J.** Functional analysis of p53 in AIDS-related non-Hodgkin's lymphomas by immunohistochemistry and biological assay in yeast. *Blood.* 1995;86:932.

46. **Pizzolato J, Greenberg D, Streeter G, et al.** P53 status in AIDS-lymphoma cell lines correlates with sensitivity to chemotherapy and radiation-induced apoptosis. *Blood.* 1995;86:739.

47. **Corn BW, Donahue BR, Rosenstock JG, et al.** Palliation of AIDS-related primary lymphoma of the brain: observations from a multi-institutional database. *Int J Radiat Oncol Biol Phys.* 1997;38:601–5.

48. **Van Kuyk R, Mosier DE.** Lack of pseudotype formation between HIV type 1 and Epstein–Barr virus in productively coinfected B-lymphoblastoid cell lines. *Virology.* 1995;209:643–8.

49. **Horenstein MG, Nador RG, Chadburn A, et al.** Epstein–Barr virus latent gene expression in primary effusion lymphomas containing Kaposi's sarcoma–associated herpesvirus/human herpesvirus-8. *Blood.* 1997;90:1186–91.

50. **Anonymous.** Epstein–Barr virus and AIDS-associated lymphomas. *Lancet.* 1991;338:979–81.

51. **Grant JW, Isaacson PG.** Primary central nervous system lymphoma. *Brain Pathol.* 1992;2:97–109.

52. **Li SL, Biberfeld P, Ernberg I.** DNA of lymphoma-associated herpesvirus (HVMF1) in SIV-infected monkeys (*Macaca fascicularis*) shows homologies to EBNA-1, -2 and -5 genes. *Int J Cancer.* 1994;59:287–95.

53. **Morgello S, Tagliati M, Ewart MR.** HHV-8 and AIDS-related CNS lymphoma. *Neurology.* 1997;48:1333–5.

54. **Arvanitakis L, Mesri EA, Nador RG, et al.** Establishment and characterization of a primary effusion (body cavity–based) lymphoma cell line (BD-3) harboring Kaposi's sarcoma–associated herpesvirus (KSHV/HHV-8) in the absence of Epstein–Barr virus. *Blood.* 1996;88:2648–54.

55. **Ambinger R, Harrington M.** HHV-8/KSHV and the mysteries of KS pathogenesis. In *Summaries of the First National AIDS Malignancy Conference.* Bethesda, MD: National Cancer Institute; 1997:2–5.

56. **Otsuki T, Kumar S, Ensoli B, et al.** Detection of HIV/8/KSHV DNA sequences in AIDS-associated extranodal lymphoid malignancies. *Leukemia.* 1996;10:1358–62.

57. **Chadburn A, Cesarman E, Nador RG, et al.** Kaposi's sarcoma–associated herpesvirus sequences in benign lymphoid proliferations not associated with HIV. *Cancer.* 1997;80:788–97.

58. **Ng VL, Komanduri KV, Luce JA.** Clinical and laboratory features of HIV-associated body cavity–based lymphomas: American Society of Hematology abstract 1506. *Blood.* 1995;86:379a.

59. **Sepkowitz KA, Telzak EE, Carrow M, Armstrong D.** Fever among outpatients with advanced HIV infection. *Arch Intern Med.* 1993;153:1909–12.

60. **Bissuel F, Leport C, Perronne C, et al.** Fever of unknown origin in HIV-infected patients: a critical analysis of a retrospective series of 57 cases. *J Intern Med.* 1994;236:529–35.

61. **Klatt EC, Nichols L, Noguchi TT.** Evolving trends revealed by autopsies of patients with AIDS: 565 autopsies in adults with AIDS, Los Angeles, California, 1982–1993. *Arch Pathol Lab Med.* 1994;118:884–90.

62. **Powitz F, Bopgner JR, Sandor P, et al.** Gastrointestinal lymphomas in patients with AIDS. *Zeitschr Gastroenterol.* 1997;35:179–85.

63. **Heise W, Arasteh K, Mostertz P, et al.** Malignant gastrointestinal lymphomas in patients with AIDS. *Digestion.* 1997;58:218–24.

64. **Straus DJ.** HIV-associated lymphomas. *Med Clin North Am.* 1997;81:495–510.

65. **Karcher DS, Alkan S.** Human herpesvirus-8–associated body cavity–based lymphoma in HIV-infected patients: a unique B-cell neoplasm. *Hum Pathol.* 1997;28: 801–8.

66. **Zakoswki MF, Ianuale-Shanerman A.** Cytology of pericardial effusions in AIDS patients. *Diagn Cytopathol.* 1993;9:266–9.

67. **Purtilo DT, Strobach RS, Okano M, Davis JR.** Epstein–Barr virus–associated lymphoproliferative disorders. *Lab Invest.* 1992;67:5–23.

68. **Horenstein MG, Nador RG, Chadburn A, et al.** Epstein–Barr virus latent gene expression in primary effusion lymphomas containing Kaposi's sarcoma–associated herpesvirus/human herpesvirus-8. *Blood.* 1997;90:1186–91.

69. **Cesarman E, Nador RG, Bai F, et al.** Kaposi's sarcoma–associated herpesvirus contains G-protein–coupled receptor and cyclin-D homologs which are expressed in Kaposi's sarcoma and malignant lymphoma. *J Virol.* 1996;70:8218–23.

70. **Maksymiuk AW, Haines C, Tan LK, Skinnider LF.** Age-related prognostic factor analysis in non-Hodgkin's lymphoma. *Can J Oncol.* 1996;6:435–442.

71. **Kaplan LD, Straus DJ, Test MA, et al.** Low-dose compared with standard-dose m-BACOD chemotherapy for non-Hodgkin's lymphoma associated with HIV infection: National Institute of Allergy and Infectious Diseases AIDS Clinical Trials Group. *N Engl J Med.* 1997;336:1641–8.

72. **Weyand M, Frye K, Fahrenkamp A, et al.** Cyclophosphamide as an adjunct to maintenance immunosuppression in cardiac transplantation. *Transplant Proc.* 1995;27:1967–8.

73. **van Wyk CW, van der Bijl P, Cooper RC.** Induced resistance to *Candida albicans* in BALB/c mice during short-term immunosuppression with cyclophosphamide. *Lab Anim Sci.* 1995;45:101–6.

74. **Neuhaus TJ, Fay J, Dillon MJ, et al.** Alternative treatment to corticosteroids in steroid sensitive idiopathic nephrotic syndrome. *Arch Dis Child.* 1994;71:522–6.

75. **Hall S, Conn DL.** Immunusuppressive therapy for vasculitis. *Curr Opin Rheumatol.* 1995;7:25–9.

76. **Umesue M, Mayumi H, Nishimura Y, et al.** Xenogeneic (rat to mouse) skin tolerance induced by monoclonal antibodies, xenogeneic cells, and cyclophosphamide. *Transplant Proc.* 1995;27:315–6.

77. **Breitkreuz A, Ulrichs K, Eckstein V, et al.** Long-term suppression of natural and graft-induced xenophile antibodies by short-term antigen-cyclophosphamide treatment. *Transplant Proc.* 1993;25:416–8.

78. **Schmader KE, Rahiga R, Porter KR, et al.** Aging and reactivation of latent murine cytomegalovirus. *J Infect Dis.* 1992;166:1403–7.

79. **Koptopoulos G, Papanastasopoulou M, Lekkas S, et al.** Immunosuppression in goats by dexamethasone and cyclophosphamide. *Comp Immunol Microbiol Infect Dis.* 1992;15:235–42.

80. **Kondratyeva TK, Fontalin LN, Mikheeva NV.** T-cell immunodeficiency induced by T-cell mitogens combined with cyclophosphamide injection. *Immunol Lett.* 1992;34:71–7.

81. **Sparano JA, Hu X, Wiernik PH, et al.** Opportunistic infection and immunologic function in patients with HIV-associated non-Hodgkin's lymphoma treated with chemotherapy. *J Natl Cancer Inst.* 1997;89:301–7.

82. **Mastino A, Grelli S, Premrov MG, Favalli C.** Susceptibility to influenza A virus infection in mice immunosuppressed with cyclophosphamide. *J Chemother.* 1991;3:156–61.

83. **Smee DF, Burger RA, Coombs J, et al.** Progressive murine cytomegalovirus disease after termination of ganciclovir therapy in mice immunosuppressed by cyclophosphamide treatment. *J Infect Dis.* 1991;164:958–61.

84. **Manoharan A.** Targeted immunosuppression with vincristine infusion in the treatment of immune thrombocytopenia. *Austr N Z J Med.* 1991;21:405–7.

85. **Renner C, Trumper L, Pfreundschuh M.** Monoclonal antibodies in the treatment of non-Hodgkin's lymphoma: recent results and future prospects. *Leukemia.* 1997;11(Suppl 2):S55-9.

86. **Gherlinzoni F, Tosi P, Mazza P, et al.** Association of zidovudine and methotrexate for the treatment of HIV-related high-grade non-Hodgkin's lymphomas. *Blood.* 1995;86:381.

87. **Tosi P, Gherlinzoni F, Massa P, et al.** 3'-Azido 3'-deoxythymidine plus methotrexate as a novel antineoplastic combination in the treatment of HIV-related non-Hodgkin's lymphomas. *Blood.* 1997;89:419–25.

88. **Levine AM, Iles F, Kaplan L, et al.** Two sequential prospective, multi-institutional phase II clinical trials of mitoguazone (MGBG) in refractory or relapsed AIDS-related lymphoma. *Blood.* 1995;86;381.

89. **Rizzo J, Levine AM, Weiss GR, et al.** Pharmacokinetic profile of mitoguazone (MGBG) in patients with AIDS-related non-Hodgkin's lymphoma. *Invest N Drugs.* 1996;14:227–34.

90. **Bernstein ZP, Porter MM, Gould M, et al.** Prolonged administration of low-dose interleukin-2 in HIV-associated malignancy results in selective expansion of innate immune effectors without significant clinical toxicity. *Blood.* 1995;86:3287–94.

91. **Byrnes JJ, Harrington WJ, Cabral L, et al.** Treatment of AIDS-associated large cell lymphoma and determinants of outcome: American Society of Hematology Abstract 199. *Blood.* 1996;88:53a.

92. **Veugelers PJ, Strathdee SA, Tindall B, et al.** Increasing age is associated with faster progression to neoplasms but not opportunistic infections in HIV-infected homosexual men. *AIDS.* 1994;8:1471–5.

93. **Levine AM, Pieters AS.** AIDS-related lymphoma: clinical aspects. In *Summaries of the First National AIDS Malignancy Conference.* Bethesda, MD: National Institute; 1997:26–28.

ANOGENITAL SQUAMOUS CELL CANCER
John Doweiko, MD

Malignancies are diagnosed in approximately 40% of HIV-infected patients at some time during their clinical course, with the incidence expected to increase as survival improves (1,2). The relative risk of squamous cell carcinomas is 5.6 to 11.5 times that of the general population (3). Among these malignancies are carcinomas of the anus and uterine cervix, which are AIDS-defining diagnoses (2). Squamous cell carcinomas of the vulva, penis, oral cavity, and skin also occur with increased frequency in HIV-infected patients (4–6).

Pathogenesis

Human papillomavirus (HPV) plays a major role in the pathogenesis of anogenital squamous cell cancers (4,7–10). However, infection with HPV alone does not give rise to these neoplasms. Immunosuppression from HIV infection is a major factor in their genesis and progression (7,8,11–14).

Alterations in the local immune response and cytokine expression of the anal and genital mucosa caused by HIV infection may result in altered susceptibility for HPV infection and increased expression of HPV oncogenes (11,13,15–18).

Squamous Cell Dysplasia and Carcinoma of the Anus

Squamous cell carcinoma of the anal canal accounts for only 2% to 3% of all malignancies of the lower gastrointestinal tract (19), but 90% of these tumors occur in HIV-positive patients (11). Over 15% of HIV-infected men have high-grade squamous cell dysplasia of the anus (16). As with uterine cervical carcinoma in HIV-infected women, squamous cell cancers of the anus tend to be more aggressive than in the general population (15,20,21).

Most often, anal squamous cell dysplasia is asymptomatic. As these lesions become malignant, early symptoms may include burning, pruritus, or other local irritation (22). Bleeding may develop, and bacterial infection of the anal canal or perirectal area may result from disruption of the integrity of the mucosa. Mass lesions and ulcers of the anal canal occur late in the course of progression of these neoplasms.

Brush cytology provides a relatively easy way to screen for dysplasia of the anal canal (23). The sensitivity of this procedure is 70% to 83% (23,24). Although there is no consensus about this issue, performing the procedure every 6 months seems reasonable.

The optimal management of invasive squamous cell cancers of the anal canal is unclear (21,25,26). Some studies have used low-dose radiotherapy along with chemotherapy, most often 5-fluorouracil, mitomycin C, or both (25,27). However, HIV disease imposes certain limitations on administration of therapies for this condition (19). HIV infection is associated with an increased risk of damage to normal tissues and delayed healing, and limited bone marrow reserve may attenuate the administration of standard doses of chemotherapy (19).

Squamous Cell Cancer of the Uterine Cervix

Worldwide, over 40% of HIV-seropositive individuals are women, and cancer of the uterine cervix is a major oncologic problem in this group (4,9,28). Approximately 95% of these neoplasms are squamous cell carcinomas, which usually arise at the squamocolumnar junction of the cervix. HPV infection in the setting of immunosuppression is a major factor in their pathogenesis (29,30). Only approximately one half of women with cervical neoplasms have a previous history of clinically apparent genital condylomata (31).

These lesions begin as squamous cell dysplasias that advance to carcinoma *in situ*. There is no association between the stage of HIV disease and the presence or degree of cervical dysplasia (31). Eventually, malignant cells become invasive by breaking through the basement membrane and entering the cervical stroma. Immunosuppression from HIV infection is associated with more aggressive disease than in the general population (11,15,20,32).

Squamous cell dysplasia can be detected easily by the Pap smear. The positive predictive value of an abnormal Pap smear in an HIV-infected woman is approximately 95%, with a negative predictive value of approximately 39% (29,33). Although this test has an overall sensitivity of only 57% to 81% compared with biopsy, the false-negative rate decreases with repeated testing (29,33). The CDC recommends annual Pap smears in most women. However, the more rapid progression of cervical dysplasia in an HIV-infected woman may warrant Pap smears every 6 months (33).

Patients with Pap smears showing cellular atypia or squamous intraepithelial neoplasia should be referred to a gynecologist for colposcopy and biopsy if indicated. High-grade lesions are managed with cryotherapy, loop excision, laser therapy, or conization.

REFERENCES

1. **Krown SE.** AIDS-associated malignancies. *Cancer Chemother Biol Response Modif.* 1996;16:441–61.

2. **Rabkin CS.** Epidemiology of AIDS-related malignancies. *Curr Opin Oncol.* 1994;6:492–6.

3. **Levine AM, Pieters AS.** Non–AIDS-defining cancer. In *Summaries of the First National AIDS Malignancy Conference.* Bethesda, MD: National Cancer Institute; 1997:18–20.

4. **Wright TC, Koulos JP, Liu P, Sun XW.** Invasive vulvar carcinoma in two women infected with HIV. *Gynecol Oncol.* 1996;60:500–3.

5. **Langford A, Langer R, Lobeck H, et al.** HIV-associated squamous cell carcinomas of the head and neck presenting as oral and primary intraosseous squamous cell carcinomas. *Quintessence Int.* 1995;26:635–54.

6. **Wang CY, Brodland DG, Su WP.** Skin cancers associated with AIDS. *Mayo Clin Proc.* 1995;70:766–72.

7. **Adimora AA, Quinlivan EB.** Human papillomavirus infection: recent findings on progression to cervical cancer. *Postgrad Med.* 1995;98:109–12.

8. **Klein RS, Ho GY, Vermund SH, et al.** Risk factors for squamous intraepithelial lesions on Pap smear in women at risk for HIV infection. *J Infect Dis.* 1994;170;1404–9.

9. **Maiman M.** Cervical neoplasia in women with HIV infection. *Oncology* 1994;8: 83–94.

10. **Henry-Stanley MJ, Simpson M, Stanley MW.** Cervical cytology findings in women infected with the HIV. *Diagn Cytopathol.* 1993;9:508–9.

11. **Unger ER, Vernon SD, Lee DR, et al.** Human papillomavirus type in anal epithelial lesions is influenced by HIV. *Arch Pathol Lab Med.* 1997;121:820–4.

12. **Maiman M, Fruchter RG, Guy L, et al.** HIV infection and invasive cervical carcinoma. *Cancer.* 1993;71:402–6.

13. **Northfelt DW, Swift PS, Palesfsky JM.** Anal neoplasia: pathogenesis, diagnosis, and management. *Hematol Oncol Clin North Am.* 1996;10:1177–87.

14. **Metcalf AM, Dean T.** Risk of dysplasia in anal condyloma. *Surgery.* 1995:118: 724–6.

15. **Unger ER, Vernon SD, Lee DR, et al.** Human papillomavirus type in anal epithelial lesions is influenced by HIV. *Arch Pathol Lab Med.* 1997;121:820–4.

16. **Critchlow CW, Surawicz CM, Holmes KK, et al.** Prospective study of homosexual men: influence of HIV infection, immunosuppression, and human papillomavirus infection. *AIDS.* 1995;9:1255–62.

17. **Stratton P, Ciacco KH.** Cervical neoplasia in the patient with HIV infection. *Curr Opin Obstet Gynecol.* 1994;6:86–91.

18. **Carter PS, de Ruiter A, Whatrup C, et al.** HIV infection and genital warts as risk factors for anal intraepithelial neoplasia in homosexual men. *Br J Surg.* 1995;82:473–4.

19. **Harrison M, Tomlinson D, Stewart S.** Squamous cell carcinoma of the anus in patients with AIDS. *Clin Oncol.* 1995;7:50–51.

20. **Northfelt DW.** Cervical and anal neoplasia and HPV infection in persons with HIV infection. *Oncology.* 1994;8:33–40.

21. **Monoz-Jimenz F, Louredo-Mendez AM, Turegano-Fuentes F, et al.** Squamous cell carcinomas of the anus and infection with human papillomavirus in patients with AIDS. *Eur J Surg.* 1996;162:251–3.

22. **Forti RL, Medwell SJ, Aboulafia DM, et al.** Clinical presentation of minimally invasive *in situ* squamous cell carcinoma of the anus in homosexual men. *Clin Infect Dis.* 1995;21:603–7.

23. **Palefsky JM, Holly EA, Hogeboom CJ, et al.** Anal cytology as a screening tool for anal squamous intraepithelial lesions. *J Acquir Immune Defic Syndr Hum Retrovirol.* 1997;14:415–22.

24. **Sherman ME, Friedman HB, Busseniers AE, et al.** Cytologic diagnosis of anal intraepithelial neoplasia using smear and thin-preps. *Modern Pathol.* 1995;8:270–4.

25. **Bottomley DM, Aqel N, Selvaratnam G, Phillips RH.** Epidermoid anal cancer in HIV-infected patients. *Clin Oncol.* 1996;8:319–22.

26. **Weiss EG, Wexner SD.** Surgery for anal lesions in HIV-infected patients. *Ann Med.* 1995;27:467–75.

27. **Peddada AV, Smith DE, Rao AR, et al.** Chemotherapy and low-dose radiotherapy in the treatment of HIV-infected patients with carcinoma of the anal canal. *Int J Radiat Oncol Biol Phys.* 1997;37:1101–5.

28. **Tearily U, Vaccher E, Spina M.** Other cancers in HIV-infected patients. *Curr Opin Oncol.* 1994;6:508–11.

29. **Wright TC Jr, Ellerbrock TV, Chaisson MA, et al.** Cervical intraepithelial neoplasia in women infected with HIV: prevalence, risk factors, and validity of Papanicolaou smears. *Obstet Gynecol.* 1994;84:591–7.

30. **Fruchter RG, Maiman M, Sillman FH, et al.** Characteristics of cervical intraepithelial neoplasia in women infected with HIV. *Am J Obstet Gynecol.* 1994;171:531–7.

31. **Murphy M, Pomeroy L, Tynan M, et al.** Cervical cytological screening in HIV-infected women in Dublin: a six-year review. *Int J STD AIDS.* 1995;6:262–6.

32. **Palefsky J.** Human papillomavirus–associated malignancies in HIV-positive men and women. *Curr Opin Oncol.* 1995;7:437–44.

33. **Del Priore G, Maag T, Bhattacharya M, et al.** The value of cervical cytology in HIV-infected women. *Gynecol Oncol.* 1995;56:395–8.

■   ▓   ▒

Key Points

- Thirty to forty percent of HIV-infected individuals will develop a malignancy. This incidence is expected to rise as survival lengthens. The most common cancers include KS, lymphoma, and squamous cell carcinomas of the anus and uterine cervix.

- The clinical manifestations of KS range from cutaneous lesions to visceral involvement, which occurs with advanced HIV disease. Skin lesions are generally papular and appear most often on the lower extremities, face, oral mucosa, and genitalia. KS is caused by KSHV/HHV8, a newly identified human herpesvirus. Treatment modality is determined by extent of disease.

- In HIV-infected patients, Hodgkin's disease is usually more advanced (stage III or IV) at the time of presentation than in HIV-seronegative individuals.

- In the treatment of AIDS-related lymphomas, complete responses are seen less often with some of the cancer regimens used in HIV-seronegative patients. Chemotherapy is believed to induce further immunosuppression, and several anticancer agents induce or enhance the expression of HIV.

- Squamous cell cancers of the anus and uterine cervix tend to be more aggressive in HIV-infected individuals.

10

■   ■   ■

Infection Control and Risk Reduction for Healthcare Workers

Kenneth Sands, MD

even percent of the U.S. labor force is employed in health services, and each year approximately one half million health care workers (HCWs) experience a percutaneous exposure to blood (1). For at least several dozen of these individuals, such an episode has resulted in transmission of HIV infection. Even in the absence of pathogen transmission, blood exposures lead to tremendous emotional strain and substantial expense from laboratory testing, medication use, and time lost from work. Because these events are largely preventable, it is incumbent on health care institutions to provide the systems and resources that allow for the safest possible environment for its employees.

Epidemiology of Occupational HIV Exposure

The term *health care worker* is used here to refer to individuals at risk for occupational HIV exposure, including physicians and nurses but also other allied professions, such as security guards, emergency response personnel, laboratory personnel, and morticians. Measuring the true incidence of occupational exposures is complicated by the fact that an estimated 30% to 70% of events go unreported. The best information comes from a handful of studies in which HCWs were observed directly over time. Not surprisingly, these show that exposures occur in direct proportion to the frequency with which exposure-prone procedures are performed (Table 10.1). Although surgeons have approximately one dozen blood percutaneous exposures per person-year, inpatient nurses average one exposure. Because nurses represent such a large proportion of the HCW population, more than half of all reported exposures occur in this group. Nurses also may be more likely to report exposures than other HCWs. Most reported percutaneous exposures are related to either phlebotomy or manipulation of an intravenous catheter. Most reported mucocutaneous exposures have involved the eyes, which likely reflects, in part, the bias to report the most dramatic events.

As of December 1998, there were 54 cases of documented occupational HIV transmission known to the Centers for Disease Control and Prevention (CDC) (2). There were an additional 134 cases of "possible" occupational transmission, i.e., occupational acquisition of HIV was reported (with no other risk factor acknowledged) but a specific exposure was not documented. Nurses and laboratory technicians (a category that includes phlebotomists) represent the majority of these cases (Table 10.2). Forty-eight (86%) of the documented cases were related to "sharps," the large majority of which were hollow-bore needles. All seroconversions involved blood, visibly bloody fluids, or concentrated viral preparations in the laboratory setting. Ninety-five percent of exposed HCWs who seroconverted did so within 6 months of exposure. The CDC has received reports from other countries of

Table 10.1   Annual Frequency of Blood Contact in Healthcare Workers*

Occupation	Blood Contacts Per Year	Percutaneous Blood Contacts Per Year
Surgeon	81–135	8–13
Obstetrician	77	4
Dentist	—	4
Medical ward physician	31.2	1.8
Nurse on medical ward	—	0.98
Surgical scrub assistant	7–12	0.6–1.0
Hospital emergency department worker	24.2	0.4
Prehospital emergency medical worker	12.3	0.2

* Data from various prospective studies.
Adapted from Bell DM. Occupational risk of HIV infection in healthcare workers: an overview. *Am J Med.* 1997;102:9–15

an additional 40 documented and 38 possible cases that have a similar profile to those reported in the United States.

The risk of HIV transmission from a percutaneous exposure has been estimated from prospective studies in several countries involving thousands of HCWs. Pooled together, these studies suggest an overall seroconversion rate of 0.3% (95% confidence interval, 0.20-0.50). The risk from a mucous membrane exposure is less well defined because there have been many fewer associated seroconversions, but it is certainly less than percutaneous exposure and is likely approximately 0.1%. Conjunctival exposures may present a higher risk than other mucous membranes. No prospective study has identified a seroconversion in association with isolated skin exposure, but exposure to nonintact skin or large areas of intact skin is thought to represent a risk of transmission on a theoretical basis.

Why does a small fraction of exposures lead to seroconversion? The answer is not really known, but an understanding of the pathogenesis of HIV infection may shed light on this issue. Following a percutaneous or mu-

Table 10.2   Cases of Occupational Transmission of HIV Infection

Occupation	Documented Transmission	Possible Transmission
Nurse	22	33
Clinical laboratory technician	16	16
Physician	6	18
Nonclinical laboratory technician	3	0
Surgical technician	2	2
Health aide	1	14
Housekeeper	1	12
Dialysis technician	1	3
Respiratory therapist	1	2
Embalmer/morgue technician	1	2
Emergency medical personnel	0	12
Other technician/therapist	0	10
Dentist/dental worker	0	6
Other healthcare occupations	0	4
Total	**54**	**134**

Adapted from Centers for Disease Control and Prevention. *HIV/AIDS Surveillance Report.* 1998;10:1–44.

cosal exposure, the most likely targets of HIV virions are immunologically competent cells of the epidermis, dermis, and submucosa known as dendritic cells. After infection, dendritic cells probably migrate to regional lymph nodes, where T-cell infection occurs. Even though seroconversion occurs just 0.3% of the time, an HIV-specific cytotoxic T-cell response can be demonstrated in as many as 35% of exposed individuals. One hypothesis for this observation is that if the viral inoculum is small, transient HIV infection may occur, but protective cellular immunity is adequate to prevent sustained propagation of infection to new cells. Clinical data support this concept. For example, even though suture needles are a common cause of percutaneous exposure, the large majority of documented HIV seroconversions involve hollow-bore needles, which result in an inoculum approximately twice the size.

The most definitive information on risk factors for seroconversion comes from a case-control study performed by the CDC that examined data from three countries and compared 33 HCWs with a documented seroconversion to 665 controls that had been exposed to blood but did not seroconvert (3). Significant risk factors related to the source patient, nature of the exposure, and postexposure intervention were identified (Table 10.3). Once again, the importance of blood inoculum is reflected by the strong relationship between seroconversion and deep injuries, injuries involving a visibly bloody object, and injuries involving needles used to access an artery or vein. "Terminal illness in source patient" is likely a surrogate marker for high viral load, which could influence the size of the inoculum. However, no studies to date have examined directly the relationship between HIV viral load in the source patient and risk of occupational transmission.

Table 10.3   Risk Factors for HIV Transmission after Exposure to HIV-Infected Blood

Risk Factor	Adjusted OR	95% CI
Deep injury	15.0	6.0–41.0
Visible blood on device	6.2	2.2–21.0
Procedure involving needle in artery or vein	4.3	1.7–12.0
Terminal illness in source patient	5.6	2.0–16.0
Postexposure use of zidovudine	0.19	0.06–0.52

CI = confidence interval; OR = odds ratio.
Adapted from Cardo DM, Culver DH, Ciesielski CA, et al. A case-control study of HIV seroconversion in health care workers after percutaneous exposure: CDC Needlestick Surveillance Group. *N Engl J Med.* 1997;337:1485–90.

The CDC study also showed an 80% reduction in transmission in association with zidovudine (ZDV) chemoprophylaxis. This finding has been scrutinized but seems robust and cannot be dismissed easily as resulting from bias inherent in the case-control study design. Data from a randomized trial likely will never be available; one had been initiated in 1987 but was abandoned when it became evident that enrollment would not be adequate to draw meaningful conclusions. Other findings, however, support that ZDV has activity as a prophylactic agent. First, there is the demonstrated ability of ZDV to prevent perinatal transmission. Second, there are studies in animals, although these must be interpreted with caution because they involve non-HIV retroviruses and artificial means of virus inoculation. The most relevant studies have been done in nonhuman primates inoculated with simian immunodeficiency virus (SIV). ZDV prophylaxis in this setting usually leads to a delay, decrease, or both in antigenemia but has prevented infection in a few instances. Finally, there are *in vitro* data from exposed HCWs showing that those not taking ZDV are more likely to have memory cell recall for HIV antigens than those who do take it. This observation suggests that ZDV prevents transient infection to the point that cellular immunity is not activated. Another important implication of this hypothesis is that maximal effect requires that a therapeutic level of the antiretroviral agent be obtained as early as possible after exposure.

Although the above data are encouraging, it is clear that ZDV does not offer absolute protection. In primate models, infection was prevented only when ZDV was given within 1 hour of exposure, and even then protection did not occur in all cases. Among HCWs, there have been at least 11 HIV seroconversions despite the use of ZDV prophylaxis. In seven of these cases, it was initiated within 2 hours. In two cases, HIV strains were available for resistance testing, one of which demonstrated ZDV resistance.

Management of Potential Exposures

When a blood exposure does occur, appropriate management demands that a system for prompt and knowledgeable intervention already be in place. The Occupational Safety and Health Administration (OSHA) Bloodborne Pathogen Standard requires 1) that all HCWs receive training that covers what to do following a blood exposure; and 2) that the facility have a mechanism to provide prompt medical evaluation, testing, and treatment. Immediate management begins with simple first aid. For percutaneous injuries, forced bleeding should be attempted. Wounds should then be washed thoroughly with plain soap and water or a disinfectant. Mucous membranes should be irrigated copiously with tap water or a sterile irrigant.

The HCW should then report the event to a supervisor, who can arrange coverage while the individual receives further evaluation. Most facilities handle these events through a designated occupational health service or an urgent care facility. A rapid response time is vital because chemoprophylaxis for HIV infection, if elected, should be started as soon as possible. Management should involve an experienced clinician who is cognizant of the anxiety that the HCW is likely to be experiencing. Consultation is also available nationally through the "National Clinicians' Post-Exposure Prophylaxis Hotline" (*see* Occupational HIV Exposure Resources and Registries below). Potential exposure to *all* bloodborne infections should be addressed. A discussion of other important pathogens including hepatitis B and C is beyond the scope of this chapter, but excellent reviews have been published (4,5).

Before the publication of studies defining specific factors associated with occupational transmission, recommendations about HIV chemoprophylaxis had to be made on an almost entirely theoretical basis. Now, even though the available data have limitations, there is at least some foundation on which one can assess risk of transmission and advise about the use of antiretroviral therapy. However, the rapid expansion in HIV therapeutics creates a new quandary: given the myriad available agents, which ones have a role in prophylaxis? Currently, the only drug for which there are data to support a preventive effect in this setting is ZDV; thus, most experts feel it should remain part of any proposed regimen. However, there are several theoretical reasons to consider using other agents as well. First, there is the possibility of decreased effectiveness of ZDV monotherapy in the setting of exposure to a resistant strain. Second, combination regimens (e.g., ZDV and lamivudine [3TC]) may demonstrate synergy. Third, there is concern that nucleoside analogs, such as ZDV, require activation by cellular phosphorylation and thus may take several hours for the active metabolite to reach peak intracellular levels (6). In contrast, nonnucleoside reverse-transcriptase inhibitors (NNRTIs) require no intracellular metabolism. Protease inhibitors (PIs) have such dramatic potency that their potential application in prophylaxis cannot be ignored.

In the absence of large experience with agents other than ZDV, decisions about HIV chemoprophylaxis must be made on the basis of extrapolation from currently available data about transmission risk, drug effectiveness, and drug toxicity. The most comprehensive synthesis of this information was published by the CDC in May 1998 (7). In this report, current knowledge of occupational HIV exposure is reviewed exhaustively and distilled into a three-step algorithm for determining appropriate postexposure prophylaxis (Fig. 10.1). Step 1 of the algorithm categorizes the exposure based on severity and extent, step 2 categorizes the source patient's transmission risk, and step 3 suggests an approach to chemoprophylaxis. For most exposures, a basic regimen of ZDV 600 mg/d and 3TC 300 mg/d (in two divided doses) should be either "considered" (if the exposure was negligible) or "recommended" (if the exposure was significant but of a type in which transmission risk is unproven). For exposures with any elements associated with an increased transmission risk, an expanded regimen that includes

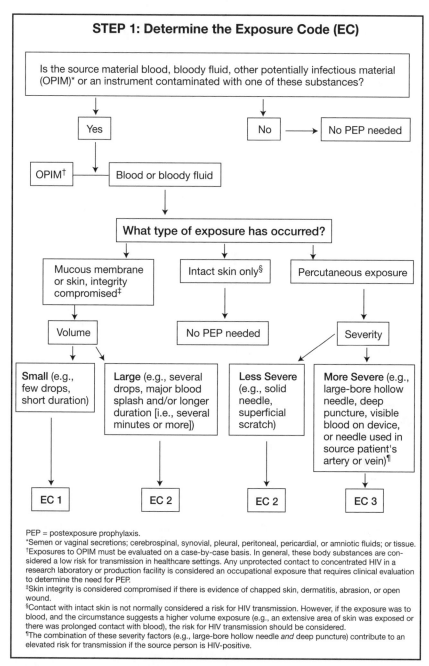

STEP 1: Determine the Exposure Code (EC)

Is the source material blood, bloody fluid, other potentially infectious material (OPIM)* or an instrument contaminated with one of these substances?

Yes

No ⟶ No PEP needed

OPIM† — Blood or bloody fluid

What type of exposure has occurred?

Mucous membrane or skin, integrity compromised‡

Intact skin only§

Percutaneous exposure

Volume

No PEP needed

Severity

Small (e.g., few drops, short duration)

Large (e.g., several drops, major blood splash and/or longer duration [i.e., several minutes or more])

Less Severe (e.g., solid needle, superficial scratch)

More Severe (e.g., large-bore hollow needle, deep puncture, visible blood on device, or needle used in source patient's artery or vein)¶

EC 1

EC 2

EC 2

EC 3

PEP = postexposure prophylaxis.
*Semen or vaginal secretions; cerebrospinal, synovial, pleural, peritoneal, pericardial, or amniotic fluids; or tissue.
†Exposures to OPIM must be evaluated on a case-by-case basis. In general, these body substances are considered a low risk for transmission in healthcare settings. Any unprotected contact to concentrated HIV in a research laboratory or production facility is considered an occupational exposure that requires clinical evaluation to determine the need for PEP.
‡Skin integrity is considered compromised if there is evidence of chapped skin, dermatitis, abrasion, or open wound.
§Contact with intact skin is not normally considered a risk for HIV transmission. However, if the exposure was to blood, and the circumstance suggests a higher volume exposure (e.g., an extensive area of skin was exposed or there was prolonged contact with blood), the risk for HIV transmission should be considered.
¶The combination of these severity factors (e.g., large-bore hollow needle *and* deep puncture) contribute to an elevated risk for transmission if the source person is HIV-positive.

Figure 10.1   Determining the need for HIV postexposure prophylaxis after an occupational exposure. This algorithm is intended to guide initial decisions about postexposure prophylaxis and should be used in conjunction with other guidance provided in this chapter. (Adapted from Centers for Disease Control and Prevention. Public Health Service guidelines for the management of health-care worker exposures to HIV and recommendations for postexposure prophylaxis. *Morbid Mortal Wkly Rep MMWR.* 1998;47:1–33.)

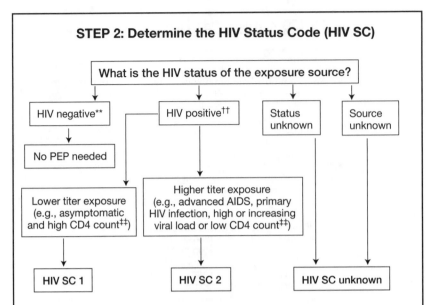

STEP 2: Determine the HIV Status Code (HIV SC)

What is the HIV status of the exposure source?

- HIV negative**
  - No PEP needed
- HIV positive††
- Status unknown
- Source unknown

Lower titer exposure (e.g., asymptomatic and high CD4 count‡‡)

Higher titer exposure (e.g., advanced AIDS, primary HIV infection, high or increasing viral load or low CD4 count‡‡)

HIV SC 1

HIV SC 2

HIV SC unknown

**A source is considered negative for HIV infection if there is laboratory documentation of a negative HIV antibody, HIV polymerase chain reaction (PCR), or HIV p24 antigen test result from a specimen collected at or near the time of exposure and there is no clinical evidence of recent retroviral-like illness.
††A source is considered infected with HIV (HIV-positive) if there has been a positive laboratory result for HIV antibody, HIV PCR, or HIV p24 antigen or physician-diagnosed AIDS.
‡‡Examples are used as surrogates to estimate the HIV titer in an exposure source for purposes of considering PEP regimens and do not reflect all clinical situations that may be observed. Although a high HIV titer (HIV SC 2) in an exposure source has been associated with an increased risk for transmission, the possibility of transmission from a source with a low HIV titer also must be considered.

Figure 10.1   *Continued*

ZDV and 3TC in combination with either indinavir 800 mg every 8 hours or nelfinavir 750 mg three times daily is "recommended."

The use of basic and expanded regimens reflects the need to strike a balance between the risk of HIV transmission and the potential for drug toxicity. ZDV is the only agent for which there is a large experience in HCWs, and it seems to be safe. In earlier studies in which ZDV was given at a dosage of 1.2 g/d, 50% to 75% of HCWs had side effects, and one third discontinued therapy (8). Toxicity is less frequent at the currently recommended dosage. 3TC is well tolerated, and preliminary data suggest that occurrence of side effects in HCWs receiving ZDV and 3TC is similar to that seen with ZDV alone. Among the recommended agents for prophylaxis, protease inhibitors have the greatest potential for serious toxicity. Drug interactions are also common. The NNRTIs were not included in any of the standard regimens suggested by the CDC. However, because of their rapid action, these agents may prove to be useful for prophylaxis and should receive consideration in special situations.

STEP 3: Determine the PEP Recommendation

EC	HIV SC	PEP recommendation
1	1	**PEP may not be warranted.** Exposure type does not pose a known risk for HIV transmission. Whether the risk for drug toxicity outweighs the benefit of PEP should be decided by the exposed healthcare worker and treating clinician.
1	2	**Consider basic regimen** (4 weeks of zidovudine, 600 mg per day in two or three divided doses *and* lamivudine 150 mg twice daily). Exposure type poses a negligible risk for HIV transmission. A high HIV titer in the source may justify consideration of PEP. Whether the risk for drug toxicity outweighs the benefit of PEP should be decided by the exposed healthcare worker and treating clinician.
2	1	**Recommended basic regimen** (4 weeks of zidovudine, 600 mg per day in two or three divided doses *and* lamivudine 150 mg twice daily). Most HIV exposures are in this category; no increased risk for HIV transmission has been observed but use of PEP is appropriate.
2	2	**Recommended expanded regimen** (basic regimen plus *either* indinavir, 800 mg every 8 hours *or* nelfinavir, 750 mg three times daily). Exposure type represents an increased HIV transmission risk.
3	1 or 2	**Recommended expanded regimen** (basic regimen plus *either* indinavir, 800 mg every 8 hours *or* nelfinavir, 750 mg three times daily). Exposure type represents an increased HIV transmission risk.
	Unknown	If the source or, in the case of an unknown source, the setting where the exposure occurred suggests a possible risk for HIV exposure and the EC is 2 or 3, consider PEP basic regimen.

Figure 10.1   *Continued*

The options for postexposure management should be communicated effectively to the HCW. This decision is time sensitive. CDC guidelines state that therapy is warranted if initiated within 36 hours of exposure but only indicated for higher-risk exposures beyond this time. The optimal duration of therapy is not established, but 4 weeks seems to be effective. If chemoprophylaxis is a consideration but the HCW is having difficulty with the decision, one potential strategy is to begin therapy with plans to reassess in 1 to 2 days. The risk of serious drug toxicity is minimal in the short term.

Exposed HCWs should have a baseline HIV antibody test performed to document that any subsequent positive test represented an occupational seroconversion. Follow-up HIV antibody testing should be performed at 6 weeks, 12 weeks, and 6 months. Additional testing beyond this time period generally is not warranted. Screening for hematologic, renal, and hepatic function should be performed at baseline and at 2 weeks for individuals electing to receive chemoprophylaxis. The exposed individual should be counseled to take measures to prevent secondary transmission, which would include either sexual abstinence or condom use and refraining from donating blood or tissues. The HCW also should be informed that there is a confidential registry sponsored by the CDC, Merck Inc., and Glaxo Wellcome Inc., which is gathering data on antiretroviral prophylaxis and associated toxicity (*see* Occupational HIV Exposure Resources and Registries below).

Certain complex situations deserve special mention. One is the management of exposures in which the source patient is suspected to have a strain of HIV that is resistant to one or more antiretroviral drugs. In such a setting, it would be appropriate to *add* an agent to the regimens outlined above, preferably of a class that the source patient has not yet received. Substituting another agent for ZDV is *not* recommended because it is the only drug for which prophylaxis is supported by clinical data. Another situation is the use of chemoprophylaxis in the setting of known or suspected pregnancy. Clinical data from HIV-infected patients suggest no increased rate of complications in pregnancy from either ZDV or 3TC. There is limited information on the use of PIs. Thus, although pregnancy is by no means a contraindication to postexposure prophylaxis, the HCW needs to be counseled as to the risks, benefits, and gaps in knowledge about the use of these agents. Many antiretroviral drugs are known to pass into breast milk, so breastfeeding should be suspended during this time.

Preventing Blood Exposures

Standard Precautions

In 1985, as occupational transmission of HIV was being appreciated, the CDC introduced universal precautions as a new approach to patient isolation. Universal precautions were based on the concept that one cannot presume the infectious status of any fluid potentially capable of transmitting HIV, and therefore precautions are uniformly necessary. However, some confusion ensued because of overlap between universal precautions and body substance isolation, which was meant to address other pathogens in addition to those transmitted by blood exposure. In 1996, the CDC revised their isolation guidelines and introduced *standard precautions* as a more coherent synthesis of both universal precautions and body substance isolation (9). Key elements of standard precautions are presented in Table 10.4.

In 1991, OSHA issued the Final Rule on Occupational Exposure to Bloodborne Pathogens, which mandates that employers provide the materials and training necessary for protection from bloodborne pathogens (10). Specifically, it requires employers to supply the necessary protective equipment (e.g., gowns, sharps disposal boxes), to instruct HCWs about bloodborne pathogens and the appropriate precautions, and to provide postexposure evaluation and therapy. Although important, standard precautions do not confer full protection. The use of barriers is more effective at preventing skin and mucous membrane exposures than higher-risk percutaneous exposures.

Table 10.4   Key Elements of Standard Precautions

Handwashing

• Wash hands after touching blood, body fluids, secretions, excretions, and contaminated items whether or not gloves are worn

Gloves

• Wear gloves when touching blood, body fluids, mucous membranes, nonintact skin, and contaminated items

• Remove gloves promptly after use

Masks, Eye Protection, Face Shields, and Gowns

• Wear a mask, gown, and eye protection or a face shield to protect mucous membranes of the eyes, nose, and mouth during activities that are likely to generate splashes or sprays of body fluids

Sharp Instruments

• Take care to prevent injuries when using, cleaning, or disposing of sharp instruments

• Never recap used needles or use another technique that involves directing the point of the needle toward any part of the body

• Do not remove used needles from disposable syringes by hand

• Place used disposable sharp items in appropriate puncture-resistant containers

Linen

• Handle linen soiled with blood or body fluids in a manner that prevents skin and mucous membrane exposures and contamination of clothing

Resuscitation Equipment

• Use a mouthpiece or resuscitation bag as an alternative to mouth-to-mouth resuscitation

Adapted from Garner JS. Hospital Infection Control Practices Advisory Committee guidelines for isolation precautions in hospitals. *Infect Control Hosp Epidemiol.* 1996;17:53–80.

Gloves reduce the blood inoculum from a needlestick but do not eliminate it. Furthermore, compliance with precautions is not optimal. For example, recapping of needles is still common, and certain barriers (e.g., eye protection) are underused.

Safety Devices

Perhaps the best hope for reducing percutaneous injuries comes from technological efforts to replace conventional sharp instruments with safer alternatives. The quest to develop such devices has spawned a mini-industry and the filing of thousands of patents in the United States. One approach is to eliminate sharps altogether with the needleless intravenous access systems. Blunt suture needles are another example; these devices have been piloted in specific surgical settings with good acceptance. Another approach is improved methods for sheathing the sharp object after use. Examples of these include safety syringes with a shield that locks over the needle after use and self-retracting lancets. Theoretically, over 80% of percutaneous injuries could be eliminated by fully deploying these devices. However, there are some practical concerns. First, the safety device must have good acceptance by HCWs. If not, it may be either misused or not used and actually might lead to an increase in blood exposures. Second, there are cost considerations because these devices may be several times more expensive than their conventional counterparts. Successful introduction of new safety devices requires careful product evaluation, including consultation with users, cost-benefit analysis, extensive in-servicing, and pilot implementation.

■   ■   ■

Occupational HIV Exposure Resources and Registries

National Clinicians' Postexposure Hotline: 888-448-4911
HIV Postexposure Prophylaxis Registry: 888-737-4448 or 888-PEP-4HIV
Antiretroviral Pregnancy Registry: 800-258-4263
Food and Drug Administration: 800-332-1088
Centers for Disease Control and Prevention: 800-332-1088 (to report HIV seroconversions in HCWs who received chemoprophylaxis)

■   ■   ■

Key Points

- Each year, approximately one half million HCWs are at risk for HIV transmission from a percutaneous exposure; of these, however, only a small percentage become infected. The average risk of seroconversion is 1 in 350.

- Blood inoculum through deep injury carries the greatest risk of occupational HIV transmission.

- All HCWs should receive training on what action to take after a blood exposure. Treatment given should be immediate because prompt administration of prophylactic antiretroviral therapy is crucial to its effectiveness.

- Zidovudine is the only drug shown to be effective for prophylaxis, although it generally is administered in combination with other agents.

■   ■   ■

REFERENCES

1. **Bell DM.** Occupational risk of HIV infection in healthcare workers: an overview. *Am J Med.* 1997;102:9–15.
2. **Centers for Disease Control and Prevention.** *HIV/AIDS Surveillance Report.* 1998;10:1–44.
3. **Cardo DM, Culver DH, Ciesielski CA, et al.** A case-control study of HIV seroconversion in health care workers after percutaneous exposure: CDC Needlestick Surveillance Group. *N Engl J Med.* 1997;337:1485–90.
4. **Bolyard EA, Tablan OC, Williams WW, et al.** Guideline for infection control in healthcare personnel, 1998. *Infect Control Hosp Epidemiol.* 1998;19:407–63.
5. **Centers for Disease Control and Prevention.** Recommendations for follow-up of health care workers after occupational exposure to hepatitis C virus. *Morbid Mortal Wkly Rep MMWR.* 1997;46:603–6.
6. **Flexner CW.** Principles of clinical pharmacology in postexposure prophylaxis. *Am J Med.* 1997;102:32–8.
7. **Centers for Disease Control and Prevention.** Public Health Service guidelines for the management of health-care worker exposures to HIV and recommendations for postexposure prophylaxis. *Morbid Mortal Wkly Rep MMWR.* 1998;47:1–33.
8. **Tokars JI, Marcus R, Culver DH, et al.** Surveillance of HIV infection and zidovudine use among health care workers after occupational exposure to HIV-infected blood: CDC Needlestick Surveillance Group. *Ann Intern Med.* 1993;118:913–9.
9. **Garner JS.** Hospital Infection Control Practices Advisory Committee guidelines for isolation precautions in hospitals. *Infect Control Hosp Epidemiol.* 1996;17:53–80.
10. **Occupational Safety and Health Administration.** Occupational exposure to bloodborne pathogens. *Federal Register.* 1991;56:64004–5182 [29CFR Part 1910.1030].

Clinical

Vignettes

HIV Infection in Pregnancy

A woman 24 years of age who is a graduate student recently missed her menstrual period and had a positive home pregnancy test. As part of follow-up at her health clinic, HIV counseling is performed. She had always been monogamous but was with several partners over the past few years and did not always use condoms. The patient agrees to HIV antibody testing, which is positive. She is clearly distressed by the results but indicates her desire to maintain the pregnancy.

■ QUESTION

How will HIV infection affect the course of her pregnancy?

The main risk of HIV infection during pregnancy is transmission from mother to child, which occurs in 25% to 30% of cases without the interventions described below. In general, the presence of HIV disease itself does not seem to enhance the likelihood of other adverse pregnancy outcomes. However, if an opportunistic infection develops, there may be an increased risk of complications, such as miscarriage, intrauterine fetal death, and premature labor and delivery. Fetal well-being is usually promoted by optimal medical management of the mother.

■ QUESTION

How will pregnancy affect the course of her HIV infection?

There is no evidence that pregnancy alters the course of HIV disease or is associated with an increased risk of opportunistic infections. Some studies have suggested that CD4 cell counts in women decrease modestly during pregnancy and rise around the time of delivery. However, these changes do not seem to have an impact on the long-term course of HIV infection.

■ QUESTION

How would you advise the patient to minimize the likelihood of transmitting HIV to her baby?

The HIV-infected woman who chooses to continue her pregnancy should be advised to begin antiretroviral therapy and to avoid breast feeding. Zidovudine (ZDV) has been demonstrated to reduce the risk of vertical transmission from 25% to 8% when given 1) to the mother throughout the second and third trimester of pregnancy, 2) intrapartum, and 3) to the baby for 6 weeks postpartum. Early data suggest that other agents also may be useful in this setting. Experience with combination antiretroviral therapy has shown that low viral loads are associated with a dramatic decrease in vertical transmission. However, the safety of administering these drugs during pregnancy remains to be established. If the patient is not already receiving antiretroviral therapy, some clinicians defer starting it until the second trimester. Because breast feeding is associated with an increased risk of vertical transmission in HIV disease, it should be discouraged in women who live in countries where safe alternatives are available.

■ QUESTION

Should cesarean section be considered?

Yes. The mode of delivery seems to have a significant effect on the likelihood of vertical transmission of HIV infection. An elective cesarean delivery in pregnant women not receiving ZDV decreases the transmission rate from 25% to 4% compared with those undergoing vaginal delivery. However, cesarean section may be associated with an increased risk of operative complications in patients with HIV disease. The role of this procedure in pregnant women on effective combination antiretroviral therapy remains controversial.

■ COMMENT

The risk of transmitting HIV infection to the newborn can be decreased significantly by the use of antiretroviral therapy during pregnancy, consideration of elective cesarean section, and avoidance of breast feeding if feasible.

Centers for Disease Control and Prevention. Update—Perinatally acquired HIV/AIDS: United States, 1997. *Morbid Mortal Wkly Rep MMWR.* 1997;46:1086-92.

Centers for Disease Control and Prevention. Public Health Service Task Force recommendations for the use of antiretroviral drugs in pregnant women infected with HIV-1 for maternal health and for reducing perinatal HIV-1 transmission in the United States. *Morbid Mortal Wkly Rep MMWR.* 1998;47:1-30.

Connor EM, Sperling RS, Gelber R, et al. Reduction of maternal-infant transmission of HIV type 1 with zidovudine treatment. *N Engl J Med.* 1994;331:1173-80.

The European Mode of Delivery Collaboration. Elective cesarean section versus vaginal delivery in prevention of vertical HIV-1 transmission: a randomised clinical trial. *Lancet.* 1999;353:1035-9.

The International Perinatal HIV Group. The mode of delivery and the risk of vertical transmission of HIV type 1. *N Engl J Med.* 1999;340:977-87.

Mofenson L. Short-course zidovudine for prevention of perinatal infection. *Lancet.* 1999;353:765-7.

Shaffer N, Chuachoowong R, et al. for the Bangkok Collaborative Perinatal HIV Transmission Study Group. Short course zidovudine for perinatal transmission in Bangkok, Thailand: a randomized controlled trial. *Lancet.* 1999;353:773-80.

Stringer JSA, Rouse DJ, Goldenberg RL. Prophylactic cesarean delivery for the prevention of perinatal HIV transmission: the case for restraint. *JAMA.* 1999;281:1946-9.

UNAIDS. HIV and infant feeding: a review of HIV transmission though breast feeding. In *UNAIDS/WHO Joint United Nations Programme on HIV/AIDS (UNAIDS).* Geneva, Switzerland: World Health Organization; Jun 1998.

Raymond Powrie, MD

CASE 2

Initiation of Antiretroviral Therapy

A man 58 years of age with a history of blood transfusion in 1983 recently underwent HIV antibody testing for a life insurance application. The test came back positive. He feels healthy, reports no significant past medical history, and has a normal physical examination and baseline laboratory studies. His CD4 count is 450 cells/mm^3, and his viral load titer (bDNA assay) is 8340 copies/mL.

■ QUESTION

What might explain the stability of the course of his HIV disease, and what is his prognosis?

This patient was likely infected with HIV through the blood transfusion, which was administered before the use of routine antibody screening. He has no history of opportunistic diseases and a borderline low CD4 cell count, which is explained by his relatively low viral load titer. The viral load "set point," which is thought to be established soon after HIV seroconversion, varies widely between patients and correlates directly with CD4 count decline and risk of disease progression. Based on this patient's close-to-normal CD4 count over many years in the absence of antiretroviral therapy, he would be considered a "long-term nonprogressor." His prognosis for continued preservation of immune function seems good, but he will need to be monitored on a regular basis.

■ QUESTION

Would you recommend that the patient start antiretroviral therapy?

Published recommendations are to initiate combination antiretroviral therapy if the patient has significant HIV-related symptoms, a CD4 count of fewer than 500 cells/mm^3 or a viral load greater than 10,000 copies/mL. However, some authorities would defer starting it in patients with CD4 count between 350-500 cells/mm^3 in the context of a low viral load. In general, the initial CD4 count and viral load titer should be repeated to establish a baseline before initiating therapy.

Combination antiretroviral therapy is difficult to take on a long-term basis. Regimens consist of at least three drugs with different dosing requirements and may be associated with side effects and adverse drug interactions. Medication adherence is important because erratic dosing invariably leads to the development of viral resistance over time.

This patient was diagnosed recently with HIV infection, so addressing any mental health concerns and educating him about HIV disease are essential before dealing with the issue of antiretroviral therapy. Because he has had a relatively stable CD4 cell count, there is some question about whether the benefit of complete viral suppression is worth the cost in terms of the impact of antiretroviral therapy on his quality of life. Answering this question requires patient participation in the decision-making process. In this setting, either the initiation of antiretroviral therapy (perhaps using two nucleoside reverse-transcriptase inhibitors [NRTIs] in combination with a non-NRTI [NNRTI] for simplicity) or monitoring the patient off of therapy (with CD4 counts and viral load titers taken every 3 months) would be reasonable management strategies.

■ COMMENT

Initiation of combination antiretroviral therapy should be considered in an HIV-infected patient with significant symptoms, a CD4 count of fewer than 500 cells/mm³, or a viral load titer (bDNA assay) greater than 10,000 copies/mL. Given the complexity of drug regimens and need for long-term adherence, patient participation in the decision-making process is essential.

Carpenter CC, Fischl MA, Hammer SM, et al. Antiretroviral therapy in adults: updated recommendations of the International AIDS Society, USA Panel. *JAMA.* 2000;283:381–90.

Centers for Disease Control and Prevention. Report of the NIH panel to define principles of therapy of HIV infection and guidelines for the use of antiretroviral agents in HIV-infected adults and adolescents. *Morbid Mortal Wkly Rep MMWR.* 1998;47:1-82. (Available as "living document" on DHHS HIV/AIDS Treatment Information Service Web site at http://www.hivatis.org.)

Mellors JW, Munoz A, Giorgi JV, et al. Plasma viral load and CD4+ lymphocytes as prognostic markers of HIV-1 infection. *Ann Intern Med.* 1997;126:946-54.

Jennifer Adelson Mitty, MD

CASE 3

Lipodystrophy Syndrome

The patient is a man 45 years of age with HIV infection dating back to at least 1987. He was started on ZDV monotherapy, which was continued for a few years, but then went on a "drug holiday." In 1997, he was started on the combination of stavudine (d4T), lamivudine (3TC), and indinavir because of declining CD4 cell count. Since that time, he has done well, with a stable CD4 count of 450 cells/mm^3 and a viral load titer of fewer than 50 copies/mL. Over the past year, although his weight is unchanged, he has experienced rather disturbing changes in his body shape with thinning of his extremities and an increase in his belt and shirt collar size. Physical examination is noteworthy for a "buffalo hump" and a very prominent abdomen.

■ QUESTION

What is known about body morphology changes in HIV disease?

The patient has manifestations of lipodystrophy syndrome, which has been described for several years in HIV-infected patients but seems to be more frequent since the advent of combination antiretroviral therapy. It is characterized by some or all of the following features:

1. Central adiposity with a "protease paunch," gynecomastia, cervicodorsal fat pad ("buffalo hump"), and lipomatosis

2. Peripheral wasting with loss of subcutaneous fat in the face, extremities, and buttocks

3. Ectodermal dysplasia manifested by ingrown toenails, dry skin, and hair loss

4. Metabolic abnormalities, including hypercholesterolemia, hypertriglyceridemia, and glucose intolerance

Premature coronary artery disease has been described in some HIV-infected patients, but its association with lipodystrophy syndrome is uncertain.

The epidemiology of lipodystrophy syndrome is controversial. It has been estimated to affect 50% of patients on combination antiretroviral therapy for 1 year. The protease inhibitors (PIs) ritonavir, indinavir, and nelfinavir (especially when given in combination) and the nucleoside reverse-transcriptase inhibitor (NRTI) d4T have been linked most closely with this syndrome. However, it also has been described in patients receiving other drugs and in patients not on antiretroviral therapy.

The pathogenesis of lipodystrophy syndrome is unknown. One hypothesis is that HIV protease shares homology with enzymes important in lipid metabolism and that PI therapy interferes with their action. The optimal management of lipodystrophy syndrome is also uncertain. Recommending common sense health measures, such as eating a well-balanced diet and getting regular exercise, are likely useful in HIV-infected patients, but their role in preventing and managing lipodystrophy syndrome is unclear. Pharmacologic treatment of hyperlipidemia with an HMG-CoA reductase inhibitor (e.g., atorvastatin) is recommended. Case reports have indicated that human growth hormone may be effective in ameliorating some of the body morphology changes, and metformin may be useful in managing the metabolic abnormalities. Preliminary information also suggests improvement in some patients who are switched from a PI-containing regimen to one not including this class of drugs.

■ QUESTION

How should the patient be managed?

It is difficult to know the best course of action in this patient, who is on a stable antiretroviral regimen. One option would be to substitute an NNRTI, such as efavirenz, for indinavir. The potential risk of this approach is that the new regimen may cause side effects or may not be suppressive. A second option would be to maintain the *status quo* and encourage good nutrition and regular exercise. A third option would be to see if the patient is interested in participating in a clinical trial to examine the role of experimental therapies in the management of lipodystrophy syndrome.

Patients with lipodystrophy syndrome should have their weight and anthropomorphic measurements monitored, and glucose and lipid studies should be performed on a regular basis. Referral to a nutritionist with expertise in HIV disease management is recommended. Bioelectric impedance analysis (BIA) can be used to monitor changes in body shape and composition.

■ COMMENT

Lipodystrophy syndrome, which is manifested by characteristic body morphology changes, hyperlipidemia, and glucose intolerance, has become more common since the advent of combination antiretroviral therapy. Its epidemiology, pathophysiology, and management remain under active investigation.

Carr A, et al. A syndrome of peripheral lipodystrophy, hyperlipidaemia, and insulin resistance in patients receiving HIV-protease inhibitors. *AIDS.* 1998;12:F51-8.

Carr A, Samaras K, Chisholm DJ, Cooper DA. Pathogenesis of HIV-1-protease inhibitor-associated peripheral lipodystrophy, hyperlipidaemia, and insulin resistance. *Lancet.* 1998;351:1881-3.

Saint Marc T, Partisani M, Poizot-Martin I, et al. A syndrome of fat wasting (lipodystrophy) in patients receiving long-term nucleoside analogue therapy. *AIDS.* 1999;13: 1659–67.

Howard Libman, MD

CASE 4

Co-infection with Hepatitis C Virus

A woman 45 years of age with a remote history of injection-drug use and prostitution presents to a nurse practitioner with vaginal itching, which is diagnosed as *Candida* infection. Given her medical history, HIV antibody testing is performed and is positive. Physical examination is otherwise normal. Laboratory evaluation is noteworthy for mildly increased liver function tests, CD4 count of 230 cells/mm^3, HIV viral load of 12,420 copies/mL, and positive antibody to hepatitis C virus (HCV).

■ QUESTION

How does HIV infection affect the course of HCV infection, and vice versa?

Although there are conflicting data, most studies suggest that co-infected patients are more likely to progress to chronic liver disease and cirrhosis than are HIV-seronegative controls and may do so more rapidly. Liver disease progression is especially common in patients with low CD4 cell counts. One study of hemophiliacs with HCV infection also showed increased mortality in patients with HIV disease. The presence of HCV infection does not seem to hasten the progression of HIV infection to AIDS.

■ QUESTION

How would you manage this patient?

The initial evaluation of this patient should include serologic tests for hepatitis A and B, and she should be vaccinated if not previously infected with these pathogens or immunized against them. Confirmatory testing for HCV infection using the recombinant immunoblot assay (RIBA) or polymerase chain reaction (PCR) for RNA is also indicated. Patients with chronic hepatitis should be cautioned about the use of alcohol, acetaminophen, and other potentially hepatotoxic agents.

Given the patient's CD4 count of 230 cells/mm^3, attention should be directed toward improving her immunologic function through HIV-replication control by initiating antiretroviral therapy. The choice of drugs in this setting is based on the understanding that, although all are potentially hepatotoxic, they can be administered safely to most patients with careful monitoring of liver function tests. Among the nucleoside reverse-transcriptase inhibitors (NRTI), zidovudine (ZDV) has a somewhat higher rate of hepatotoxicity than other agents. Increased serum transaminase levels have been associated with abacavir (ABC) as part of its hypersensitivity syndrome. Rarely lactic acidosis with hepatomegaly and steatosis has been described with NRTIs. The nonnucleoside reverse-transcriptase inhibitors (NNRTIs) can cause liver function test abnormalities but seem to have a low risk of serious toxicity. The protease inhibitors (PIs) are metabolized by the hepatic cytochrome P450 enzyme system. Based on limited data, the risk of hepatotoxicity in a patient with HCV infection seems highest with ritonavir, followed by indinavir, and then nelfinavir and saquinavir.

Unfortunately, liver function tests and HCV viral load titers do not correlate well with the degree of hepatic dysfunction. Liver biopsy may be necessary to establish the extent of disease and to identify patients who are candidates for treatment. A number of studies have shown an initial response to interferon-α therapy in HIV-infected patients with HCV, but long-term benefit is not common. Studies to assess the role of interferon-α with ribavirin are in progress. Interferon can have significant side effects, including constitutional complaints, neuropsychiatric symptoms, and gastrointestinal intolerance. Ribavirin causes anemia and has potential antagonism with ZDV, stavudine (d4T), and possibly other NRTIs.

■ **COMMENT**

The patient with HIV disease who is infected with HCV is more likely to progress to chronic liver disease over a shorter period of time. Antiretroviral therapy may be problematic because of hepatotoxicity. The role of interferon with ribavirin in the management of HCV infection in this population remains under investigation.

Orenstein R, LeGall-Salmon E. HIV treatment-associated hepatitis. *AIDS Reader.* 1999;9:339-46.

Spengler U, Rockstroh JK. Hepatitis C in the patient with HIV infection. *J Hepatol.* 1998;29:1023-30.

Sulkowski MS, Thomas DL, Chaisson RE, Moore RD. Hepatotoxicity associated with antiretroviral therapy in adults infected with human immunodeficiency virus and the role of hepatitis C or B virus infection. *JAMA.* 2000;283:74-80.

Daniel B. Levy, MD

Postexposure Prophylaxis

A homosexual man 23 years of age presents to the emergency room after having unprotected receptive anal intercourse. He does not know the partner well and is not sure whether he is HIV-infected. The patient recently broke up with his steady partner of several years. His HIV antibody test 6 months ago was negative. The patient is interested in taking a "drug cocktail" to prevent his acquiring HIV infection.

■ **QUESTION**

What do you advise this patient?

Although there are data supporting the use of postexposure prophylaxis (PEP) in health care workers following an occupational exposure to HIV, it is unclear whether this intervention is effective in patients after a sexual exposure. Nevertheless, given that risks of percutaneous and sexual exposure to HIV are similar, PEP would seem reasonable under certain circumstances. The Centers for Disease Control and Prevention (CDC) has published recommendations, but not firm guidelines, on this subject. Identification of candidates for PEP requires assessment of 1) frequency of exposure, 2) type of exposure, 3) HIV status of the source person, and 4) timing of exposure.

PEP should be considered for isolated HIV exposures but not repeated ones. The patient discussed in this case presumably had a single high-risk exposure. However, if he had presented on several occasions after episodes of unsafe sex or injection drug use, the risks and cost of repeated courses of antiretroviral drug prophylaxis would outweigh any potential benefit.

The type of exposure is important information to obtain. The risk of HIV transmission from one episode of receptive penile-anal sexual intercourse with a seropositive partner is 0.5% to 3.0%. For receptive penile-vaginal intercourse, it is estimated to be 0.1%. The risk of transmission among injection drug users is approximately 0.4% to 3.0% per shared injection with a seropositive individual. Oral sex is known to transmit HIV infection but at a rate that has not been quantified. In comparison, the risk of transmission after percutaneous exposure to HIV in health care workers is approximately 0.25%; after mucous membrane exposure, it is approximately 0.09%. Based on these data, it is reasonable to recommend PEP for high-risk exposures (e.g., unprotected receptive anal and vaginal intercourse and shared injection drug use in which the source patient has or is at high risk for HIV infection). Some authors also recommend PEP for unprotected insertive vaginal and anal intercourse and receptive fellatio with ejaculation, although the risk of HIV transmission in these situations seems lower.

As much information as possible about the source person should be obtained to determine risk for HIV infection. If possible, the source should be HIV antibody tested. If the source is already known to be HIV infected, knowledge of his or her disease status and antiretroviral therapy experience may be helpful in designing a rational PEP regimen.

Finally, the timing of exposure should be obtained. Immediate initiation of PEP is optimal based on our understanding of the pathophysiology of HIV infection. Antiretroviral therapy started more than 72 hours following exposure is not likely to be effective.

■ QUESTION

How is postexposure prophylactic antiretroviral therapy given?

The treatment regimen for nonoccupational PEP is generally the same as that used for occupational exposure: zidovudine (ZDV) and lamivudine (3TC) are prescribed for 4 weeks. A protease inhibitor, nelfinavir or indinavir, can be added if the source patient is known to have a high viral load, advanced disease, or history of therapy with nucleoside reverse-transcriptase inhibitors. A second possible nucleoside combination is didanosine (ddI) and stavudine (d4T). If the source patient has a complicated antiretroviral history, a more individualized regimen, which is best determined in consultation with an expert HIV clinician, may be necessary.

The CDC recommends documentation of the patient's understanding of 1) the need to initiate or resume HIV risk-reduction behaviors, 2) limited knowledge about the effectiveness of antiretroviral therapy for nonoccupational exposure, 3) potential side effects of medications, 4) symptoms and signs of HIV seroconversion syndrome, and 5) importance of adherence to prescribed medications. The patient should undergo baseline laboratory studies, including an HIV antibody test; HIV viral load titer (if the patient has had several episodes of unsafe sex in the past 6 months); hepatitis B and C virus serologies; screening for gonorrhea, syphilis, and chlamydia infection; and a pregnancy test in women. A complete blood count and kidney and liver function tests also should be ordered at baseline and at 2 weeks into treatment. Follow-up HIV antibody testing should be performed at 6 weeks, 3 months, and 6 months.

The CDC is collecting anonymous information on nonoccupational PEP through the Nonoccupational HIV Postexposure Prophylaxis Registry. Further information can be obtained by telephone (877-HIV-1PEP) or via the Internet (www.hivpepregistry.org).

■ **COMMENT**

Postexposure prophylactic antiretroviral therapy should be considered in the patient who has a single or limited number of high-risk exposures through sexual or injection-drug use behaviors. Information about the nature and timing of exposure and the source patient is important in making this decision. The effectiveness of nonoccupational PEP is unknown.

Centers for Disease Control and Prevention. Management of possible sexual, injecting-drug-use, or other nonoccupational exposure to HIV, including considerations related to antiretroviral therapy: Public Health Service statement. *Morbid Mortal Wkly Rep MMWR.* 1998;47(RR-17):1-14.

Katz MH, Gerberding JL. The care of persons with recent sexual exposure to HIV. *Ann Intern Med.* 1998;128:306-12.

Lurie P, Miller S, Hecht F, et al. Postexposure prophylaxis after nonoccupational HIV exposure: clinical, ethical, and policy considerations. *JAMA.* 1998;280:1769-73.

Sara E. Cosgrove, MD

CASE 6

Antiretroviral Therapy Failure

The patient is a man 52 years of age with HIV infection diagnosed in the late 1980s. He received several different antiretroviral regimens over the years, with the most recent being didanosine (ddI), stavudine (d4T), saquinavir, and ritonavir. He has some gastrointestinal side effects and has not been taking the medications reliably. He also reports feeling depressed and has started drinking alcohol again. His last CD4 count was 330 cells/mm^3, which is stable, and his HIV viral load was 15,320 copies/mL, which compares to a previous value of 2520.

■ QUESTION

What factors contribute to antiretroviral therapy failure?

This patient has a significant increase in his viral load titer, indicating that his antiretroviral regimen is no longer effective. The three main factors that may contribute to drug failure are 1) poor adherence to medications, 2) viral mutations leading to resistance, and 3) pharmacokinetic issues (e.g., absorption, drug interactions, metabolism), which lead to subtherapeutic drug levels.

Based on history, the patient's lack of adherence to medical therapy is a significant problem, with depression and alcoholism clearly important contributing factors. Furthermore, his virus may have developed mutations that confer resistance to specific drugs. This finding would likely be related to poor adherence, which leads to resistance through selective pressure on replication, and previous sequential monotherapy, which was the standard of care in early years of the epidemic. Medication toxicity also may contribute to poor adherence and adversely affect pharmacokinetics. For example, if the patient is having diarrhea or is vomiting, this may diminish drug absorption. It is also important to assess for drug interactions. For example, the protease inhibitors are metabolized by the hepatic cytochrome P450 enzyme system, and, as such, there are many possible drug interactions that could decrease serum levels of these medications.

■ QUESTION

Should this patient's antiretroviral therapy be modified?

This patient's regimen will likely need to be changed. However, his depression and alcohol use, as well as any other remediable factors that might affect the ability to take medications, need to be addressed first. Mental health counseling and addiction treatment should be offered. There is little use in modifying antiretroviral therapy if the likelihood of adherence remains low.

■ QUESTION

What is the role of HIV genotypic or phenotypic testing in this setting?

Given this patient's extensive antiretroviral drug history, genotypic or phenotypic testing may be helpful in choosing a rational drug combination. Genotypic testing provides a genetic blueprint of the predominant viral strain, showing where mutations are present compared with a sensitive "wild type" strain, along with an explanation of what those mutations may mean clinically. Each antiretroviral medication is listed with an interpretation as to whether the virus is sensitive, resistant, or possibly resistant. Phenotypic testing compares the inhibitory effect of each antiretroviral medication on the patient's virus with a "wild type" strain and provides a clinical interpretation of the results. However, the limitation of both genotypic and phenotypic testing is that they give information on the predominant viral strain but not ones present in small numbers. Because of this shortcoming, these tests may not detect resistant background strains and are better in predicting which drugs are not likely to be beneficial rather than which ones are. The role of genotypic and phenotypic testing in clinical practice continues to evolve.

■ COMMENT

Antiretroviral failure can be attributed to poor adherence, drug resistance, and pharmacokinetic issues. Optimizing adherence to medications by addressing depression, alcoholism, and other remediable factors is essential. If the patient is taking medications reliably, a sustained increase in the HIV viral load necessitates changing the antiretroviral regimen. Genotypic or phenotypic analysis of the viral strain may facilitate selection of new agents.

Altice FL, Friedland GH. The era of adherence to HIV therapy. *Ann Intern Med.* 1998;129:503-5.

Carpenter CC, Fischl MA, Hammer SM, et al. Antiretroviral therapy in adults: updated recommendations of the International AIDS Society, USA Panel. *JAMA.* 2000;283: 381–90.

Centers for Disease Control and Prevention. Report of the NIH panel to define principles of therapy of HIV infection and guidelines for the use of antiretroviral agents in HIV-infected adults and adolescents. *Morbid Mortal Wkly Rep MMWR.* 1998;47(RR-5):1-82. (Available as "living document" on DHHS HIV/AIDS Treatment Information Service Web site at http://www.hivatis.org.)

Hirsch MS, Conway B, D'Aquila RT, et al. Antiretroviral drug-resistance testing in adults with HIV infection: implications for clinical management: International AIDS Society, USA Panel. *JAMA.* 1998;279:1984-91.

Lucas GM, Chaisson RE, Moore RD. Highly active antiretroviral therapy in a large urban clinic: risk factors for virologic failure and adverse drug reactions. *Ann Intern Med.* 1999;131:81-7.

Jennifer Adelson Mitty, MD

Appendix

■ ▓ ■

Drugs Used in the
Treatment of HIV Infection

Compiled by
Sara E. Cosgrove, MD
David B. Levy, MD, PhD
Howard Libman, MD

Antiretroviral Therapy

Nucleoside Reverse Transcriptase Inhibitors (NRTIs)

Abacavir (ABC, Ziagen)

Indications   Treatment of HIV infection in combination with other agents.

Contraindications Known or suspected hypersensitivity.

Dosage   300 mg po bid.

Toxicity   Four percent of patients develop a *hypersensitivity reaction* within 6 weeks of initiating therapy. It is manifested by fever, constitutional or respiratory symptoms, gastrointestinal intolerance, and/or rash. Stopping the drug leads to rapid resolution of symptoms. *Note: Never rechallenge a patient thought to have had a hypersensitivity reaction to abacavir because severe reactions and death have been reported.*

Other side effects include nausea, vomiting, diarrhea, headache, malaise, and lactic acidosis (rare).

Pregnancy category C.

Pregnancy Categories: A = controlled studies show no risk; B = no evidence of risk in humans; C = risk cannot be excluded; D = positive evidence of risk; X = contraindicated in pregnancy.

Didanosine (ddI, Videx)

Indications	Treatment of HIV infection in combination with other agents.
Contraindications	Known hypersensitivity, history of pancreatitis or significant peripheral neuropathy.
Dosage	Tablets for patients ≥60 kg: 200 mg po bid or 400 mg po qd.
	Tablets for patients <60 kg: 125 mg po bid or 250 mg po qd.
	Buffered powder for patients ≥60 kg: 250 mg po bid.
	Buffered powder for patients <60 kg: 167 mg po bid.
	Tablets must be chewed or dissolved in water and both formulations taken on an empty stomach (>30 minutes before a meal or >2 hours after a meal).
	Co-administration of hydroxyurea 500 mg po bid may enhance the effectiveness of ddI by increasing intracellular level of drug.
Toxicity	Peripheral neuropathy, acute pancreatitis, gastrointestinal intolerance, and abnormal liver function tests.
	Pregnancy category B.

Lamivudine (3TC, Epivir)

Indications	Treatment of HIV infection in combination with other agents. Also has activity against hepatitis B virus.
Contraindications	Known hypersensitivity.
Dosage	150 mg po bid. Also available as Combivir, a fixed-dose combination of zidovudine 300 mg and 3TC 150 mg.
Toxicity	Uncommon; headache, gastrointestinal intolerance, insomnia, and lactic acidosis (rare) have been reported.
	Pregnancy category C.

Stavudine (d4T, Zerit)

Indications	Treatment of HIV infection in combination with other agents.
Contraindications	Known hypersensitivity, concurrent ZDV use because of pharmacologic antagonism.

Pregnancy Categories: A = controlled studies show no risk; B = no evidence of risk in humans; C = risk cannot be excluded; D = positive evidence of risk; X = contraindicated in pregnancy.

Dosage	For patients ≥60 kg: 40 mg po bid.
	For patients <60 kg: 30 mg po bid.
	Dosage adjustment for peripheral neuropathy: 20 mg po bid.
Toxicity	Peripheral neuropathy, abnormal liver function tests, and lactic acidosis (rare).
	Pregnancy category C.

Zalcitabine (ddC, HIVID)

Indications	Treatment of HIV infection in combination with other agents.
Contraindications	Known hypersensitivity, significant peripheral neuropathy.
Dosage	0.75 mg po tid.
Toxicity	Peripheral neuropathy, aphthous ulcers of mouth and esophagus, abnormal liver function tests, and lactic acidosis (rare).
	Pregnancy category C.

Zidovudine (ZDV, AZT, Retrovir)

Indications	Treatment of HIV infection in combination with other agents. In addition, ZDV may have specific benefits for patients who have HIV-related thrombocytopenia or encephalopathy.
	Prevention of perinatal transmission when given prenatally and during delivery to HIV-infected mother and to the infant postpartum.
Contraindications	Known hypersensitivity.
Dosage	Treatment of HIV infection in adults: 300 mg po bid. Also available as Combivir, a fixed-dose combination of ZDV 300 mg with lamivudine 150 mg.
	Prevention of perinatal transmission: during pregnancy (weeks 14–34), give 100 mg po 5 times daily; during labor, give 2 mg/kg IV loading dose over 30 minutes to 1 hour, then 1 mg/kg/h IV through delivery; to infant, give 2 mg/kg syrup every 6 hours for 6 weeks.
Toxicity	Gastrointestinal intolerance, headache, anemia, leukopenia, myopathy, abnormal liver function tests, macro-

Pregnancy Categories: A = controlled studies show no risk; B = no evidence of risk in humans; C = risk cannot be excluded; D = positive evidence of risk; X = contraindicated in pregnancy.

cytosis, fingernail discoloration, insomnia, asthenia, neutropenia, and lactic acidosis (rare).

Recommended for pregnant women after the first trimester to prevent vertical transmission.

Nonnucleoside Reverse Transcriptase Inhibitors (NNRTIs)

Delavirdine (Rescriptor)

Indications	Treatment of HIV infection in combination with other agents.
Contraindications	Known hypersensitivity.
Dosage	400 mg po tid. Two tablets must be dissolved in ≥3 oz water to produce a slurry. Antacids and didanosine should not be taken 1 hour before or after the dose. *Note: There are many potential drug interactions, some of which require dosage modification;* see *Chapter 5,* Physicians Desk Reference, *or package insert for more information.*
Toxicity	Rash is common and does not require discontinuation of the drug unless accompanied by fever, mucous membrane involvement, or other systemic manifestations. Stevens–Johnson syndrome has been reported infrequently. Pregnancy category C.

Efavirenz (Sustiva)

Indications	Treatment of HIV infection in combination with other agents.
Contraindications	Known hypersensitivity.
Dosage	600 mg po qhs. Avoid taking with high fat meals. *Note: There are many potential drug interactions, some of which require dosage modification;* see *Chapter 5,* Physicians Desk Reference, *or package insert for more information.*
Toxicity	Rash is common; it does not require discontinuation of the drug unless accompanied by fever, mucous membrane involvement, or other systemic manifestations.

Pregnancy Categories: A = controlled studies show no risk; B = no evidence of risk in humans; C = risk cannot be excluded; D = positive evidence of risk; X = contraindicated in pregnancy.

Other side effects include neurocognitive dysfunction (confusion, somnolence, difficulty concentrating, depersonalization, insomnia, vivid dreams and nightmares), hyperlipidemia, and abnormal liver function tests.

Pregnancy category C; teratogenic in nonhuman primates.

Nevirapine (Viramune)

Indications   Treatment of HIV infection in combination with other agents.

Contraindications   Known hypersensitivity.

Dosage   200 mg po qd for 2 weeks; 200 mg po bid thereafter. Patients who develop rash during the first 2 weeks should not increase the dose until the rash resolves. *Note: There are many potential drug interactions, some of which require dosage modification; see Chapter 5,* Physicians Desk Reference, *or package insert for more information.*

Toxicity   Rash is common (~17% of patients; fewer with dose escalation regimen) and does not require discontinuation of the drug unless accompanied by fever, mucous membrane involvement, or other systemic manifestations. Stevens–Johnson syndrome has been reported infrequently. Other side effects include nausea, headache, and abnormal liver function tests.

Pregnancy category C.

Protease Inhibitors (PIs)

Amprenavir (Agenerase)

Indications   Treatment of HIV infection in combination with other agents.

Contraindications   Known hypersensitivity.

Dosage   1200 mg po bid. *Note: There are many potential drug interactions, some of which require dosage modification; see Chapter 5,* Physicians Desk Reference, *or package insert for more information.*

Toxicity   Nausea, diarrhea, rash, headache, and oral paresthesias.

Pregnancy category C.

Pregnancy Categories: A = controlled studies show no risk; B = no evidence of risk in humans; C = risk cannot be excluded; D = positive evidence of risk; X = contraindicated in pregnancy.

Indinavir (Crixivan)

Indications	Treatment of HIV infection in combination with other agents.
Contraindications	Known hypersensitivity.
Dosage	800 mg po every 8 hours on an empty stomach or with a nonfat meal. Didanosine should not be taken 1 hour before or after dose. Patients should drink at least 48 oz/d of fluid. Of note, twice-daily dosing has decreased efficacy and should be avoided. When co-administered with ritonavir, dosage is 400 mg po bid. *Note: There are many potential drug interactions, some of which require dosage modification; see Chapter 5, Physicians Desk Reference, or package insert for more information.*
Toxicity	Nephrolithiasis, gastrointestinal intolerance, hyperbilirubinemia, fat redistribution, hyperlipidemia, and glucose intolerance.
	Pregnancy category C.

Nelfinavir (Viracept)

Indications	Treatment of HIV infection in combination with other agents.
Contraindications	Known hypersensitivity.
Dosage	1250 mg po bid or 750 mg po every 8 hours with food. *Note: There are many potential drug interactions, some of which require dosage modification; see Chapter 5, Physicians Desk Reference, or package insert for more information.*
Toxicity	Diarrhea, fat redistribution, hyperlipidemia, and glucose intolerance.
	Pregnancy category B.

Ritonavir (Norvir)

Indications	Treatment of HIV infection in combination with other agents.
Contraindications	Known hypersensitivity.
Dosage	600 mg po every 12 hours with food, following 2-week dose-escalation regimen (days 1–2: 300 mg po bid; days

Pregnancy Categories: A = controlled studies show no risk; B = no evidence of risk in humans; C = risk cannot be excluded; D = positive evidence of risk; X = contraindicated in pregnancy.

3–5: 400 mg po bid; days 6–13: 500 mg po bid). When co-administered with saquinavir or indinavir, dosage is 400 mg po bid. Didanosine should not be taken within 2 hours of dose. *Note: There are many potential drug interactions, some of which require dosage modification;* see *Chapter 5,* Physicians Desk Reference, *or package insert for more information.*

Toxicity   Gastrointestinal intolerance, circumoral and extremity paresthesias, asthenia, taste perversion, abnormal liver function tests, increased creatinine phosphokinase and uric acid, fat redistribution, hyperlipidemia, and glucose intolerance.

Pregnancy category B.

Saquinavir (Fortovase)

Indications   Treatment of HIV infection in combination with other agents. Fortovase (soft gel cap formulation) is preferred to Invirase (hard gel cap) because of its enhanced absorption and bioavailability.

Contraindications   Known hypersensitivity.

Dosage   Fortorase dosage is 1200 mg po tid with food. When co-administered with ritonavir, dosage is 400 mg po bid. *Note: There are many potential drug interactions, some of which require dosage modification;* see *Chapter 5,* Physicians Desk Reference, *or package insert for more information.*

Toxicity   Gastrointestinal intolerance, abnormal liver function tests, fat redistribution, hyperlipidemia, and glucose intolerance.

Pregnancy category B.

ABT-378/Ritonavir (Lopinavir)

Indications   Treatment of HIV infection in combination with other agents for patients not responding to or intolerant of other regimens.

ABT-378 is a new protease inhibitor combined with ritonavir that significantly augments its blood level. The drug is not FDA approved but is available through the

Pregnancy Categories: A = controlled studies show no risk; B = no evidence of risk in humans; C = risk cannot be excluded; D = positive evidence of risk; X = contraindicated in pregnancy.

pharmaceutical company expanded-access program; contact Abbott Early Access Program at 1-888-711-7193.

Contraindications   Known hypersensitivity and concurrent use of riton-avir or delavirdine.

Dosage   Three (133 mg ABT-378/33 mg ritonavir) po bid.

Toxicity   Nausea, diarrhea, rash, abnormal liver function tests, and hyperlipidemia.

Tenofovir

Indications   Treatment of HIV infection in combination with other agents for patients not responding to or intolerant of other regimens.

Tenofovir is a new nucleotide agent; it is not FDA approved but is available through the pharamceutical company expanded-access program; contact Gilead Compassionate Access Study at 1-800-GILEAD-5.

Contraindications   Known hypersensitivity.

Dosage   300 mg po qd.

Toxicity   Renal dysfunction, increased serum creatine phospho-kinase, and abnormal liver function tests.

Antifungal Therapy

Pneumocystis carinii Pneumonia (PCP): Treatment and Prophylaxis

Atovaquone (Mepron)

Indications   Treatment and prophylaxis of PCP (mild to moderate infection) in patients unable to tolerate trimethoprim-sulfamethoxazole or dapsone.

Contraindications   Known hypersensitivity.

Dosage   750 mg of suspension po bid with food for 21 days. Same dosage for treatment and prophylaxis.

Toxicity   Gastrointestinal intolerance, rash, headache, fever.

Pregnancy category C.

Pregnancy Categories: A = controlled studies show no risk; B = no evidence of risk in humans; C = risk cannot be excluded; D = positive evidence of risk; X = contraindicated in pregnancy.

Clindamycin/Primaquine

Indications   Treatment of PCP in patients unable to tolerate trimethoprim-sulfamethoxazole.

Contraindications   Known hypersensitivity; glucose 6-phosphate dehydrogenase (G6PD) deficiency is contraindication to primaquine use.

Dosage   Clindamycin 600 mg IV every 8 hours (or 300–450 mg po qid) and primaquine 15 mg/d base po for 21 days.

Toxicity   Clindamycin: diarrhea, nausea, rash

Primaquine: nausea, dyspepsia, hemolytic anemia (G6PD deficiency).

Pregnancy categories B (clindamycin) and C (primaquine).

Dapsone

Indications   Treatment of PCP (mild to moderate infection) in combination with trimethoprim; prophylaxis of PCP in patients unable to tolerate trimethoprim-sulfamethoxazole; primary prophylaxis of toxoplasmosis in combination with pyrimethamine.

Contraindications   Known hypersensitivity, G6PD deficiency.

Dosage   PCP treatment: dapsone 100 mg po qd and trimethoprim 15 mg/kg po qd for 21 days.

PCP prophylaxis: 100 mg po qd.

Toxoplasmosis prophylaxis: add pyrimethamine 50 mg/wk with folinic acid 25 mg.

Toxicity   Rash, fever, gastrointestinal intolerance, neutropenia, methemoglobinemia.

Pregnancy category C.

Pentamidine (NebuPent [aerosol], Pentam [intravenous])

Indications   Treatment and prophylaxis of PCP in patients unable to tolerate trimethoprim-sulfamethoxazole or dapsone.

Contraindications   Severe asthma or bronchospasm, active pulmonary tuberculosis.

Dosage   Prophylaxis (aerosol): 300 mg via Respirgard II nebulizer once per month.

Treatment (intravenous): 3–4 mg/kg/d for 21 days.

Pregnancy Categories: A = controlled studies show no risk; B = no evidence of risk in humans; C = risk cannot be excluded; D = positive evidence of risk; X = contraindicated in pregnancy.

Toxicity	Aerosol: bronchospasm (particularly in patients with history of asthma or chronic obstructive pulmonary disease), pharyngeal irritation, metallic taste.

Intravenous: hypotension, nephrotoxicity, hypoglycemia, hyperglycemia, leukopenia, thrombocytopenia, hypokalemia, hypocalcemia.

Pregnancy category C.

Trimethoprim-sulfamethoxazole (TMP-SMX, Bactrim, Septra)

Indications Treatment and prophylaxis of PCP; primary prophylaxis of toxoplasmosis.

Contraindications Known hypersensitivity to trimethoprim or sulfonamides, megaloblastic anemia.

Dosage Treatment of PCP: 5 mg/kg po or IV every 8 hours of trimethoprim component (equivalent to two tablets po tid of double-strength (DS) TMP-SMX for a 65-kg patient).

Prophylaxis of PCP and toxoplasmosis: one DS tablet po daily (one single-strength [SS] tablet po daily *or* one DS tablet po 3 d/wk also seems to be effective for PCP prophylaxis.).

Toxicity Side effects are common in HIV-infected patients and include gastrointestinal intolerance, rash, urticaria, photosensitivity, Stevens–Johnson syndrome, fever, leukopenia, thrombocytopenia, hemolytic anemia, abnormal liver function tests, renal dysfunction, interstitial nephritis, aseptic meningitis.

Patients with history of mild to moderate drug toxicity should be given retrial of TMP-SMX or desensitized using an established protocol (*see* Table 6.2).

Pregnancy category C; avoid use at term because of risk of kernicterus in newborn.

Other Fungal Infections: Treatment and Prophylaxis

Amphotericin B

Indications Suspension for treatment of oral candidiasis; intravenous drug for treatment of systemic fungal infections.

Pregnancy Categories: A = controlled studies show no risk; B = no evidence of risk in humans; C = risk cannot be excluded; D = positive evidence of risk; X = contraindicated in pregnancy.

Contraindications	Known hypersensitivity.
Dosage	Oral candidiasis: 1–5 mL of suspension po qid for 14 days.
	Systemic fungal infections: intravenous dosages range from 0.3–1.0 mg/kg/d depending on the pathogen and type of infection. Lipid complex preparations are less toxic but very expensive.
Toxicity	Oral suspension: nausea, vomiting, diarrhea, rash; intravenous drug: infusion-related chills, hypotension, nausea, vomiting, nephrotoxicity, hypokalemia, hypomagnesemia, hypocalcemia, anemia.
	Pregnancy category B.

Clotrimazole

Indications	Treatment of mucosal candidiasis.
Contraindications	Known hypersensitivity.
Dosage	Oral candidiasis treatment: 10-mg lozenge dissolved in the mouth five times daily.
	Vaginal candidiasis treatment: 100-mg tablet intravaginally bid for 3 days.
Toxicity	Nausea, abnormal liver function tests.
	Pregnancy category C.

Fluconazole (Diflucan)

Indications	Treatment and secondary prophylaxis of mucosal candidiasis; secondary prophylaxis of cryptococcal infection.
Contraindications	Known hypersensitivity.
Dosage	Oral candidiasis treatment: 50–100 mg po qd for 7–14 days.
	Candida esophagitis treatment: 100–200 mg po qd for 14–21 days.
	Vaginal candidiasis: 150 mg po (one-time dose).
	Secondary prophylaxis of mucosal candidiasis: 50–200 mg/d po. *Note: There are many potential drug interactions, some of which require dosage modification;* see *text,* Physicians Desk Reference, *or package insert for more information.*

Pregnancy Categories: A = controlled studies show no risk; B = no evidence of risk in humans; C = risk cannot be excluded; D = positive evidence of risk; X = contraindicated in pregnancy.

Cryptococcal infection maintenance therapy (secondary prophylaxis): 200 mg po qd indefinitely. Most experts recommend initial treatment of cryptococcal infection with amphotericin B; if using fluconazole, dosage is 400 mg po qd po for 8 weeks.

Toxicity   Nausea, headache, hepatotoxicity.

Pregnancy category C.

Nystatin

Indications   Treatment of mucosal candidiasis.

Contraindications Known hypersensitivity.

Dosage   Oral candidiasis treatment: 5 mL suspension to be gargled and swallowed five times daily for 7–14 days.

Vaginal candidiasis treatment: 100,000-U tablet intravaginally once or twice daily for 7–14 days.

Toxicity   Nausea, vomiting, diarrhea

Pregnancy category C.

Antibacterial Therapy

Mycobacterium avium Complex (MAC) Infection and Tuberculosis (TB): Treatment and Prophylaxis*

Amikacin (Amikin)

Indications   Treatment of MAC infection in combination with other agents.

Contraindications Known hypersensitivity to aminoglycoside antibiotics.

Dosage   7.5–15 mg/kg/d IV for first 4 weeks of MAC therapy.

Toxicity   Ototoxicity, especially with larger total dose and longer duration (more auditory than vestibular and usually irreversible); nephrotoxicity.

Pregnancy category D.

Azithromycin (Zithromax)

Indications   Treatment of MAC infection in combination with other agents; prophylaxis of MAC infection.

---

* Drugs for TB also can be administered as directly observed therapy (DOT) in different dosage regimens. Consultation with an expert clinician in this area is recommended.
Pregnancy Categories: A = controlled studies show no risk; B = no evidence of risk in humans; C = risk cannot be excluded; D = positive evidence of risk; X = contraindicated in pregnancy.

Contraindications Known hypersensitivity to macrolide antibiotics.

Dosage MAC treatment: 500 mg po qd; prophylaxis: 1200 mg/wk po.

Toxicity Gastrointestinal intolerance.

Pregnancy category B.

Ciprofloxacin (Cipro)

Indications Treatment of MAC infection in combination with other agents; treatment of TB in combination with other agents.

Contraindications Known hypersensitivity.

Dosage 500–750 mg po bid.

Toxicity Gastrointestinal intolerance, central nervous system dysfunction, rash.

Pregnancy category C.

Clarithromycin (Biaxin)

Indications Treatment of MAC infection in combination with other agents; prophylaxis of MAC infection.

Contraindications Known hypersensitivity to macrolide antibiotics, concurrent use of terfenadine.

Dosage MAC treatment and prophylaxis: 500 mg po bid.

Toxicity Gastrointestinal intolerance, abnormal liver function tests.

Pregnancy category C; teratogenic in animals.

Ethambutol (Myambutol)

Indications Treatment of MAC infection in combination with other agents; treatment of TB in combination with other agents.

Contraindications Known hypersensitivity, history of optic neuritis.

Dosage 25 mg/kg/d po for the first 2 months, followed by 15 mg/kg/d.

Toxicity Optic neuritis, rash, gastrointestinal intolerance, hepatotoxicity.

Pregnancy category C; teratogenic in animals.

Pregnancy Categories: A = controlled studies show no risk; B = no evidence of risk in humans; C = risk cannot be excluded; D = positive evidence of risk; X = contraindicated in pregnancy.

Isoniazid (INH)

Indications   Treatment of TB in combination with other agents; prophylaxis of TB in context of positive skin test.

Contraindications   Known hypersensitivity, significant hepatic disease.

Dosage   Treatment: 300 mg po qd; prophylaxis: 300 mg po qd for 9 months. Pyridoxine should be given concurrently for prevention of peripheral neuropathy.

Toxicity   Hepatotoxicity, especially in alcoholics and in people over 50 years of age; peripheral neuropathy; fever; rash.

Pregnancy category C.

Pyrazinamide

Indications   Treatment of TB in combination with other agents.

Contraindications   Known hypersensitivity, significant hepatic disease.

Dosage   25 mg/kg/d po.

Toxicity   Abnormal liver function tests, hyperuricemia, rash.

Pregnancy category C.

Rifabutin (Mycobutin)

Indications   Treatment of MAC infection in combination with other agents; treatment of TB in combination with other agents; prophylaxis of MAC infection in patients unable to tolerate clarithromycin or azithromycin.

Contraindications   Known hypersensitivity.

Dosage   Treatment and prophylaxis: 300 mg po qd. *Note: There are many potential drug interactions, some of which require dosage modification;* see *text,* Physicians Desk Reference, *or package insert for more information.*

Toxicity   Orange discoloration of body secretions, gastrointestinal intolerance, rash, abnormal liver function tests. Acute uveitis has been reported when used in association with clarithromycin.

Pregnancy category C.

Rifampin

Indications   Treatment of TB in combination with other agents.

Contraindications   Known hypersensitivity.

Pregnancy Categories: A = controlled studies show no risk; B = no evidence of risk in humans; C = risk cannot be excluded; D = positive evidence of risk; X = contraindicated in pregnancy.

Dosage	600 mg/d po. *Note: There are many potential drug interactions, some of which require dosage modification; see text,* Physicians Desk Reference, *or package insert for more information.*
Toxicity	Orange discoloration of body secretions, gastrointestinal intolerance, abnormal liver function tests, rash.
	Pregnancy category C.

Streptomycin

Indications	Treatment of TB in combination with other agents.
Contraindications	Hypersensitivity to aminoglycoside antibiotics.
Dosage	15 mg/kg/d IM.
Toxicity	Ototoxicity, vestibular toxicity.
	Pregnancy category D.

Antiparasitic Therapy

Toxoplasmosis: Treatment and Prophylaxis[†]

Clindamycin

Indications	Treatment of toxoplasmic encephalitis (for patients unable to tolerate sulfadiazine) in combination with pyrimethamine.
Contraindications	Known hypersensitivity.
Dosage	Initial therapy: 900 mg IV every 6 hours or 300–450 mg po every 6 hours.
	Maintenance therapy (secondary prophylaxis): 300–450 mg po every 6 hours.
Toxicity	Diarrhea, nausea, rash.
	Pregnancy category B.

Dapsone

See section on *Pneumocystis carinii* Pneumonia above.

Pyrimethamine

Indications	Treatment of toxoplasmic encephalitis in combination with sulfadiazine or clindamycin.

[†] For primary prophylaxis, *see* section on *Pneumocystic carinii* pneumonia.
Pregnancy Categories: A = controlled studies show no risk; B = no evidence of risk in humans; C = risk cannot be excluded; D = positive evidence of risk; X = contraindicated in pregnancy.

Contraindications   Known hypersensitivity.

Dosage   Initial therapy: 100–200 mg po qd (loading dose), followed by 50–100 mg po qd for 6 weeks in conjunction with folinic acid 10 mg po qd.

Maintenance therapy (secondary prophylaxis): 25–75 mg po qd with folinic acid 10 mg po qd.

Toxicity   Reversible bone marrow suppression, gastrointestinal intolerance.

Pregnancy category C; teratogenic in animals.

Sulfadiazine

Indications   Treatment of toxoplasmic encephalitis in combination with pyrimethamine.

Contraindications   Known hypersensitivity to sulfonamides.

Dosage   Initial therapy: 1–2 g po qid for 6 weeks.

Maintenance therapy (secondary prophylaxis): 0.5–1.0 g po qid.

Toxicity   Fever, rash, pruritus, bone marrow suppression.

Pregnancy category C; avoid use at term because of risk of kernicterus in newborn.

Trimethoprim-sulfamethoxazole

See section on *Pneumocystis carinii* Pneumonia above.

Other Antiviral Therapies

Cytomegalovirus (CMV) Infection: Treatment and Prophylaxis

Cidofovir (Vistide)

Indications   Treatment of CMV infection, including ganciclovir-resistant strains.

Contraindications   Known hypersensitivity, significant renal dysfunction, use of other nephrotoxic medications.

Dosage   Initial therapy: 5 mg/kg IV once weekly for 2 weeks.

Maintenance therapy (secondary prophylaxis): 5 mg/kg IV once every other week.

Pregnancy Categories: A = controlled studies show no risk; B = no evidence of risk in humans; C = risk cannot be excluded; D = positive evidence of risk; X = contraindicated in pregnancy.

Probenecid 2 g po 3 hours before, 1 g po 2 hours before, and 1 g po 8 hours after infusion should be administered to prevent nephrotoxicity; 1 L normal saline also given before cidofovir dosing.

Toxicity   Nephrotoxicity, neutropenia.

Probenecid is associated with fever, chills, headache, rash, nausea.

Pregnancy category C.

Foscarnet (Foscavir)

Indications   Treatment of CMV infection, including ganciclovir-resistant strains.

Contraindications   Known hypersensitivity, significant renal dysfunction.

Dosage   Initial therapy: 60 mg/kg IV every 8 hours *or* 90 mg/kg IV every 12 hours for 14–21 days.

Maintenance therapy (secondary prophylaxis): 90–120 mg/kg/d IV.

Toxicity   Nephrotoxicity, hypocalcemia, hypophosphatemia, hypokalemia, headache, fatigue, nausea, anemia, seizure.

Pregnancy category C.

Ganciclovir (Cytovene)

Indications   Treatment and prophylaxis of CMV infection.

Contraindications   Known hypersensitivity, neutropenia, thrombocytopenia.

Dosage   Initial therapy: 5 mg/kg IV every 12 hours for 14–21 days.

Maintenance therapy (secondary prophylaxis): 5 mg/kg/d IV.

Primary and secondary prophylaxis: 1 gm po tid.

Toxicity   Neutropenia, thrombocytopenia, anemia, nausea, diarrhea, abdominal pain, headache, confusion.

Pregnancy category C; teratogenic in animals.

Pregnancy Categories: A = controlled studies show no risk; B = no evidence of risk in humans; C = risk cannot be excluded; D = positive evidence of risk; X = contraindicated in pregnancy.

Herpes Simplex Virus (HSV) and Varicella-Zoster Virus (VZV) Infections: Treatment and Prophylaxis[‡]

Acyclovir (Zovirax)

Indications	Treatment of HSV and VZV infections.
Contraindications	Known hypersensitivity.
Dosage	HSV treatment: 400 mg po tid for 5–7 days.
	Secondary prophylaxis: 400 mg po bid is standard dose, but larger doses may be necessary in advanced HIV disease. For extensive or disseminated disease, intravenous therapy (5–10 mg/kg every 8 hours) is given.
	VZV treatment: 800 mg po every 4 hours while awake (five times daily) for 7 days. For disseminated zoster or ophthalmic involvement, intravenous therapy (10–12 mg/kg every 8 hours) is given. Secondary prophylaxis generally is not indicated.
Toxicity	Nausea, renal dysfunction.
	Pregnancy category C.

Famciclovir

Indications	Treatment of HSV and VZV infections.
Contraindications	Known hypersensitivity.
Dosage	HSV treatment: 125 mg po bid for 5–7 days.
	HSV secondary prophylaxis: 125–250 mg po bid.
	VZV treatment: 500 mg po tid for 7 days. Secondary prophylaxis generally is not indicated.
Toxicity	Headache, nausea.
	Pregnancy category B.

Miscellaneous Therapeutic Agents

Dronabinol (Marinol)

Indications	Appetite stimulant for treatment of AIDS wasting syndrome.

[‡] Cidofovir and foscarnet also have activity against HSV and VZV and may have a role in the treatment of resistant strains. Valacyclovir, an acyclovir analogue, has been associated with cases of thrombotic thrombocytopenic purpura in patients with advanced HIV disease.
Pregnancy Categories: A = controlled studies show no risk; B = no evidence of risk in humans; C = risk cannot be excluded; D = positive evidence of risk; X = contraindicated in pregnancy.

Contraindications   Known hypersensitivity, significant cognitive dysfunction.

Dosage   2.5–5.0 mg po bid.

Toxicity   Neuropsychiatric symptoms, gastrointestinal intolerance.

Pregnancy category C.

Erythropoietin (Procrit)

Indications   Treatment of HIV- or ZDV-associated anemia (hematocrit ≤30) in patients with serum erythropoietin levels ≤500 mU/mL.

Contraindications   Known hypersensitivity to mammalian cell–derived products or human albumin; uncontrolled hypertension.

Dosage   100 U/kg IV or SC three times weekly; response usually seen between 2 and 4 weeks. Maximal dosage is 300 U/kg three times weekly.

Toxicity   Headache, nausea, arthralgia, hypertension, seizures.

Pregnancy category C; teratogenic in animals.

Granulocyte Colony–Stimulating Factor (G-CSF, Filgrastim)

Indications   Treatment of neutropenia, defined as absolute neutrophil count (ANC) <500–750/mm^3, as a result of HIV disease, chemotherapy, or other drugs (hydroxyurea, ganciclovir, zidovudine, trimethoprim-sulfamethoxazole).

Contraindications   Known hypersensitivity to drug or *Escherichia coli*–derived products.

Dosage   5–10 µg/kg/d SC. Complete blood count should be checked twice weekly, and ANC should be maintained at >1000–2000 cells/mL. G-CSF should be stopped if there is no response after 7 days at a dosage of 10 µg/kg/d.

Toxicity   Bone pain.

Pregnancy category C.

Human Growth Hormone (Somatropin, Serostim)

Indications   Hormonal treatment of AIDS wasting syndrome.

Contraindications   Known hypersensitivity or presence of an actively growing intracranial tumor.

Pregnancy Categories: A = controlled studies show no risk; B = no evidence of risk in humans; C = risk cannot be excluded; D = positive evidence of risk; X = contraindicated in pregnancy.

Dosage	For patients >55 kg: 6 mg SC at bedtime.
	For patients 45–55 kg: 5 mg SC at bedtime.
	For patients 35–45 kg: 4 mg SC at bedtime.
Toxicity	Arthralgia, edema, hypertension, hyperglycemia.
	Pregnancy category B.

Hydroxyurea (Hydrea)

Indications	Has been shown to act synergistically with didanosine and possibly stavudine (*see* section on Nucleoside Reverse-Transcriptase Inhibitors above); not FDA-approved for management of HIV infection.
Contraindications	Known hypersensitivity, significant bone marrow suppression, pregnancy.
Dosage	500 mg po bid.
Toxicity	Bone marrow suppression, stomatitis, nausea, vomiting, rash; severe pancreatitis has been described rarely when administered with didanosine.
	Pregnancy category D.

Megestrol Acetate (Megace)

Indications	Appetite stimulant for treatment of AIDS wasting syndrome.
Contraindications	Known hypersensitivity, pregnancy.
Dosage	Oral suspension: 400–800 mg po qd.
	Tablets: 80 mg po qid up to 800 mg po qd.
Toxicity	Hypogonadism, adrenal insufficiency, diarrhea, impotence, hyperglycemia, rash.
	Pregnancy category D.

Nandrolone (Deca-Durabolin)

Indications	Anabolic steroid for treatment of AIDS wasting syndrome.
Contraindications	Known hypersensitivity, history of breast or prostate cancer, significant hepatic dysfunction, nephrosis, pregnancy.
Dosage	Men: 100–200 mg IM every 1–2 weeks.
	Women: 25 mg/wk IM *or* 50 mg IM every 2 weeks.

Pregnancy Categories: A = controlled studies show no risk; B = no evidence of risk in humans; C = risk cannot be excluded; D = positive evidence of risk; X = contraindicated in pregnancy.

| Toxicity | Edema, hypertension, virilization, hypoglycemia, hyperlipidemia, abnormal liver function tests. |
| | Pregnancy category X. |

Oxandrolone (Oxandrin)

Indications	Anabolic steroid for treatment of AIDS wasting syndrome.
Contraindications	Known hypersensitivity, history of breast or prostate cancer, significant hepatic dysfunction, nephrosis, pregnancy.
Dosage	Men: 10–20 mg po bid *or* 20 mg po qd.
	Women: 5–20 mg po qd.
Toxicity	Edema, hypertension, virilization, glucose intolerance, hyperlipidemia, abnormal liver function tests.
	Pregnancy category X.

Testosterone

Indications	Treatment of hypogonadism; treatment of AIDS wasting syndrome.
Contraindications	Known hypersensitivity, history of breast or prostate cancer, pregnancy.
Dosage	200–400 mg IM every 2 weeks
	Alternative transdermal system: Androderm-2 system and Testoderm TTS both supply 5 mg of testosterone once daily via nonscrotal patch.
Toxicity	Coagulopathy, cholestatic jaundice, increased libido, edema, flushing, priapism, local reaction with patches.
	Pregnancy category X.

Thalidomide (Thalomid)

Indications	Treatment of refractory aphthous ulcers; treatment of refractory AIDS wasting syndrome.
Contraindications	Known hypersensitivity, pregnancy.
Dosage	200 mg po every day *or* twice daily. Physicians and pharmacists must be registered in the STEPS program to prescribe thalidomide. (Call the System for Thalidomide Education and Prescribing Safety at 888-423-5436.) Female patients must 1) have a negative pregnancy test

Pregnancy Categories: A = controlled studies show no risk; B = no evidence of risk in humans; C = risk cannot be excluded; D = positive evidence of risk; X = contraindicated in pregnancy.

within 24 hours of starting therapy, 2) have weekly pregnancy tests in the first month of therapy, 3) have monthly pregnancy tests thereafter, and 4) agree to use two forms of contraception. Male patients must use a condom for contraception.

Toxicity   Peripheral neuropathy, drowsiness, orthostatic hypotension, fever, rash, neutropenia.

Pregnancy category X.

Pregnancy Categories: A = controlled studies show no risk; B = no evidence of risk in humans; C = risk cannot be excluded; D = positive evidence of risk; X = contraindicated in pregnancy.

Index

■   ■   ■

Note: "f" following page number indicates figure; "t" indicates table.

A

Abacavir
  characteristics of, 98t, 105
  indications, dosage, and toxicity
      of, 275
  manifestations of toxicity, 159t
ABT-378/Ritonavir, 108, 281
Abuse, substance, 52-53, 52t, 91
Acyclovir
  for herpes simplex virus infection,
      202
  indications, dosage, and toxicity
      of, 292
  for varicella-zoster virus infection,
      204
Adherence, 97, 111
Adjustment disorder, 86
Aerosol pentamidine. *See* Pentamidine
Age
  incidence of HIV infection and, 7
  risk for HIV infection and, 48
Agenerase, 100t
AIDS, progression to, 35
AIDS surveillance case definition, 3t
Alitretinoin, 219
Amikacin
  characteristics of, 170, 171, 172t
  indications for, dosage of, and tox-
      icity of, 286
Amphotericin B
  for candidiasis, 183t
  for cryptococcosis, 184-185, 186t
  for histoplasmosis, 187
  indications, dosage, and toxicity
      of, 284-285
Amprenavir
  characteristics of, 100t, 107-108
  drugs contraindicated with, 102t-
      103t

indications, dosage, and toxicity
    of, 279
  interactions with, 104t
Anal intercourse, 70
Angiomatosis, bacillary, 147t, 166t
Anogenital malignancy, 237-239
Antibacterial therapy, 286-289
Antibody, monoclonal, for lymphoma,
    230
Antibody testing, 63-66, 251
Antifungal therapy, 282-286
Antigen
  cryptococcal, 184
  cytomegalovirus, 198
Antiparasitic therapy, 289-290
Antiretroviral therapy, 95-113, 275-
    296. *See also Specific drug*
  antibacterial, 286-289
  antifungal, 282-286
  antiparasitic, 289-290
  categories of, 97
  CD4 lymphocytes and, 136
  clinical guidelines for, 109-111
  clinical vignettes about, 261-262,
      271-273
  cryptosporidial infection and, 194
  drug failure and, 96-97, 112t
  dual-protease inhibitors, 108
  future directions of, 112-113
  goals of, 96
  hydroxyurea, 108-109
  Kaposi's sarcoma and, 214
  lipodystrophy syndrome and, 109
  miscellaneous, 292-296
  nonnucleoside reverse-transcriptase
      inhibitors. *See* Nonnucleoside
      reverse-transcriptase inhibitor
  nucleoside reverse-transcriptase
      inhibitors. *See* Nucleoside
      reverse-transcriptase inhibitor

Antiretroviral therapy—*continued*
  opportunistic infection and, 117-118
  other antiviral, 290-292
  in pregnancy, 88-91, 88t, 111-112
  for primary disease, 75-78
  protease inhibitors, 100t, 106-108
  quality of life and, 34
Aphthous ulcer, 149t
Arthralgia, 31
Arthropod Infestation, 156t
Aspergillus infection, respiratory, 141,
  142t-143t
Asthma, symptoms of, 142t-143t
Asymptomatic patient, long-term, 35-36
Atovaquone, 119t, 121, 282
At-risk populations, 48
Azithromycin
  indications, dosage, and toxicity
    of, 286-287
  for *Mycobacterium avium* com-
    plex, 81, 123-125, 124t, 170-
    171

B

B cell in lymphoma, 227
Bacillary angiomatosis, 147t, 166t
Bacterial opportunistic infection. *See*
  Opportunistic infection, bacterial
Bactrim. *See* Trimethoprim-
  sulfamethoxazole
Bartonellosis, 165-168, 167f
Biaxin (Clarithromycin), 81, 123-125,
  124t, 170m, 172t, 287
Blastocystis hominis infection, 191, 193t
Blood count, 71-72
Blood transmission of HIV, 10. *See*
  also Occupational HIV expo-
  sure
Body habitus, change in, 149-150
Breast feeding, 11, 90-91

C

Cancer. *See* Malignancy
Candidiasis, 180-183, 182f, 183t

  esophageal, 148
  prophylaxis for, 127
CCR5 molecule, 22-23
CD4 lymphocyte
  cell count of, 72-73
  classification of HIV and, 2
  cytomegalovirus infection and, 128
  diarrhea and, 144-145
  fever and, 138-139
  immune destruction and, 23-26
  immune reconstitution and, 28
  interaction with HIV, 22f
  long-term asymptomatic patient
    and, 36
  management of HIV stratified by, 74t
  opportunistic infection and, 117-118
  oral lesions and, 148
  progression of disease and, 34
  risk of developing AIDS and, 25f
  symptoms and, 135-136
  transmission of HIV and, 22-23
  tuberculosis and, 178
  viral reservoir and, 26-27
Cell
  B, in lymphoma, 227
  CD4 lymphocyte. *See* CD4 lym-
    phocyte
  peripheral blood mononuclear, 31
Central nervous system lymphoma,
  225-226, 228-229, 231
Cerebrospinal fluid in cryptococcosis,
  184
Cervical cancer, 83, 238-239
Cervical dysplasia, 70
Cesarean section, 54, 90
Chemotherapy for Kaposi's sarcoma,
  220
Cholangiopathy, 147t
Chronic obstructive pulmonary dis-
  ease, 142t-143t
Cidofovir, 199t, 200, 290-291
Ciprofloxacin, 170, 171, 172t, 287
Clarithromycin, 81, 123-125, 124t, 170,
  172t, 287
Classification of HIV, 2-4, .2t
Clindamycin
  indications, dosage, and toxicity
    of, 283, 289

for *Pneumocystis carinii* pneumonia, 189t
for toxoplasmosis, 196-197, 196t
Clostridium difficile infection, 145, 145t
Clotrimazole
  for candidiasis, 181, 183t
  indications, dosage, and toxicity of, 285
  for prevention of fungal infection, 127
Coccidioides infection, 141, 142t-143t
Combivir, 105
Community-acquired pneumonia, 168-169
Computed tomography, 137
  cryptococcosis and, 184
  fever and, 140
  toxoplasmosis and, 195-196
Condom, appropriate use of, 51-52
Congestive heart failure, 142t-143t
Corticosteroid, 189t, 216
Cough, 140
Crixivan, 100t. *See* Indinavir
Cryptococcosis, 127, 183-186, 185f, 186t
Cryptosporidium infection, 145t, 190-194, 192f, 193t
Cyclospora infection, 191, 193t
Cytokine, 226
Cytomegalovirus
  diarrhea with, 145t
  drugs for, 290-291
  fever and, 138
  incidence of, 128-129
  liver function and, 147t
  neurologic symptoms of, 154t
  oral lesions from, 149t
  prophylaxis for, 81-82, 128-130
  screening for, 72
Cytovene. *See* Gancyclovir

D

Dapsone
  indications, dosage, and toxicity of, 283, 289-290
  for *Pneumocystis carinii* pneumonia, 80, 119t, 120

skin disorder caused by, 159t
for toxoplasmosis prophylaxis, 122
Daunorubicin, 220
Deca-Durabolin, 294-295
Delavirdine, 106
  characteristics of, 99t
  drugs contraindicated with, 102t-103t
  indications, dosage, and toxicity of, 278
  interactions with, 104t
Delivery of infant
  clinical vignette about, 258-260
  testing of neonate and, 91
  transmission of HIV during
    mechanism of, 10-11
    prevention of, 53-55, 54t
Dementia, 154t
Demographics, 48
Dermatitis, seborrheic, 160
Dermatologic manifestations. *See* Skin disorder
Diarrhea
  as common symptom, 144-146, 145t
  Cryptosporidium infection causing, 191
Didanosine, 101
  characteristics of, 98t
  indications, dosage, and toxicity of, 276
Differential diagnosis, 33t
Diflucan. *See* Fluconazole
Discharge, vaginal, 154-155
Doxil, 220
Doxorubicin, 220
Doxycycline, 176, 177t
Dronabinol, 292-293
Drug abuse, 52-53, 52t, 91
Drug failure, 96-97
  modification of therapy and, 110, 112t
Drug therapy. *See* Antiretroviral therapy; *specific drug*
Drug-induced disorder
  dermatologic, 158-159, 159t
  diarrhea as, 145t, 146t
  hepatitis as, 146
  liver function and, 147t

Dual-protease inhibitors, 108
Dysphagia, 148
Dysplasia
   cervical, 70
   squamous cell, 237-238
Dyspnea, 140

E

Efavirenz, 106
   characteristics of, 99t
   drugs contraindicated with, 102t-
      103t
   indications, dosage, and toxicity
      of, 278-279, 106278
   interactions with, 104t
Effusion lymphoma, 229
ELISA, 65
Encephalitis
   cytomegalovirus, 154t, 197, 198
   toxoplasmosis, 121-122
Encephalitozoon infection, 191, 192-193
Endocrine disorder, 139t
Entamoeba histolytica, 193t
Enterocytozoon infection, 193t
Enterovirus infection, 145t
Enzyme-linked immunosorbent assay,
   65
Eosinophilic folliculitis, 160
Epidemiology, 1-8
   classification and, 2-4, 2t
   of hepatitis, 204-205
   of occupational HIV exposure,
      243-247, 244t, 245t, 246t
   prevalence and, 8
   in United States, 4-8, 5f, 6f
   for women, 87
   worldwide, 11-12
Epivir, 98t. See Lamivudine
Epstein-Barr virus, 34t
Equipment, transmission of HIV via, 10
Erythropoietin, 293
Esophageal candidiasis, 148, 181
Esophageal ulcer, 30
Ethambutol
   indications, dosage, and toxicity
      of, 287

   for Mycobacterium avium com-
      plex, 172t
Ethnic minority
   incidence of HIV infection n, 7
   as population at risk, 48
Exchange, needle, 45, 53
Extremity pain, 152-154
Eye, 70

F

Famciclovir
   indications, dosage, and toxicity
      of, 292
   for varicella-zoster virus infection,
      204
Female
   gynecologic symptoms in, 154-155
   incidence of HIV infection in, 5-6
   as population at risk, 48
Female condom, 51-52
Female-to-male transmission, 49-50
Fever, 138-140, 139t
Filgrastim, 293
Financial issues, 92
Fluconazole, 127, 128
   for candidiasis, 182, 183t
   for cryptococcosis, 185-186, 186t
   for esophagitis, 148
   indications, dosage, and toxicity
      of, 285-286
Folliculitis, eosinophilic, 160
Food safety, 92
Fortovase. See Saquinavir
Foscarnet
   cutaneous manifestations of, 159t
   for cytomegalovirus infection, 199t,
      200
   indications, dosage, and toxicity
      of, 291
Fungal infection
   candidiasis, 180-183, 182f, 183t
   cryptococcosis, 183-186, 185f, 186t
   drugs for
      other infections, 284-286
      Pneumocystis carinii pneumonia,
         79-91, 80t, 118-121, 282-284

fever and, 139t
histoplasmosis, 186-187
Pneumocystis carinii pneumonia.
  See Pneumocystis carinii
  pneumonia
prophylaxis for, 127-128
respiratory, 141, 142t-143t
of skin, 156t

G

Gancyclovir
  for cytomegalovirus infection, 81-
    82, 129, 199t, 200
  indications, dosage, and toxicity
    of, 291
Gastrointestinal disorder, 144-150
  diarrhea as, 144-146, 145t
  dysphagia as, 148
  hepatitis causing, 146, 147t,
    148
  Kaposi's sarcoma and, 216-217
  lymphoma and, 228
  natural history of, 30
  odynophagia as, 148
  oral ulcers and, 149t
  parasitic, 190-192, 192f, 193t,
    194
  in review of systems, 69t
  weight loss as, 149-150
Genital squamous cell carcinoma,
  237-239
Genital tract infection, 9
Genitourinary symptoms, 69t
Genotype test, 96-97
Geographic variation in incidence of
  HIV infection, 7-8
Giardia lamblia infection
  diagnosis and treatment of,
    193t
  diarrhea with, 145t
Gonorrhea, 9
Gram-negative bacteria, 142t-143t
Granulocyte colony-stimulating factor,
  293
Growth hormone, human, 293-294
Gynecologic symptoms, 154-155

H

Habitus, change in, 149-150
Haemophilus influenzae infection,
  141, 142t-143t
Haemophilus influenzae vaccine, 84t
Hairy leukoplakia, 70
Headache, 150-152
Health care maintenance issues, 82-86
  age-appropriate screening as, 86
  cervical cancer screening as, 83
  immunizations as, 82-83, 84t
  sexually transmitted disease as, 85-
    86
  tuberculosis as, 83, 85
Health care worker. *See* Occupational
  HIV exposure
Hepatitis
  characteristics of, 146-148
  clinical manifestations of, 205
  diagnosis of, 205
  epidemiology of, 204-205
  history of, 68
  HIV infection with, 266-267
  immunization against, 84t
  liver function tests and, 147t
  management of, 205-206
  symptoms of, 146, 147t, 148
  testing for, 72
Herpes simplex virus infection
  clinical features of, 201, 201f
  diagnosis of, 201-202
  drugs for, 292
  epidemiology of, 200-201
  management of, 202, 202t
  oral, 149t
  treatment of, 202t
Heterosexual transmission
  increasing, 48
  sexually transmitted disease and,
    50-51
Histoplasma capsulatum infection,
  141, 142t-143t
Histoplasmosis, 186-187
History-taking, 67-68, 67t
HIVID (zalcitabine), 98t
Hodgkin's lymphoma, 222-224, 224t

Homosexual
   Kaposi's sarcoma in, 213-214
   as population at risk, 48
Host immune response, 23
Human growth hormone, 293
Hydroxyurea
   characteristics of, 108-109
   indications, dosage, and toxicity
      of, 294
Hypoadrenalism, 139t

I

Imaging, radiologic, 137
   cryptococcosis and, 184
   fever and, 140
   respiratory infection and, 141
Immune destruction, 23-26
Immune reconstitution, 28
Immune response, 23
Immunization, 82-83, 84t
Indinavir, 107
   characteristics of, 100t
   drugs contraindicated with, 102t-103t
   indications, dosage, and toxicity
      of, 280
   interactions with, 104t
Infant. See Neonate
Infection. See also Opportunistic
      infection
   diarrhea with, 144-145
   fever and, 139t
   odynophagia and dysphagia with,
      148
   respiratory, 140-141, 142t-143t, 144
   skin disorder caused by, 155, 156t-
      157t, 158
   vaginal, 70-71
   viral
      cytomegalovirus. See
         Cytomegalovirus
      drugs for, 290-292
      hepatitis as. See Hepatitis
      herpes simplex, 149t, 200-202,
         201f, 202t
      liver function and, 147t
      skin disorder from, 156t

      varicella-zoster, 202-204, 202t,
         203f
Influenza vaccine, 84t
Injected-drug use, 52-53, 52t, 57
Intercourse, receptive anal, 70
Interferons for Kaposi's sarcoma, 220
Interleukins for lymphoma, 230
Invirase, 100t, 107
Isoniazid
   indications, dosage, and toxicity
      of, 288
   for *Mycobacterium avium* com-
      plex, 172t
   as prophylaxis, 85
   for tuberculosis, 126, 179-180
Isosporiasis
   clinical manifestations of, 191
   treatment of, 194
Itraconazole, 128

K

Kaposi's sarcoma, 213-221
   bacillary angiomatosis *vs.*, 166t
   clinical manifestations of, 216-217,
      217f
   cutaneous manifestations of, 160
   diagnosis of, 218
   epidemiology of, 213-214
   pathogenesis of, 214-216
   respiratory symptoms with, 142t-
      143t
   staging and prognosis of, 218, 219t
   treatment of, 218-221
Kidney disorder, 30

L

Laboratory findings, 31-33
Lamivudine (3TC)
   characteristics of, 98t, 103
   indications, dosage, and toxicity
      of, 276
   in pregnancy, 111, 90
   resistance to, 101
Latex condom, appropriate use of,
   51-52

Legal issues, 92
Legionella infection, respiratory, 141, 142t-143t
Leukoencephalopathy, progressive multifocal, 154t
Leukoplakia, hairy, 70
Lipodystrophy syndrome
    clinical vignette about, 263-264
    combination drug therapy causing, 78, 109
    management of, 149-150
Liver disorder, 140
Lopinavir, 108
Lumbar puncture in syphilis, 176
Lung disorder
    Kaposi's sarcoma and, 217
    in natural history of HIV, 30
    symptoms of, 69t, 140-141, 142t-143t, 144
Lymph node, 70
Lymphocyte
    B, 227
    CD4. *See* CD4 lymphocyte
    T, 32
        Hodgkin's lymphoma and, 224
        primary infection and, 32
Lymphocytic interstitial pneumonitis, 142t-143t
Lymphoma, 222-232
    central nervous system, 225-226
    clinical manifestations of, 228-229, 229t
    diagnosis of, 229
    histology of, 227-228
    Hodgkin's, 222-224, 224t
    liver function and, 147t
    non-Hodgkin's, 224
    pathogenesis of, 226-227
    prognosis of, 231-232, 231t
    respiratory symptoms of, 142t-143t
    toxoplasmosis *vs.*, 226t
    treatment of, 230-231

M

Magnetic resonance imaging, 137
    cryptococcosis and, 184
    fever and, 140

toxoplasmosis and, 195-196
Male, incidence of HIV infection in, 5
Male-to-female transmission, 49-50
Male-to-male transmission, 49-50
Malignancy, 213-241
    anogenital, 237-239
    Kaposi's sarcoma, 213-221. *See also* Kaposi's sarcoma
    lymphoma, 222-232. *See also* Lymphoma
    screening for, 86
    skin and, 160
Marinol, 292-293
Megestrol acetate, 294
Menstrual abnormality, 155
Mental status
    altered, 152, 153t
    screening of, 71
Mepron, 282
MGBG, for lymphoma, 230
Microsporidia infection
    clinical manifestations of, 191
    diagnosis and treatment of, 193t
    diarrhea with, 145t
    management of, 192, 194
Minority, racial/ethnic
    incidence of HIV infection and, 7
    as population at risk, 48
Mitoguazone, 230
Modification of antiretroviral therapy, 110-111
Monitoring of antiviral therapy, 96
Monoclonal antibody for lymphoma, 230
Mononuclear cell, peripheral blood, 31
Mortality in United States, 4
Mother-to-child transmission
    clinical vignette about, 258-260
    mechanism of, 10-11
    prevention of, 53-55, 54t
    testing of neonate and, 91
Mouth lesion, 148, 149t
Multifocal leukoencephalopathy, progressive, 154t
Myambutol. *See* Ethambutol
Mycobacterium avium complex, 169-171, 172t, 173

Mycobacterium avium complex—
    continued
  CD4 lymphocyte count and, 73
  diarrhea with, 145t
  drugs for, 286-289
  fever and, 138
  incidence of, 123
  liver function and, 147t
  prophylaxis for, 81, 123-125, 124t
  recommendations for, 125
Mycobacterium tuberculosis. See
    Tuberculosis
Mycobutin. *See* Rifabutin

N

Nandrolone, 294-295
National Health and Nutrition
    Examination survey, 8
National Institute of Health, 45
Natural history, 35f
  differential diagnosis of, 33t
  long-term nonprogression, 35-36
  of primary infection
    clinical features of, 28-31, 29t
    laboratory findings and, 31-33,
      34t
  of progression
    to AIDS, 35
    to symptomatic disease, 33-34
Needle, transmission of HIV via, 9
Needle exchange program, 45, 53
Needle-stick exposure. *See also*
    Occupational HIV exposure
  zidovudine after, 55
Nelfinavir, 107
  characteristics of, 100t
  drugs contraindicated with, 102t-
    103t
  indications, dosage, and toxicity
    of, 280-281
  interactions with, 104t
Neonate
  clinical vignette about, 258-260
  testing of, 91
  transmission of HIV to
    mechanism of, 10-11
    prevention of, 53-55, 54t

Nephrosis, 30
Neurocognitive disorder, 86
Neurologic disorder, 30-31, 150-154
  altered mental status as, 152, 153t
  cytomegalovirus encephalitis caus-
    ing, 154t
  dementia and, 154t
  fever and, 140
  headache as, 150-152
  painful extremities as, 152-154
  progressive multifocal leukoen-
    cephalopathy causing, 154t
  syphilis causing, 175, 176
  toxoplasmosis causing, 194-197.
    See also Toxoplasmosis
Neurologic symptoms, 69t
Nevirapine, 106
  characteristics of, 99t
  cutaneous manifestations of, 159t
  indications, dosage, and toxicity
    of, 279
  interactions with, 104t
  in pregnancy, 90
Nodule, in bartonellosis, 166, 167f
Non-Hodgkin's lymphoma, 224
  clinical manifestations of, 228-229
Nonnucleoside reverse-transcriptase
    inhibitor, 97, 104t, 105-106
  cross resistance and, 112-113
  indications, dosage, and toxicity of
    delavirdine, 278
    efavirenz, 278-279
    nevirapine, 279
    tenofovir, 279
Nonprogression to HIV disease, 35-36
Norcardia asteroides infection, respi-
    ratory, 141, 142t-143t
Norvir. *See* Ritonavir
Nucleoside reverse-transcriptase
    inhibitor, 77
  action of, 99, 101
  characteristics of, 98t, 99t
  indications, dosage, and toxicity
    of, 275-282
    abacavir, 275
    didanosine, 276
    lamivudine, 276
    stavudine, 276-277
    zalcitabine, 277

zidovudine, 277-278
types of, 101-103, 105
Nystatin
for candidiasis, 181-182, 183t
indications, dosage, and toxicity
of, 286

O

Occupational HIV exposure, 243-255
clinical vignette about, 268-270
epidemiology of, 243-247, 244t,
245t, 246t
management of, 247-248, 249f-
251f, 250-252
prevention of, 252-254, 253t
prophylaxis after, 55, 57
resources and registries for, 254
Occupational Safety and Health
Administration, 247, 252
Odynophagia, gastrointestinal symptoms, 148
Ophthalmoscopy, 70
Opportunistic cancer, 213-241. *See
also* Cancer
Opportunistic infection
bacterial
bartonellosis, 165-168, 166t,
167f
community-acquired pneumonia, 168-169
Mycobacterium avium complex. *See Mycobacterium
avium* complex
salmonellosis, 173-174
syphilis, 174-177, 175f, 177t
tuberculosis, 177-180, 179f
CD4 lymphocyte count and, 73
as clinical symptom, 31
cytomegalovirus. *See*
Cytomegalovirus
epidemiology of, 4
fungal, 127-128
candidiasis, 180-183, 182f, 183t
cryptococcosis, 183-186, 185f,
186t
histoplasmosis, 186-187
liver function and, 147t

parasitic
gastrointestinal, 190-192, 192f,
193t, 194
toxoplasmosis, 194-197, 196t
Pneumocystis carinii pneumonia.
See Pneumocystis carinii
pneumonia
prevention of, 117-131
cytomegalovirus, 81-82, 128-130
drug profiles for, 282-292
fungal, 127-128
Mycobacterium avium complex, 81, 123-125, 124t
Pneumocystis carinii pneumonia, 78-81, 79f, 80t, 118-
121, 119t, 120t
toxoplasmosis, 81, 121-123
tuberculosis, 125-126
toxoplasmosis. *See* Toxoplasmosis
tuberculosis. *See* Tuberculosis
viral
cytomegalovirus, 197-200, 198f,
199t
hepatitis, 204-206
herpes simplex virus, 200-202,
201f, 202t
varicella-zoster, 202-204, 202t,
203f
Oral lesion
candidiasis, 181
types of, 70
ulcerated, 30, 148, 149t
Oxandrolone, 295

P

Paclitaxel, 220
Pain
extremity, 152-154
pelvic, 154-155
Papanicolaou smear, 83
Parasitic infection
fever and, 139t
gastrointestinal, 190-192, 192f,
193t, 194
toxoplasmosis. *See* Toxoplasmosis
Parenteral transmission of HIV,
9-10

Pathogenesis, 21-28
  host immune response and, 23
  immune destruction and, 23-26,
    25f, 26f
  immune reconstitution and, 28
  transmission and, 22-23
  viral phenotype and, 27-28
  viral reservoirs and, 26-27
Pelvic examination, 83
Pelvic pain, 154-155
Penicillin for syphilis, 177t
Penis, herpes infection of, 201f
Pentamidine
  cost of, 119t
  disadvantages of, 120-121
  dosage of, 189t, 283-284
  indications for and toxicity of, 283-
    284
  trimethoprim-sulfamethoxazole *vs.,*
    80
  tuberculosis and, 80-81
Pentoxifylline for tuberculosis, 180
Perinatal transmission of HIV
  clinical vignette about, 258-260
  mechanism of, 10-11
  prevention of, 53-55
  testing of neonate and, 91
Peripheral blood mononuclear cell, 31
Phenotype, viral, 27
Phenotype test, 97
Physical examination, 68-71
Physician's role in prevention of HIV
    transmission, 46
Plasma viremia, 22-23
Pneumococcal vaccine, 84t
Pneumocystis carinii pneumonia,
    187-190, 189t
  algorithm for prophylaxis of, 79t
  CD4 lymphocyte count and, 73
  drugs for, 79-91, 80t, 118-121, 119t,
    120t
    indications for, dosage of, and
      toxicity of, 282-284
  incidence of, 118
  liver function and, 147t
  recommendations for, 121
Pneumonia, community-acquired,
    168-169

Pneumonitis, 142t-143t
Polio vaccine, 84t
Polymerase chain reaction, 136-137
Polyradiculopathy, 197, 198
Polyurethane condom, 51
Population, at-risk, 48
Postexposure prophylaxis. *See*
    Occupational HIV exposure
Posttest counseling, 64-65
PPD test for tuberculosis, 125-126,
    178-179
Precautions, standard, 252-253, 253t
Prednisone, 189t
Pregnancy
  antiretroviral therapy in, 87-91, 88t
    guidelines for, 111-112
  clinical vignette about, 258-260
  perinatal transmission and, 10-11,
    53-55
  zidovudine in, 88-91, 88t
Pretest counseling, 64-65
Prevention of HIV infection, 45-59.
    See also Prophylaxis
  barriers to, 46
  definition of, 47-48
  of drug-use transmission, 52-53,
    52t
  of perinatal transmission, 53-55,
    54t
  populations at risk and, 48
  risk assessment in, 47t
  sexual transmission and, 49-52, 49t
    condom use in, 51-52
    high-risk activities and, 49-50
    postexposure prophylaxis in,
      55-57
    treatment of sexually transmit-
      ted disease and, 50-51
Primary care
  antibody testing in, 63-66, 64t
  clinical evaluation in, 66-71
    history taking and, 67-68, 67t
    physical examination in, 68-71,
      69t
  clinical trials and, 91
  complementary medical therapy
    and, 91
  financial issues and, 92

food safety and, 92
health care maintenance issues in,
    82-86
    age-appropriate screening and,
        86
    cervical cancer screening an, 83
    immunizations and, 82-83, 84t
    sexually transmitted disease
        and, 85-86
    tuberculosis and, 83, 85
laboratory studies in, 71-73, 71t
legal issues and, 92
management in, 73-82
    antiviral therapy and, 75-78
    CD4 cell count and, 74t
    general approach to, 73-75
    prophylaxis of opportunistic
        infection, 78-82, 79f, 80t
psychiatric disorders and, 86
risk-reduction counseling in, 65t
substance abuse and, 91
for women, 87-91
    clinical manifestations and, 87
    epidemiology and transmission
        and, 87
    pregnancy and, 87-91, 88t
Primary effusion lymphoma, 229
Primary infection, 28-33
    clinical features of, 29-31, 29t
    laboratory findings in, 31-33
Procrit, 293
Progression of HIV infection, 33-35
Progressive multifocal leukoen-
    cephalopathy, 154t
Prophylaxis
    for occupational exposure
        clinical vignette about, 268-270
        exposure code for, 249f-251f
        zidovudine for, 55, 57
    for opportunistic infection, 78-83,
        117-131. See also
        Opportunistic infection, pre-
        vention of
Protease inhibitor, 97
    characteristics of, 100t
    combination therapy with, 77
    cross resistance and, 112-113
    cutaneous manifestations of, 159t

indications, dosage, and toxicity
    of, 280-282
types of, 106-108
Pseudomonas infection, respiratory,
    141, 142t-143t
Psychiatric disorder, 86
Psychosocial issues, 68
Pulmonary symptoms. See Respiratory
    disorder
Pyrazinamide
    indications, dosage, and toxicity
        of, 288
    for Mycobacterium avium com-
        plex, 172t
    as prophylaxis, 85
    for tuberculosis, 126
Pyridoxine, 126
Pyrimethamine, 122

R

Racial minority
    incidence of HIV infection and, 7
    as population at risk, 48
Radiation therapy for lymphoma, 231
Radiologic imaging, 137
    cryptococcosis and, 184
    fever and, 140
    respiratory infection and, 141
Rash, 30
Receptive anal intercourse, 70
Registry, occupational exposure, 254
Renal symptoms, 30
Reporting
    of HIV infection, 3-4
    of occupational exposure, 248
Rescriptor, 99t, 278
Reservoir, viral, 26-27
Resistance
    to antiviral therapy, 77
    cross, 112-113
Resource, occupational exposure, 254
Respiratory disorder
    Kaposi's sarcoma and, 217
    in natural history of HIV, 30
    symptoms of, 69t, 140-141, 142t-
        143t, 144

Retinitis, cytomegalovirus, 197, 198
Retonavir, 281
Retrovir. *See* Zidovudine
Review of systems, 69t
Rifabutin
    indications, dosage, and toxicity
        of, 288
    for *Mycobacterium avium* com-
        plex, 81, 123-125, 124t, 171,
        172t
    for tuberculosis, 180
Rifampin
    indications, dosage, and toxicity
        of, 288-289
    as prophylaxis, 85
    for tuberculosis, 126, 179-180
Risk assessment, 47-48, 47t
Risk behavior
    counseling about, 65t
    incidence of HIV infection and, 7
Ritonavir, 107
    characteristics of, 100t
    drugs contraindicated with, 102t-103t
    interactions with, 104t
RNA, immune destruction and, 25-26

S

Safer sex, attitude toward, 56
Safety, food, 92
Safety device, 254
Salmonella infection, 173-174
    diarrhea with, 145
Saquinavir
    characteristics of, 100t, 107
    drugs contraindicated with, 102t-
        103t
    indications, dosage, and toxicity
        of, 281
    interactions with, 104t
Sarcoma, Kaposi's. *See* Kaposi's
        sarcoma
Scabies, 156t
Screening
    age-appropriate, 86
    for cervical cancer, 83
    for cytomegalovirus, 72

mental status, 71
    for sexually transmitted disease,
        85-86
    syphilis, 176
    for toxoplasmosis, 72
    for tuberculosis, 72, 83, 85
Seborrheic dermatitis, 160
Septra. *See* Trimethoprim-sul-
        famethoxazole
Seroconversion, 32
Serostim, 293
Sexual transmission of HIV, 9
    postexposure prophylaxis and, 55-
        56
    prevention of, 49-52, 49t
Sexually transmitted disease
    screening for, 85-86
    treatment of, 50-51
Shingles, 202-203
Skin disorder
    bartonellosis and, 166, 167f
    drug reactions causing, 158-160,
        159t
    eosinophilic folliculitis as, 160
    infectious, 155, 156t-157t, 158
    Kaposi's sarcoma. *See* Kaposi's sar-
        coma
    malignant, 160
    in natural history of HIV, 30
    seborrheic dermatitis as, 160
    syphilis causing, 174, 175f
    tuberculosis and, 179f
    types of, 69-70, 69t
Skin test for tuberculosis, 125-126,
        178-179
Somatropin, 293
Squamous cell carcinoma, cervical,
        238-239
Standard precautions, 252-253, 253t
Staphylococcus aureus, respiratory,
        141, 142t-143t
Stavudine
    characteristics of, 98t, 103
    indications, dosage, and toxicity
        of, 276-277
Steroid in Kaposi's sarcoma, 216
Streptococcus infection, respiratory,
        141, 142t-143t

Streptomycin
   indications, dosage, and toxicity
      of, 289
   for *Mycobacterium avium* com-
      plex, 172t
Strongyloides stercoralis, 193t
Substance abuse, 52-53, 52t, 91
Sulfadiazine
   indications, dosage, and toxicity
      of, 290
   for toxoplasmosis, 196-197, 196t
Surveillance case definition, 3t
Sustiva, 99t, 278
Symptomatic HIV disease, develop-
      ment of, 33-35
Symptoms
   dermatologic, 155, 156t-157t, 158-
      160, 159t
   fever as, 138-140, 139t
   gastrointestinal, 144-150
      diarrhea as, 144-146, 145t
      dysphagia as, 148
      hepatitis causing, 146, 147t, 148
      odynophagia as, 148
      oral ulcers and, 149t
      weight loss as, 149-150
   gynecologic, 154-155
   neurologic, 150-154
      altered mental status as, 152, 153t
      cytomegalovirus encephalitis
         causing, 154t
      dementia and, 154t
      headache as, 150-152
      painful extremities as, 152-154
      progressive multifocal leukoen-
         cephalopathy causing, 154t
   respiratory, 140-141, 142t-143t, 144
Syncytium-inducing virus, 27-28
Syphilis, 174-177, 175f, 177t
   screening for, 72, 176
Syringe, transmission of HIV via, 9

T

T lymphocyte
   Hodgkin's lymphoma and, 224
   primary infection and, 32

tat protein, 215
Taxol, 220
Td toxoid, 84t
Tenofovir
   characteristics of, 105
   indications, dosage, and toxicity
      of, 279
Tertiary syphilis, 175
Testosterone, 295
Thalidomide
   indications, dosage, and toxicity
      of, 295-296
   for tuberculosis, 180
3TC (lamivudine)
   characteristics of, 103
   in pregnancy, 90, 111
   resistance to, 101
Thrush, 148
   treatment of, 183t
Titer, viral load, 73
TMP-SMX. *See* Trimethoprim-sul-
      famethoxazole
Toxoplasmosis, 194-197, 195f, 196t
   drugs for, 122, 289-290
   incidence of, 121-122
   lymphoma *vs.,* 225t
   prophylaxis for, 81-82, 121-123
   recommendations for, 122-123
   screening for, 72
Transmission, 8-11, 22-23
   parenteral, 9-10
   perinatal, 10-11
   prevention of, 45-59. *See also*
      Prevention
   sexual, 9
Treponema pallidum, 174-177, 175f,
      177t
Trichomoniasis, 9
Trimethoprim-sulfamethoxazole
   cutaneous manifestations of, 159t
   indications, dosage, and toxicity
      of, 284
   for isosporiasis, 194
   oral desensitization protocol for, 120t
   for *Pneumocystis carinii* pneumo-
      nia, 79-80, 118-121, 119t,
      189-190, 189t
   for toxoplasmosis prophylaxis, 122

Trimetrexate, 189t
Triple therapy, 112
Tuberculosis, 141, 142t-143t, 177-180,
    179f
    drugs for, 286-289
    incidence of, 125-126
    prophylaxis for, 126
    respiratory infection and, 141, 144
    screening for, 72, 83, 85
    symptoms of, 142t-143t
Tumor. See Malignancy
Tumor necrosis factor inhibitor, 180

U

Ulcer
    aphthous, 149t
    gastrointestinal, 30
    oral, 148, 149t
Urethritis, 9
Uterine cervical cancer, 238-239

V

Vaccination, 82-83, 84t
Vaginal discharge, 154-155
    candidiasis and, 180
Vaginosis, 70-71
Varicella-zoster virus infection, 176,
    202-204, 202t, 203f, 292
Venereal Disease Research Laboratory
    test, 176
Ventriculoencephalitis, 197, 198
Vertical transmission of HIV
    mechanism of, 10-11
    prevention of, 53-55
Videx, 98t, 276
Vinblastine, 219
Viracept. See Nelfinavir
Viral infection
    cytomegalovirus. See
        Cytomegalovirus
    hepatitis as. See Hepatitis
    herpes simplex, 200-202, 201f, 202t
        oral, 149t
        treatment of, 202t
    liver function and, 147t

    skin disorder from, 156t
    varicella-zoster, 202-204, 202t, 203f
Viral load titer, 73
Viral phenotype, 27
Viral reservoir, 26-27
Viramune, 99t, 279
Viremia, plasma, 22-23
Virus, cytopathic, 21
Vistide (Cidofovir), 199t, 200, 290
Vulvovaginal candidiasis, 180, 181

W

Weight loss, 149-150, 150t
Women
    clinical manifestations in, 87
    gynecologic symptoms in, 154-155
    incidence of HIV infection in, 5
    as population at risk, 48
    pregnancy and. See Pregnancy
    transmission of HIV in, 87
World Health Organization, HIV epi-
    demiology and, 11-12

Z

Zalcitabine, 98t, 102, 159t, 277
Ziagen. See Abacavir
    characteristics of, 98t
Zidovudine, 101
    characteristics of, 98t
    cutaneous manifestations of, 159t
    indications, dosage, and toxicity
        of, 277-278
    for lymphoma, 230
    occupational exposure and, 247,
        252
    perinatal transmission and, 54
    for postexposure prophylaxis, 55,
        57, 250
    in pregnancy, 111
    resistance to, 101
Zithromax. See Azithromycin
Zoster, 202-204, 203f
    drugs for, 292
    treatment of, 202t
Zovirax. See Acyclovir

Color Plates

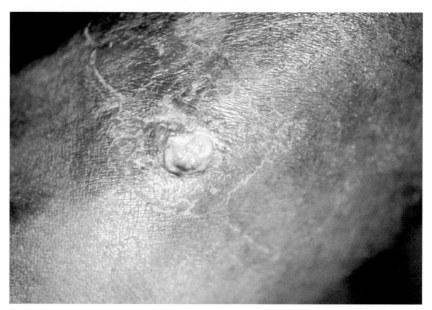

Plate 1 Cutaneous tuberculosis in patient with advanced HIV disease. For further information, see discussion of Figure 8.4 in Chapter 8 text (where Plate 1 is reproduced in black and white).

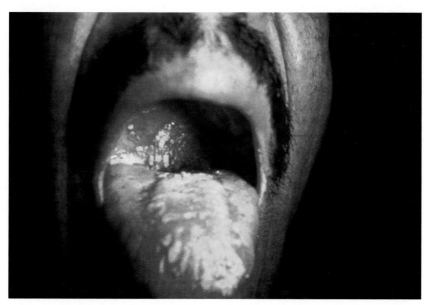

Plate 2 Pseudomembranous variant of oral candidiasis. For further information, see discussion of Figure 8.5A in Chapter 8 text (where Plate 2 is reproduced in black and white).

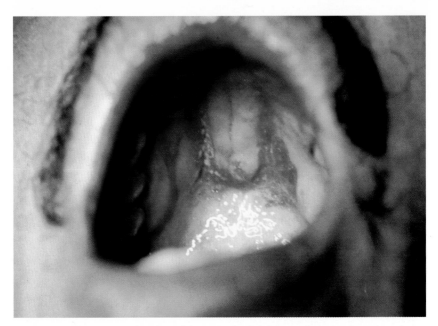

Plate 3 Atrophic variant of oral candidiasis. For further information, see discussion of Figure 8.5B in Chapter 8 text (where Plate 3 is reproduced in black and white).

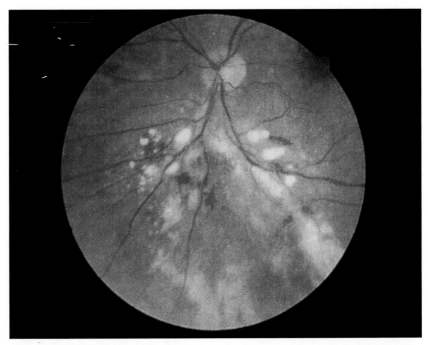

Plate 4 Retinal photograph of patient with cytomegalovirus retinitis. For further information, see discussion of Figure 8.10 in Chapter 8 text (where Plate 4 is reproduced in black and white).

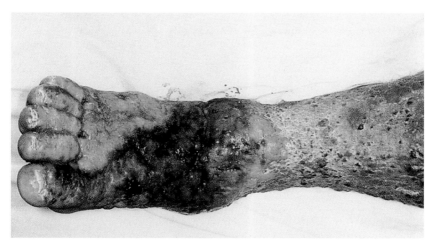

Plate 5 Plaque-like lesion on foot with breakdown of overlying skin in an AIDS patient with Kaposi's sarcoma. (Reprinted with permission from van den Brink MR, Dezube BJ. AIDS-related Kaposi's sarcoma. *J Clin Oncol.* 1997;15: 1283.) For further information, see discussion of Figure 9.1A in Chapter 9 text (where Plate 5 is reproduced in black and white).

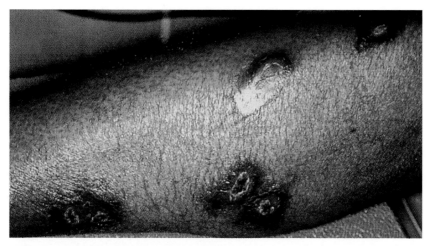

Plate 6 Multiple colored lesions on leg in an AIDS patient with Kaposi's sarcoma. (Reprinted with permission from van den Brink MR, Dezube BJ. AIDS-related Kaposi's sarcoma. *J Clin Oncol.* 1997;15:1283.) For further information, see discussion of Figure 9.1B in Chapter 9 text (where Plate 6 is reproduced in black and white).

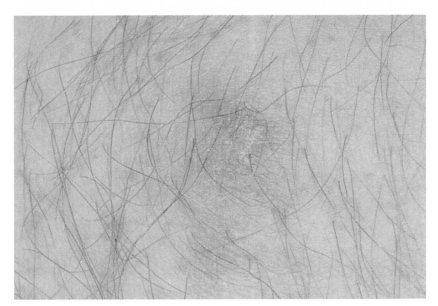

Plate 7 Yellow perilesional halo in an AIDS patient with Kaposi's sarcoma. (Reprinted with permission from van den Brink MR, Dezube BJ. AIDS-related Kaposi's sarcoma. *J Clin Oncol.* 1997;15:1283.) For further information, see discussion of Figure 9.1C in Chapter 9 text (where Plate 7 is reproduced in black and white).

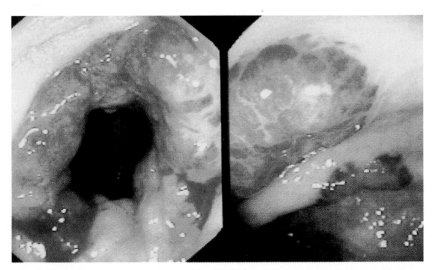

Plate 8 Kaposi's sarcoma can appear as large annular masses with circumferential infiltration and luminal obstruction in the colon and rectum. (Reprinted with permission from van den Brink MR, Dezube BJ. AIDS-related Kaposi's sarcoma. *J Clin Oncol.* 1997;15:1283.) For further information, see discussion of Figure 9.1D in Chapter 9 text (where Plate 8 is reproduced in black and white).